Cases on Psychiatric Medicine

Samet Uludag
Kastamonu City Arac Government Hospital, Turkey

Kadir Uludag
https://orcid.org/0000-0003-3713-4670
Shanghai Jiaotong University, China

IGI Global
Scientific Publishing
Publishing Tomorrow's Research Today

Vice President of Editorial Melissa Wagner
Director of Acquisitions Mikaela Felty
Director of Book Development Jocelynn Hessler
Production Manager Mike Brehm
Cover Design Jose Rosado

Published in the United States of America by
IGI Global Scientific Publishing
701 East Chocolate Avenue
Hershey, PA, 17033, USA
Tel: 717-533-8845 | Fax: 717-533-7115
Website: https://www.igi-global.com E-mail: cust@igi-global.com

Library of Congress Cataloging-in-Publication Data

LCCN: 2025945063 (CIP Data Pending)
ISBN13: 9798337330846
Isbn13Softcover: 9798337330853
EISBN13: 9798337330860

British Cataloguing in Publication Data
A Cataloguing in Publication record for this book is available from the British Library.

Table of Contents

Detailed Table of Contents

This abstract presents a case study of a 55-year-old Turkish female residing in Turkey diagnosed with Schizophrenia (SCZ) thirteen years ago, which was later compounded by a diagnosis of bipolar disorder (BD) five years following the initial diagnosis. Notably, the patient does not have any chronic disorders. Due to agranulocytosis resulting from the discontinued use of the antipsychotic clozapine, the patient currently receives lithium treatment in a dosage of 300 mg once daily. The patient's white blood cell (WBC) count and neutrophil levels remained stable for four years, but subsequently, the WBC count decreased to 3.8 and the absolute neutrophil count dropped to 1.7, a change that was linked to clozapine. Following the discontinuation of clozapine, his blood values returned to normal. It is also intriguing that both values deviated from the norm.

This chapter provides readers with a comprehensive overview of the "Schizophrenia Spectrum and Other Psychotic Disorders" chapter in the Diagnostic and Statistical Manual of Mental Disorders, Fifth edition, Text Revision (DSM-5-TR). It achieves this through the use of illustrative case studies, which provide real-life examples of psychotic disorders in clinical practice. The chapter provides background information on schizophrenia spectrum disorders, including their prevalence, symptoms, and evidence-based treatments, before detailing realistic case presentations.

Neurocognitive disorders, are becoming more common among older adults, which presents significant difficulties for individuals, those who care for them, and healthcare systems. This review emphasizes the significance of precise differentiation for effective care, highlighting the clinical features, diagnostic complexities, and treatment strategies of these conditions. While dementia and Alzheimer's involve progressive, irreversible neurodegeneration, delirium, which is frequently reversible, may indicate underlying cognitive decline. Improving patient outcomes necessitates personalized care, early diagnosis, caregiver support, and lifestyle interventions. The article also underscores the urgent need for continued research into disease-modifying therapies, early detection biomarkers, and health system improvements. To manage the growing burden of neurocognitive disorders and improve the quality of life for those who suffer from them, comprehensive strategies that integrate efforts at the policy, social, and clinical levels are essential as global populations age. (World Health Organization, 2021)

Understanding and managing anxiety, schizophrenia, depression, and bipolar disorder in children is critical for promoting their mental health and well-being. These conditions can manifest differently in younger populations, requiring tailored approaches to diagnosis and treatment. Anxiety in children often presents as excessive worry or fear, while schizophrenia may involve delusions, hallucinations, and impaired social functioning. Depression in children can lead to mood disturbances, irritability, and withdrawal from activities, while bipolar disorder is characterized by extreme mood swings, ranging from manic episodes to deep depression. Early identification and intervention, including therapy, medication, and support from caregivers, are essential to managing these disorders effectively. A comprehensive approach that includes medical, psychological, and educational strategies can help children cope with and manage these conditions, improving their overall quality of life.

The cardiorespiratory effects in mental illnesses have recently received much attention. However, the cardiovascular and respiratory effects in patients with bipolar disorder and the corresponding rehabilitation strategies have not been clearly demonstrated. This chapter aims to demonstrate exercise capacity, respiratory strength, pulmonary function, dyspnea, physical activity level and rehabilitation strategies in patient with bipolar disorder (BD). The patients had dyspnea, expiratory muscle weakness, small airway dysfunction, obesity, smoking, reduced exercise capacity and physical inactivity. Eight-week cardiopulmonary rehabilitation program were recommended to BD patient that consist of lifestyle modification training, expiratory muscle training, aerobic and resistance training.

Chronic physical illnesses frequently co-occur with mental health disorders, complicating patient care. This chapter examines the intersection of chronic illness and psychological resilience through a biopsychosocial lens. It reviews epidemiological data illustrating high rates of depression, anxiety, and trauma-related symptoms among individuals with conditions like diabetes, cancer, and rare diseases. Theoretical frameworks (biopsychosocial model, developmental, and family systems theories) inform the discussion. Three case studies (adolescent diabetes, adult cancer survivor, child with a rare disorder) demonstrate integrative psychotherapeutic interventions, cognitive-behavioral, trauma-focused, narrative, and family therapies tailored to whole-person care. Emphasis is placed on collaboration with medical teams via integrated care models to address both physical and mental needs. The chapter highlights how coordinated, holistic approaches bolster patient and family resilience, improving outcomes across the lifespan.

Neurostimulation has emerged as a significant therapeutic approach for various disabilities (e.g., emotional disability), revolutionizing the management and treatment of affected individuals. By delivering electrical impulses to the nervous system, it targets multiple types of disabilities, including those related to emotion. It has emerged as a significant therapeutic option for emotional disabilities, offering new hope for patients who do not respond adequately to traditional treatments. Emotional disabilities, such as major depressive disorder, anxiety disorders, and post - traumatic stress disorder, are characterized by dysregulated emotional states and disrupted neural circuits. Neurostimulation techniques, including deep brain stimulation (DBS), vagus nerve stimulation, transcranial magnetic stimulation (TMS), and transcranial direct - current stimulation (tDCS), target these underlying neural dysfunctions. DBS and vagus nerve stimulation, which are invasive and semi - invasive methods respectively, are often used for severe cases.

Chronic Pelvic Pain (CPP) is pain lasting over three months, classified as a biopsychosocial disorder in ICD-11. Endometriosis and interstitial cystitis/bladder pain syndrome (IC/BPS) cause CPP, linking to depression and poor life quality. The Psychoneuroimmunological (PNI) model explains CPP's involvement with immune, nervous, and psychological systems. In endometriosis, ectopic implants trigger immune cell infiltration, increasing cytokines and NGF. IC/BPS shows inflammation with immune infiltration causing sensitization. Inflammatory signals activate microglia and astrocytes, triggering neuroinflammation. Stress affects the HPA axis, reducing anti-inflammatory responses and activating NLRP3 inflammasome. The gut-brain axis links dysbiosis to inflammation, while epigenetic mechanisms maintain neuronal hyperexcitability. Treatment must target the neuroimmune axis through pharmacologic and behavioral therapy for outcomes.

Preface

I. INTRODUCTION

This book emerges from a confluence of urgent clinical realities and timeless philosophical questions. It is a curated psychological collection of case-based investigations. Yet, collectively, these contributions converge on a central, unifying theme in modern psychiatric science and practice: the essential, non-negotiable integration of biological, psychological, and social dimensions in understanding, treating, and ultimately, preventing complex mental illness (e.g., depression and anxiety).

For decades, the dominant paradigms in psychology, medicine and psychiatry have oscillated between reductionist models. We have witnessed eras where the biological—the neurochemical imbalance, the genetic polymorphism—was viewed as the sole architect of psychopathology.

Conversely, purely psychodynamic or behavioral models sometimes minimized the profound influence of the physical brain and body on our thoughts and emotions. The chapters that follow are a testament to the obsolescence of such siloed thinking. They collectively move beyond diagnostic silos to examine the complex, dynamic interfaces where psychiatric disorders (e.g., depression, bipolar disorder, and anxiety) intersect with neurocognitive decline, systemic medical comorbidity, and the powerful, often deterministic, psychosocial determinants of health across the entire developmental lifespan.

The structure of this book is therefore not merely organizational; it is philosophical. The journey begins with a granular, biological focus—the impact of a powerful antipsychotic on the cellular components of blood—and expands outward. It moves through the complex presentation of schizophrenia spectrum disorders, into the critical diagnostic territory of neurocognitive disorders in the elderly, and then descends into the vulnerable world of pediatric psychiatry.

From there, it explores the intricate dance between chronic physical illness and the psyche, before examining novel neurostimulation techniques and the fascinating, emerging field of psychoneuroimmunology as applied to conditions like pelvic pain.

II. THE CLINICAL IMPERATIVE: A LANDSCAPE OF URGENCY

The urgency of this integrative perspective is not an abstract academic concept; it is clearly underscored by current global mental health realities. The work presented in this book addresses a clinical landscape marked by profound challenges that demand a practitioner fluent in multiple disciplines.

First, we face the persistent and tragic reality of the mortality gap. Individuals with severe mental illnesses, such as the schizophrenia and bipolar disorder explored in these pages, continue to experience a lifespan shorter than the general population. This gap is not only due to suicide or accidents, but largely attributable to preventable cardiovascular, metabolic, and infectious diseases. The case study on clozapine's impact on neutrophil counts is a powerful microcosm of this larger issue. It reminds us that the most effective psychiatric medication can carry physical health risks that require medical monitoring. A psychiatrist cannot simply be a prescriber; they must be a physician attuned to the systemic health of their patient, collaborating with other specialists to manage the intertwined realities of mental and physical illness. The chapter on cardiopulmonary rehabilitation in a patient with bipolar disorder is another exemplary model of this necessary synthesis, demonstrating that recovery involves not just mood stabilization, but the active rebuilding of physical health and function.

Concurrently, our global population is aging, presenting rising rates of neurocognitive disorders. The chapter dedicated to delirium, dementia, and Alzheimer's disease tackles one of the most critical, often life-saving, diagnostic challenges in modern medicine: distinguishing between a reversible, acute confusional state (delirium) and an irreversible, progressive neurodegenerative process (dementia). This distinction cannot be made from a textbook alone. It requires a deep

understanding of neurobiology, a keen eye for the nuanced behavioral changes that signal an underlying medical crisis, and the wisdom to engage with a patient's social and environmental context, which are often the root causes of delirium. Here, the biological and social dimensions are inextricably linked.

And finally, we are confronted with the developing minds of our children. In pediatric populations, early manifestations of psychiatric illness—the anxieties, the mood dysregulations, the prodromal symptoms of thought disorders—demand vigilant, developmentally attuned intervention. The work on understanding and managing these conditions in children is not merely about treating a present disorder; it is about altering long-term trajectories, about intervening at a critical juncture to foster resilience and prevent a lifetime of suffering. This is perhaps the purest form of biopsychosocial practice, where interventions must be carefully calibrated to a child's neurodevelopmental stage, psychological maturity, and the all-important family and school systems that form their world.

This book situates itself squarely within this demanding clinical landscape. It argues, through the power of example, that advancing patient outcomes necessitates a deliberate and skilled synthesis of medical monitoring, psychopharmacology, psychotherapeutic intervention, and rehabilitative support. No single tool in the clinician's kit is sufficient on its own.

III. AN INVITATION TO THE MULTIDISCIPLINARY MIND

It is with this conviction that we have designed this book for the discerning clinician, psychologist, doctors, investigator, and trainee, addressing a fundamentally multidisciplinary audience. The complexity of the human condition, particularly in states of suffering, cannot be adequately understood from the vantage point of a single discipline.

This book, therefore, offers critical insights for a wide spectrum of professionals. For the psychiatrist, neurologist, and geriatrician, it provides nuanced perspectives on managing complex comorbid conditions where psychiatric symptoms are often the presenting face of underlying neurological or systemic illness. The chapters serve as case-based consultations, illustrating the diagnostic reasoning and collaborative care required when the boundaries between medical specialties blur.

For the psychologist, social worker, and nurse, it illuminates the biological underpinnings of the conditions they address therapeutically, reinforcing the importance of integrated treatment plans that respect both the talking cure and the physiological realities of the patient. Understanding the psychoneuroimmunology of pelvic pain, for instance, can profoundly reshape a psychotherapeutic approach, validating the patient's physical experience while exploring its potential psychological correlates.

For the researcher, these clinical narratives offer a rich source of hypotheses, grounding scientific inquiry in the complexities of real-world patients and examining the biopsychosocial mechanisms of both illness and resilience. The interplay between chronic illness and psychological resilience, explored through case-based perspectives, provides a fertile ground for investigating how the human mind can adapt and even thrive in the face of profound physical challenge.

And for the student across these disciplines, this collection offers a compelling vision of 21st- century practice. It demonstrates that true expertise is measured not only by diagnostic acumen or knowledge of the latest research, but by the ability to navigate, coordinate, and synthesize care across the full spectrum of a patient's health needs. It is a vision of the clinician as a translator, a collaborator, and a holistic healer.

IV. THE TAPESTRY OF CONTRIBUTIONS

The significance of each contribution lies in its specific lens on this integrative whole. Together, they form not a linear argument, but a comprehensive clinical mosaic. Let us briefly preview the threads that weave this tapestry.

The journey begins in Section I with a foundational exploration of core psychiatric conditions through an integrative lens.

- Dr. Samet Uludag grounds us in the biological with a meticulous case study on the impact of clozapine, a gold-standard antipsychotic, on neutrophil and white blood cell counts. This chapter is a vital reminder of the somatic vigilance required in psychiatric practice.
- Dr. Jennifer Schulz broadens the scope with case studies in schizophrenia and related disorders, illustrating the phenomenological presentation and psychosocial management of these complex conditions.
- The critical interface of neurology and psychiatry is then explored by Samruddhi Datta Thube, Pranoti Pramod Bendre, and Rohini Mahadev Chavan in their chapter on neurocognitive disorders in the elderly, a masterclass in diagnostic differentiation between delirium and dementia.
- Turning to the youngest patients, Wasswa Shafik addresses the profound challenge of understanding and managing anxiety, schizophrenia, depression, and bipolar disorder in children, linking child mental health to the broader goal of sustainable social inclusion.
- The theme of physical-mental comorbidity is powerfully advanced by Irem Huzmeli and Sabiha Bezgin, who present a case study on cardiopulmonary rehabilitation in a patient with bipolar disorder, demonstrating the power of interdisciplinary rehabilitation.
- Dr. Jennifer Marshall delves into the psychology with her chapter on interfacing chronic illness and psychological resilience, offering case-based perspectives on integrative psychotherapeutic interventions that help patients adapt and find meaning.
- Dr. Kadir Uludag then introduces us to the frontier of treatment with case studies in clinical psychiatry focusing on neurostimulation for emotional and affective disorders, a field that directly manipulates brain biology to alleviate psychological suffering.

- Finally, Prof. Issa Sulaiman Al-Amri, Hoda Doustmohammadi, and Ashkan Delavari take us to the cutting edge of psychosomatic medicine with their exploration of the psychoneuroimmunology of pelvic pain, a chapter that illustrates the bidirectional communication between the brain, the immune system, and the body.

V. A BROADER VISION: BEYOND MATERIAL PRODUCTION

As we consider the sum of these parts, a larger vision emerges, one that extends beyond the clinic and into the very fabric of how we, as a global society, define progress and well-being. The scientific rigor applied in these chapters to understand depression, anxiety, psychosis, and neurodegeneration points to a profound truth: the health of the mind is the foundation upon which a fulfilling life is built. It is the wellspring of creativity, connection, resilience, and the capacity for happiness.

In a world often fixated on material production and economic growth as the primary metrics of success, this volume serves as a quiet but persistent counter-narrative. The intricate dance between a bipolar patient's mood and their physical capacity for rehabilitation, the profound disorientation of dementia that strips away the accumulated wealth of a lifetime's memories, the crippling anxiety of a child that prevents them from learning and playing—these clinical realities starkly illustrate that material wealth is meaningless in the absence of psychological well-being.

A society can produce goods at an unprecedented rate, but if its members are suffering, isolated, and unable to experience joy or connection, what, ultimately, has been produced?

The cases within this book argue, implicitly and explicitly, for a reprioritization of values. They suggest that psychology and the pursuit of happiness should not be seen as secondary concerns to be addressed after material needs are met, but as the primary goals of a healthy society. Material production is a tool, a means to an end. That end must be human flourishing. The chapters on resilience, on the role of social work, on the importance of family systems in pediatric care, all underscore that our social fabric and our internal psychological worlds are the true determinants of a life well-lived. Investing in mental health, in understanding the complex interplay of factors that lead to suffering and recovery, is not merely a medical expense; it is a fundamental investment in the happiness and sustainability of our world.

The detailed exploration of contributors' backgrounds—the family physician, the postdoctoral researcher, the professor of social work, the community data analyst turned digital health researcher—further enriches this vision. They represent a global, interdisciplinary community dedicated to this very goal. Their diverse paths, from the clinics of Ohio to the laboratories of Brunei, from the universities of

Turkey to the research centers of China, converge on this shared commitment. Their work demonstrates that the pursuit of psychological well-being is a universal human project, transcending borders and disciplines.

VI. A NOTE ON METHOD AND CONTEXT

In presenting these case studies, we are acutely aware of the inherent tension between the uniqueness of individual experience and the search for generalizable knowledge. A case study is not a randomized controlled trial. It does not offer statistical proof. But it offers something arguably more foundational for clinical practice: context, nuance, and the messy reality of human decision-making.

Each chapter is a narrative of clinical reasoning. The authors guide us through their thought processes as they encounter diagnostic ambiguity, weigh treatment options, navigate patient preferences and values, and contend with the unpredictable course of illness and recovery. In reading these narratives, we are invited into a virtual apprenticeship, learning not just *what* the experts did, but *why* they did it, and *how* they adapted when the unexpected occurred. This is the wisdom that resides at the heart of clinical expertise, and it is this wisdom we hope to transmit. Furthermore, the references compiled at the end of this volume serve as a gateway to the broader scientific literature, grounding these clinical narratives in the evidence base that informs them.

They are an invitation for the reader to explore further, to critically evaluate the authors' conclusions, and to continue the process of lifelong learning that defines the committed clinician- scholar.

VII. CONCLUSION: TOWARD A MORE HUMANE PSYCHIATRY

Ultimately, this book is an argument for a more humane psychiatry. A psychiatry that sees the person behind the diagnosis, the life behind the symptom. It is a psychiatry that recognizes the patient not as a collection of broken circuits or maladaptive thoughts, but as a whole human being, embedded in a family, a community, and a culture, striving for meaning and connection, even in the depths of their suffering.

The case studies that follow are windows into these lives. They are stories of struggle, but also of adaptation, resilience, and the profound power of the therapeutic relationship. They remind us that our work, whether in the clinic, the laboratory, or the classroom, is ultimately a service to individual lives and to the communities they form. It is our hope that this volume serves as a meaningful resource for all those dedicated to advancing integrative, compassionate, and scientifically grounded mental health care, and in doing so, contributes, in its own small way, to a world where psychological well-being and the pursuit of happiness are truly prioritized.

Suggestions for Further Research

The case studies presented in this volume offer a rich tapestry of clinical wisdom, illuminating the complex, multifaceted nature of mental illness and its treatment. They demonstrate, with vivid detail, the power of an integrative biopsychosocial approach and the necessity of attending to the full spectrum of human suffering—biological, psychological, and social. Yet, for all their depth and insight, these clinical narratives also illuminate the vast territories of knowledge that remain unexplored. Each chapter concludes not with finality, but with questions. Each case resolves some mysteries while revealing others. It is the purpose of this section to map these territories, to articulate the questions that emerge from the preceding pages, and to propose a comprehensive agenda for future research that can advance the field toward more effective, equitable, and humane mental health care.

The research suggestions that follow are organized thematically, reflecting the major domains addressed in this book. They are not intended as an exhaustive catalog but as a strategic roadmap, prioritizing lines of inquiry that hold the greatest promise for translating the insights of case- based investigation into generalizable knowledge and improved clinical practice. They call upon investigators from all disciplines—psychiatry, psychology, neuroscience, immunology, social work, public health, and beyond—to join in a collaborative effort to deepen our understanding and expand our capacity to heal.

VIII. DEEPENING THE INTEGRATIVE MODEL: MECHANISMS OF INTERACTION

The biopsychosocial model, while widely endorsed, remains superficially understood. A critical priority for future research is to move beyond simple acknowledgment of the three domains and toward a mechanistic understanding of how they interact dynamically over time.

A. Biological-Psychological Interface

The chapters on neurostimulation and psychoneuroimmunology hint at the profound bidirectional communication between brain and body. Future research must elucidate the specific pathways through which psychological states influence biological processes, and vice versa. Key questions include:

- How do specific psychotherapeutic interventions (e.g., cognitive-behavioral therapy, mindfulness-based stress reduction) produce measurable changes in neurotransmitter systems, inflammatory markers, and neural circuitry? Neuroimaging studies combined with longitudinal biomarker assessment can map these changes in real-time, identifying the neural mediators of therapeutic response.
- What are the psychological mechanisms through which biological interventions exert their effects? For example, how does neurostimulation (TMS, tDCS) alter not only brain activity but also cognitive patterns, emotional regulation, and self-perception? Understanding these pathways can lead to synergistic treatment combinations that target both biology and psychology simultaneously.
- Can we identify psychological profiles that predict differential response to biological treatments? The case of clozapine response in schizophrenia, for instance, may be moderated by psychological factors such as insight, treatment alliance, or illness beliefs. Research integrating psychological assessment into psychopharmacology trials can move us toward personalized medicine.

B. Biological-Social Interface

The profound impact of social determinants on health is well-established epidemiologically, but the biological mechanisms remain poorly understood. The mortality gap experienced by individuals with severe mental illness, highlighted in the preface, demands urgent investigation into these pathways.

- How does chronic social adversity—poverty, discrimination, social isolation—become biologically embedded to increase disease risk? Research must explore epigenetic modifications, accelerated cellular aging, and dysregulation of stress response systems (HPA axis, autonomic nervous system) as potential mediators.
- What are the biological mechanisms linking social support to improved health outcomes? Studies can investigate how positive social relationships buffer stress responses, enhance immune function, and promote neuroplasticity.
- Can social interventions (e.g., supported housing, vocational rehabilitation, peer support) be shown to produce measurable biological changes? Demonstrating that addressing social determinants is not merely "social work" but a biological intervention could transform healthcare funding and policy.

C. Psychological-Social Interface

The intersection of individual psychology and social context is perhaps the most clinically relevant yet methodologically challenging domain for research.

- How do psychological factors—resilience, coping styles, explanatory models of illness— moderate the impact of social adversity on mental health? Longitudinal studies can identify psychological protective factors that buffer against the harmful effects of poverty, trauma, or discrimination.
- How do social interventions produce psychological change? For example, does obtaining stable housing reduce psychological distress directly, or does it operate through changes in self-efficacy, hope, or social identity? Understanding these mechanisms can optimize the design of social programs.
- Can we develop and test interventions that target the psychological-social interface directly? Family-based interventions for pediatric psychiatric disorders, as touched upon in the chapter on children's mental health, are a prime example. Research must identify the active ingredients of such interventions and test their effectiveness across diverse cultural contexts.

IX. ADVANCING EQUITY: RESEARCH ON EQUAL PSYCHOLOGICAL TREATMENT

The necessity of equal psychological treatment, argued forcefully in the preface, demands a dedicated research agenda to identify and dismantle barriers to access and to demonstrate the value of psychological interventions with the same rigor applied to somatic treatments.

A. Access and Utilization

Research must document and analyze the persistent inequities in access to psychological treatment across populations.

- What are the specific structural, financial, and cultural barriers that prevent individuals from low-income, minority, and rural communities from accessing evidence-based psychological care? Mixed-methods research combining epidemiological data with qualitative inquiry can illuminate these barriers from multiple perspectives.
- How do insurance policies, reimbursement rates, and healthcare system design create a two- tiered system that privileges somatic over psychological

treatment? Health services research can model the impact of policy changes, such as parity laws, on access and outcomes.

- Can innovative service delivery models—telehealth, collaborative care, task-sharing with community health workers—reduce inequities? Implementation research is needed to test the effectiveness, cost-effectiveness, and sustainability of these models in real-world settings.

B. Comparative Effectiveness and Value

To argue for equal treatment, psychological interventions must demonstrate their value using metrics that capture their full impact.

- How do psychological and somatic treatments compare on outcomes that matter most to patients, including quality of life, functioning, and subjective well-being, in addition to symptom reduction? Comparative effectiveness research should employ patient-centered outcome measures and longitudinal follow-up.
- What is the cost-effectiveness of psychological interventions when accounting for their long- term benefits, including reduced medical utilization, improved occupational functioning, and enhanced quality of life? Economic analyses must adopt a societal perspective and model long- term outcomes.
- Can we identify the optimal sequencing and combination of psychological and somatic treatments for specific conditions? Adaptive treatment strategies and sequential multiple assignment randomized trials (SMART designs) can guide clinical decision-making.

C. Dissemination and Implementation

Even when effective psychological treatments exist, they often fail to reach those who need them. Research on dissemination and implementation is urgently needed.

- What are the most effective strategies for training and supervising clinicians in evidence-based psychological treatments, particularly in low-resource settings? Research must compare different training models and identify the minimal training needed to achieve competency.
- How can psychological treatments be adapted for diverse cultural contexts without losing their effectiveness? Cultural adaptation research must balance fidelity to evidence-based protocols with flexibility to accommodate local beliefs, values, and practices.

- What organizational and policy-level factors facilitate or hinder the implementation of psychological treatments in routine care settings? Organizational research can identify barriers and facilitators at the level of clinics, hospitals, and healthcare systems.

X. PLACING PAIN AT THE CENTER: RESEARCH ON SUFFERING AND ITS RELIEF

Elevating pain reduction to the primary goal of treatment, as advocated in this volume, requires a fundamental reconceptualization of outcome measurement and a deepened understanding of the nature of suffering itself.

A. The Phenomenology of Pain

Research must take seriously the subjective experience of pain in all its forms—physical, psychological, and existential.

- Can we develop better instruments for assessing pain that capture its multidimensional nature, including sensory, affective, cognitive, and social dimensions? Patient-reported outcome measures must be refined to reflect the complexity of lived experience.
- How do individuals from different cultural backgrounds experience, express, and cope with pain? Cross-cultural phenomenological research can illuminate both universal and culture- specific aspects of suffering, informing culturally sensitive assessment and treatment.
- What is the relationship between different types of pain? For example, how does chronic physical pain (as in the pelvic pain chapter) relate to psychological pain (depression, anxiety) and existential pain (loss of meaning, hopelessness)? Research exploring the common and distinct mechanisms underlying different pain experiences can inform transdiagnostic treatment approaches.

B. Pain as a Transdiagnostic Treatment Target

If pain is the common currency of suffering, it may serve as a unifying outcome measure across diverse diagnostic categories.

- Can pain reduction serve as a transdiagnostic outcome in clinical trials, allowing for comparisons of treatment effects across conditions that are traditionally siloed? This would require the development of pain measures that are valid and reliable across psychiatric and medical disorders.

- Do treatments that are effective for one type of pain also reduce other types of pain? For example, does successful treatment of depression reduce not only psychic pain but also sensitivity to physical pain? Does mindfulness training reduce both anxiety and the suffering associated with chronic illness? Research exploring the cross-cutting effects of interventions can identify treatments with broad-spectrum pain-reducing properties.
- Can we develop and test interventions specifically designed to target pain as a unified construct, rather than focusing on diagnosis-specific symptoms? Transdiagnostic psychotherapies that teach skills for managing suffering, regardless of its source, hold promise and warrant rigorous investigation.

C. The Neurobiology of Suffering

Advances in neuroscience offer the potential to understand the brain mechanisms underlying the experience of pain and its relief.

- What are the neural circuits and networks that subserve the experience of suffering across different diagnostic categories? Neuroimaging studies can identify common and distinct patterns of brain activity associated with physical pain, psychological distress, and existential anguish.
- How do effective treatments—both psychological and somatic—modulate these neural circuits? Understanding the neural mechanisms of pain relief can guide the development of more targeted and efficient interventions.
- Can neuroimaging or other biomarkers be used to predict individual differences in pain sensitivity and treatment response? This could enable personalized treatment matching, directing patients to the interventions most likely to reduce their specific type of suffering.

XI. LIFESPAN PERSPECTIVES: FROM CHILDHOOD TO OLD AGE

The developmental trajectory of mental illness, from early manifestations in childhood to neurocognitive decline in old age, demands a research agenda that spans the entire lifespan.

A. Early Intervention and Prevention in Childhood

The chapter on children's mental health underscores the critical importance of early intervention. Research must focus on identifying risk factors, developing preventive interventions, and understanding the long-term impact of early treatment.

- Can we identify biomarkers—biological, psychological, or social—that predict the onset of psychiatric disorders in high-risk children? Longitudinal studies following children from birth through adolescence can identify early warning signs and targets for prevention.
- What are the most effective interventions for preventing the onset of full-blown psychiatric disorders in at-risk children? Preventive trials must test interventions targeting multiple levels— individual, family, school, and community.
- How does early intervention alter long-term trajectories? Long-term follow-up studies of children who received treatment can document the enduring effects on psychiatric morbidity, physical health, occupational functioning, and quality of life.

B. The Interface of Physical and Mental Health Across the Lifespan

The chapters on cardiopulmonary rehabilitation in bipolar disorder and chronic illness and resilience highlight the inextricable link between physical and mental health at all ages.

- How do psychiatric disorders accelerate the development of physical illness across the lifespan? Longitudinal studies can track the emergence of cardiovascular, metabolic, and inflammatory diseases in individuals with psychiatric disorders, identifying mediating mechanisms and critical windows for intervention.
- How do chronic physical illnesses increase the risk of psychiatric disorders? Research must explore the psychological, social, and biological pathways through which physical illness impacts mental health.
- Can integrated care models that address both physical and mental health simultaneously improve outcomes for patients with comorbidity? Comparative effectiveness trials are needed to test the impact of integrated care on both mental and physical health outcomes, as well as on cost and patient satisfaction.

C. Neurocognitive Disorders in Aging Populations

The chapter on delirium, dementia, and Alzheimer's disease addresses one of the most pressing challenges of our aging society. Research must focus on prevention, early detection, and improved management.

- Can we identify modifiable risk factors for neurocognitive disorders that cut across the biopsychosocial spectrum? Longitudinal studies of aging populations can investigate the role of cardiovascular health, inflammation, social engagement, cognitive stimulation, and psychological factors (e.g., depression, stress) in the development of cognitive decline.
- What are the most effective strategies for distinguishing delirium from dementia in clinical practice, and for preventing delirium in at-risk populations? Implementation research can test the impact of screening protocols, staff training, and environmental modifications on delirium recognition and prevention.
- How can we improve the quality of life for individuals with neurocognitive disorders and their caregivers? Research must develop and test psychosocial interventions that address behavioral symptoms, support caregivers, and promote dignity and well-being in the face of progressive cognitive decline.

XII. NOVEL THERAPEUTIC TARGETS AND APPROACHES

The chapters in this volume point toward several promising directions for the development of novel treatments that go beyond current paradigms.

A. Psychoneuroimmunology and Inflammation

The chapter on psychoneuroimmunology of pelvic pain opens a window onto the exciting frontier of immune-based treatments for psychiatric and psychosomatic disorders.

- Can anti-inflammatory agents be repurposed for the treatment of depression, schizophrenia, or other psychiatric disorders characterized by elevated inflammation? Clinical trials are needed to test the efficacy of specific anti-inflammatory drugs in well-defined patient subgroups.
- Do psychological interventions exert their therapeutic effects, in part, through modulation of the immune system? Research can investigate whether psycho-

therapies reduce inflammatory markers and whether these changes mediate clinical improvement.

- Can we identify biomarkers of inflammation that predict treatment response and guide personalized treatment selection? This would allow for the matching of patients with elevated inflammation to treatments targeting the immune system.

B. Neurostimulation and Neuromodulation

The chapter on neurostimulation highlights the potential of directly modulating brain activity to treat emotional and affective disorders.

- What are the optimal parameters (target, frequency, intensity, duration) for different neurostimulation modalities in specific patient populations? Dose-finding studies and comparative effectiveness trials are needed to optimize these interventions.
- Can neurostimulation be combined with psychological interventions to enhance and synergize treatment effects? For example, does TMS combined with CBT produce greater and more durable improvements in depression than either treatment alone?
- How can we identify patients most likely to respond to neurostimulation? Neuroimaging and other biomarkers may predict response and guide patient selection.

C. Psychedelic-Assisted Psychotherapy

While not directly addressed in the case studies, the resurgence of interest in psychedelic-assisted psychotherapy for conditions such as depression, PTSD, and end-of-life anxiety is highly relevant to the themes of this volume. This approach uniquely combines biological (pharmacological) and psychological (psychotherapy) interventions in a structured therapeutic context.

- What are the active mechanisms of psychedelic-assisted psychotherapy? Research must disentangle the relative contributions of the drug's pharmacological effects, the psychotherapeutic context, and the set and setting to therapeutic outcomes.
- For which patient populations and psychiatric conditions is psychedelic-assisted psychotherapy most effective and safe? Rigorous clinical trials are needed to establish efficacy and safety across diverse diagnoses.

- Can the therapeutic benefits of psychedelic-assisted psychotherapy be sustained over the long term, and what factors predict durable improvement? Longitudinal follow-up studies are essential.

XIII. SOCIAL AND STRUCTURAL INTERVENTIONS

The biopsychosocial model demands that we take seriously the social determinants of health and develop interventions that target these structural factors.

A. Housing, Employment, and Income

Research must investigate the mental health impact of interventions that address basic social needs.

- Does providing stable, affordable housing to individuals with severe mental illness improve psychiatric outcomes, reduce hospitalizations, and enhance quality of life? Longitudinal studies of housing first and other supported housing models can document these effects.
- Do supported employment programs improve not only vocational outcomes but also mental health, self-esteem, and social integration? Research must measure the full range of outcomes relevant to recovery.
- Can income support programs (e.g., basic income guarantees) reduce psychological distress and improve mental health at the population level? Natural experiments and randomized trials of income interventions can test these hypotheses.

B. Community and Social Connection

The protective effects of social connection are well-established, but interventions to enhance social connection are underdeveloped.

- What are the most effective interventions for reducing social isolation and loneliness in individuals with mental illness? Research must test peer support programs, community engagement initiatives, and social skills training.
- How can communities be designed to promote mental health and social connection? Urban planning research can investigate the impact of green space, walkability, and community centers on mental health outcomes.

- In the digital age, how do online social networks impact mental health, both positively and negatively? Research must explore the complex relationship between social media use, social connection, and psychological well-being.

C. Stigma and Discrimination

Stigma remains a powerful barrier to seeking help and achieving recovery. Research must identify effective strategies for reducing stigma at multiple levels.

- What are the most effective anti-stigma interventions targeting the general public, healthcare providers, and individuals with mental illness themselves? Comparative effectiveness trials can test different educational, contact-based, and advocacy approaches.
- How does structural discrimination—in housing, employment, healthcare, and criminal justice—impact the lives of individuals with mental illness? Research must document these inequities and advocate for policy change.
- Can interventions that empower individuals with mental illness to challenge stigma and assert their rights improve self-esteem, empowerment, and recovery outcomes?

XIV. METHODOLOGICAL INNOVATIONS: STUDYING COMPLEXITY

The complexity of the biopsychosocial model demands methodological innovations that go beyond the traditional randomized controlled trial.

A. Mixed-Methods Research

The integration of quantitative and qualitative methods is essential for understanding both the outcomes of interventions and the processes through which they work. Qualitative research can illuminate patient perspectives, contextual factors, and mechanisms of change that are invisible to quantitative measures alone. Future research should routinely incorporate qualitative components to enrich interpretation and generate hypotheses.

B. N-of-1 and Single-Case Designs

The case-based approach of this volume highlights the value of studying individuals in depth. N- of-1 trials, in which a single patient is studied repeatedly over time under different conditions, offer a rigorous method for determining causal effects at the individual level. These designs are particularly well-suited to studying rare conditions, personalizing treatment, and understanding heterogeneity of treatment effects.

C. Longitudinal and Life-Course Designs

Understanding the dynamic interplay of biological, psychological, and social factors over time requires longitudinal studies that follow individuals across the lifespan. Such studies are expensive and time-consuming but essential for identifying causal pathways and critical windows for intervention. Existing longitudinal cohorts should be leveraged, and new cohorts established, with repeated measurement of biopsychosocial variables.

D. Systems Science and Computational Modeling

The biopsychosocial system is characterized by complex, nonlinear interactions among multiple components. Systems science methods—including agent-based modeling, system dynamics, and network analysis—offer tools for understanding these complex dynamics and simulating the impact of interventions. Computational models can integrate data from multiple sources and generate testable predictions about system behavior.

XV. REDEFINING SUCCESS: OUTCOMES THAT MATTER

Finally, the vision articulated in this volume—prioritizing psychological well-being, reducing pain, and promoting human flourishing—demands a fundamental reconsideration of how we define and measure success in mental health research and practice.

A. Beyond Symptom Reduction

While symptom reduction remains important, it is insufficient as the sole measure of treatment success. Future research must routinely assess outcomes that matter to patients: quality of life, functioning in valued roles, subjective well-being, hope, meaning, and purpose. The development and validation of patient-reported outcome measures that capture these domains is a critical priority.

B. Recovery-Oriented Outcomes

The recovery movement, led by individuals with lived experience of mental illness, has articulated a vision of recovery that goes beyond clinical remission to encompass living a meaningful, satisfying, and hopeful life. Research must operationalize and measure recovery- oriented outcomes, including personal recovery, empowerment, and community integration.

C. Positive Mental Health and Flourishing

Building on the philosophical argument that psychology and happiness should be prioritized, research must investigate not only the absence of mental illness but the presence of positive mental health. What are the determinants of flourishing? Can interventions explicitly designed to promote well-being, resilience, and happiness be effective in both clinical and general populations? This positive psychology agenda is not a luxury but a fundamental component of a comprehensive approach to mental health.

XVI. CONCLUSION: A CALL TO ACTION

The suggestions for further research outlined in this section are ambitious, but the challenges they address are urgent. The mortality gap, the inequities in access to psychological treatment, the profound suffering of individuals and families affected by mental illness—these realities demand nothing less than a transformative research agenda. It is a call to action for investigators across disciplines to collaborate, to innovate, and to commit themselves to the pursuit of knowledge that can truly make a difference in the lives of those who suffer. The case studies in this volume illuminate the path; future research must walk it.

Chapter 1
Impact of Clozapine on Neutrophil and White Blood Cell Counts:
A Case Study

samet uludag
Kastamonu Arac Government Hospital, Turkey

Kadir Uludag
http://orcid.org/0000-0003-3713-4670
Capital Medical University Xuanwu Hospital, China

EXECUTIVE SUMMARY

This abstract presents a case study of a 55-year-old Turkish female residing in Turkey diagnosed with Schizophrenia (SCZ) thirteen years ago, which was later compounded by a diagnosis of bipolar disorder (BD) five years following the initial diagnosis. Notably, the patient does not have any chronic disorders. Due to agranulocytosis resulting from the discontinued use of the antipsychotic clozapine, the patient currently receives lithium treatment in a dosage of 300 mg once daily. The patient's white blood cell (WBC) count and neutrophil levels remained stable for four years, but subsequently, the WBC count decreased to 3.8 and the absolute neutrophil count dropped to 1.7, a change that was linked to clozapine. Following the discontinuation of clozapine, his blood values returned to normal. It is also intriguing that both values deviated from the norm.

DOI: 10.4018/979-8-3373-3084-6.ch001

INTRODUCTION

Schizophrenia (SCZ) is a multifaceted and enduring psychotic condition marked by various symptoms that impact the mental health (Uludag, 2024b; Uludag & Kara, 2024). Antipsychotics are commonly used to treat patients with SCZ (Bruijnzeel, Suryadevara, & Tandon, 2014; Hamina et al., 2024; Uludag, 2024a). However, it leads to certain side effects such as metabolic problems (Collares et al., 2025; De Nayer et al., 2005; Uludag, Wang, Goodman, Wang, & Zhang, 2021). Clozapine, a widely used second-generation antipsychotic, is associated with superior treatment outcomes in individuals diagnosed with SCZ (Bleich et al., 2024; Wheeler, Humberstone, & Robinson, 2009). It can be effective in managing positive (Leucht, Arbter, Engel, Kissling, & Davis, 2009) and negative symptoms (Novick, Montgomery, Treuer, Moneta, & Haro, 2017). Clozapine, a dibenzodiazepine compound first developed in 1961, is an atypical antipsychotic with activity across multiple receptors and is approved for managing treatment-resistant SCZ (De Berardis et al., 2018; Pinioti et al., 2025).

Despite its controversial history as both a highly effective and potentially dangerous treatment, recent Food Drug Administration (FDA) revisions to clozapine prescribing and monitoring guidelines present an opportunity for renewed and safer clinical adoption (Newman & Newman, 2016). Despite being the most efficacious medication for treatment-resistant SCZ, clozapine is not used to its full potential, and the commencement of its use is frequently postponed and one contributing factor to this delay is the presence of a severe and potentially lethal adverse effect known as clozapine-induced agranulocytosis (CIA) (Islam et al., 2022; Shad, 2023). CIA is a dangerous adverse drug reaction that poses a significant risk, restricting the wider use of this highly potent atypical antipsychotic in individuals with SCZ (Alvir, Lieberman, Safferman, Schwimmer, & Schaaf, 1993; Opgen-Rhein & Dettling, 2008). Previous findings suggest that the majority of patients and their caregivers lack awareness of CIA (Oloyede et al., 2025). After clozapine was first introduced, eight Finnish patients passed away due to agranulocytosis. Consequently, clozapine was removed from the market and later reintroduced (Schulte et al., 2024). The balance between its unparalleled therapeutic benefits and the potential for severe adverse reactions highlights the urgent need for predictive biomarkers and individualized monitoring strategies to enhance safety and optimize treatment outcomes.

A meta-analysis encompassing thirty-six studies with individuals treated with clozapine revealed that the occurrence rates of agranulocytosis and agranulocytosis-related fatalities were 0.4% and 0.05%, respectively (Li et al., 2020). Over time, the likelihood of clozapine causing agranulocytosis drops, although it may still be higher than that associated with non-clozapine antipsychotics (Rubio, Kane, Tanskanen, Tiihonen, & Taipale, 2024). In our specific case study, the patient did not experience agranulocytosis when they initially started using clozapine. Furthermore, unique drug-induced agranulocytosis continues to pose a significant risk due to the high incidence of severe sepsis resulting in severe deep tissue infections like pneumonia and septic shock (Andrès et al., 2011). Drug-induced agranulocytosis is a potentially fatal adverse reaction characterized by a severe reduction in white blood cell (WBC), often accompanied by fever or symptoms indicating a severe infection (Rattay & Benndorf, 2021). The clozapine screening protocols require checking the WBC count without fail (Cohen, Bogers, van Dijk, Bakker, & Schulte, 2012).

WBC in individuals with SCZ can be influenced by specific antipsychotics. Short-term treatment tends to reduce WBC levels, while long-term use can lead to increases. WBC levels can serve as an indicator of how a patient may respond to medication, with lower counts indicating a potentially more positive response to antipsychotics (Zhang et al., 2024).

Other results emphasize the importance of monitoring standard vital signs and blood total and diverse WBC counts as relevant indicators for assessing the cardiovascular disease risk in the clinical management of patients with psychosis (Moody & Miller, 2018).

In conclusion, drug-induced agranulocytosis poses a serious threat due to its potential fatality and is characterized by a significant decrease in WBC count, often accompanied by fever or signs suggestive of a severe infection. Monitoring standard vital signs and various WBC counts is crucial for evaluating cardiovascular risk in the clinical care of psychosis patients, as these parameters can also offer insights into how patients may respond to antipsychotic treatment.

Furthermore, the impact of clozapine on the immune system has become more important following a previous study that revealed a negative relationship between drug plasma levels and neutrophil counts in individuals consistently receiving treatment (Willcocks et al., 2021).

Moreover, a different study showed that a reduction in the lifespan of human neutrophils was noted during brief exposure to clozapine at a concentration of 100 μM and during prolonged exposure, even at a lower concentration of 50 μM (Goto et al., 2017). Recent studies have highlighted the increasing significance of clozapine's effects on the immune system (Liu, Zhao, & Wang, 2025; Wei & Dong, 2025), with findings indicating an inverse correlation between drug plasma levels and neutrophil counts in regularly treated individuals.

METHODOLOGY

The data was collected by interview. The findings from the case study were summarized in the abstract section. Written informed consent was obtained from the patient. We have also conducted a review of the relevant literature. Table 1 displays an overview of chosen instances involving patients diagnosed with SCZ and Agranulocytosis.

LITERATURE REVIEW

Lithium and White Blood Cell

Medical professionals have utilized lithium for managing bipolar disorder (BD) (Airainer & Seifert, 2024; Licht, 2012; Malhi, Tanious, Das, Coulston, & Berk, 2013; Young, 2009). Increasing evidence indicates that inflammation is implicated in the development of BD and that lithium possesses anti-inflammatory properties (Nassar & Azab, 2014; Zhou, Zheng, Guo, Wu, & Zhong, 2025). Lithium is linked to an elevated likelihood of decreased urinary concentration and weight increase (Ferensztajn-Rochowiak & Rybakowski, 2023; McKnight et al., 2012). The literature is limited on the relationship between Lithium and WBC and neutrophil. Moreover, the clinical implications and safety profile of concomitant administration of lithium and antipsychotic medications have not been systematically investigated, highlighting a gap in current knowledge that warrants further research.

Polydrug Use

Polydrug use is a critical factor influencing the clinical course and treatment outcomes in SCZ, particularly among patients receiving complex pharmacological regimens. The concurrent use of multiple psychoactive substances—such as antipsychotics, mood stabilizers, or other psychotropics—can alter drug metabolism, increase toxicity risks, and exacerbate adverse effects, including hematological complications like clozapine-induced agranulocytosis. Moreover, combining agents such as clozapine and lithium requires careful monitoring, as interactions between these drugs may influence WBC dynamics and immune responses. Given the multifaceted effects of polydrug use on efficacy, safety, and patient adherence, individualized treatment strategies and close hematological surveillance are essential for optimizing therapeutic outcomes and minimizing the risk of severe adverse reactions in patients with SCZ (Biso, Aringhieri, Carli, Scarselli, & Longoni, 2024).

Immunomodulatory Effects of Clozapine

Beyond its well-established antipsychotic efficacy, clozapine exerts significant immunomodulatory effects that are increasingly recognized as clinically relevant, particularly in relation to hematological safety. Clozapine interacts with multiple immune pathways and has been shown to influence both innate and adaptive immune responses, with neutrophils and total WBC counts being especially affected. Furthermore, clozapine changes the cytokines profile in SCZ patients (Drzyzga, Obuchowicz, Marcinowska, & Herman, 2006; Shao et al., 2024; Yuan et al., 2022).

Side Effects of Clozapine and Treatment Response

Clozapine is the most effective treatment for treatment-resistant schizophrenia, yet its clinical use is closely tied to a distinctive profile of side effects that can significantly influence treatment response and adherence. Clozapine therapy is accompanied by short-term hematological alterations in the initial month of treatment, but these changes do not appear to be associated with clinical treatment response (Blackman et al., 2021). There are many recently studies published on clozapine and treatment response (Tralongo, Konecki, Feliu, Kaladjian, & Djerada, 2023). A previous review discussed if Clozapine levels can be used as a predictor for therapeutic response (Siskind et al., 2021). A systematic review further indicated that favorable clinical response was associated with clozapine plasma concentrations, rather than dose, with responders showing a mean concentration 117 ng/mL higher than non-responders (Tralongo et al., 2023). Collectively, this evidence underscores the importance of therapeutic drug monitoring and individualized dosing strategies to optimize clozapine efficacy while minimizing adverse effects in patients with treatment-resistant SCZ.

Ethnic and Racial Disparities in Clozapine Use

Despite its established status as the most effective pharmacological treatment for treatment-resistant schizophrenia (TRS), clozapine remains profoundly underutilized globally. A significant and persistent factor in this treatment gap is the stark disparity in its prescription and access across ethnic and racial lines. Emerging evidence consistently shows that patients from Black, Hispanic, and other minority ethnic backgrounds are significantly less likely to be prescribed clozapine and experience longer delays before initiating therapy compared to their White counterparts.

The Evidence of Disparity

Multiple studies in the United States, the United Kingdom, and other diverse healthcare systems document this pattern. For instance, across 24 studies, robust and consistent evidence indicates that Black and Hispanic service users in the UK and the USA are markedly less likely than White/Caucasian service users to be prescribed clozapine, even after adjustment for a wide range of demographic confounding factors(Ventura, Hayes, & Fonseca de Freitas, 2022). Moreover, another study reported that, among 2,239 individuals with treatment-resistant schizophrenia, Black service users were significantly less likely than White British service users to receive clozapine after controlling for potential confounding variables (de Freitas et al., 2022). Addressing these inequities requires targeted efforts to identify structural, institutional, and clinician-level barriers to clozapine use, alongside the development of equitable prescribing guidelines and culturally informed interventions to ensure that evidence-based care is delivered consistently across ethnic groups.

Root Causes of the Disparity

The drivers of this disparity are multifactorial, stemming from a complex interplay of clinical, systemic, and socio-cultural factors:

ECONOMIC FACTORS AND RISK IN CLOZAPINE TREATMENT

The utilization of clozapine is profoundly influenced by economic factors, which interact with its risk profile to create significant barriers to access and optimal management. The decision to initiate and maintain clozapine therapy involves a complex economic and risk-benefit calculus at systemic, institutional, and individual levels.

The Direct and Indirect Economic Burden of Clozapine Management

While the drug itself is now largely available in generic form, the total cost of clozapine care is exceptionally high, primarily due to its rigorous monitoring requirements.

Monitoring Infrastructure: Mandatory weekly to monthly blood draws, associated laboratory fees, and the administrative cost of maintaining a registry (e.g., the U.S. Clozapine Risk Evaluation and Mitigation Strategy [REMS] Program) represent a sustained financial burden. Healthcare systems, especially under-resourced public clinics or those in low- and middle-income countries, may lack the infrastructure for consistent, long-term hematological monitoring.

Specialist Care and Clinic Time: Optimal clozapine management often requires consultation with psychopharmacology specialists and more frequent clinic visits, consuming more clinician time and specialized resources than standard antipsychotic regimens.

Cost of Managing Adverse Effects: The economic impact extends to managing common side effects (e.g., sedation, sialorrhea, metabolic monitoring) and, critically, the high cost of treating severe adverse events like agranulocytosis, which necessitates emergency care, hospitalization, and treatment with granulocyte colony-stimulating factors (G-CSF).

Confounding Factors

There are several confounding factors inherent in this and similar case studies that must be considered when interpreting the hematological data, including patient-specific variables such as age, genetic susceptibility, and the potential immunomodulatory effects of concomitant medications like lithium.

CONCLUSION

To summarize, antipsychotic medications can result in decreased WBC counts, and discontinuing or altering antipsychotic treatment can benefit individuals with SCZ.

Limitations

One limitation is that a case study may not be fully representative of all patients with SCZ. The duration of observation in this case study is not specified, which may affect the understanding of the long-term effects of the treatment.

Suggestions for Further Studies

Further studies can investigate how genetic variations may impact the efficacy and side effects of medications commonly used to treat SCZ and BD in patients with a dual diagnosis like the one this patient has. Understanding how genetic factors influence treatment outcomes can help tailor medication regimens to individual patients. Future research should prioritize interdisciplinary studies that elucidate the precise molecular mechanisms—including inflammatory pathways and direct myelosuppressive effects—underlying clozapine-induced hematological changes. Concurrently, well-powered prospective studies are needed to validate genetic and inflammatory biomarkers for predicting individual risk of agranulocytosis versus benign neutropenia, which could translate into personalized monitoring strategies. Furthermore, clinical trials should systematically evaluate the safety and immunological interactions of common polypharmacy regimens, particularly clozapine with lithium, and assess the real-world impact of modern, risk-based monitoring protocols on treatment adherence and patient outcomes. Ultimately, integrating mechanistic, genetic, and clinical data through longitudinal studies and advanced analytics is essential to develop safer, more precise application of this uniquely efficacious antipsychotic.

Figure 1. Therapeutic benefits and risks of Clozapine

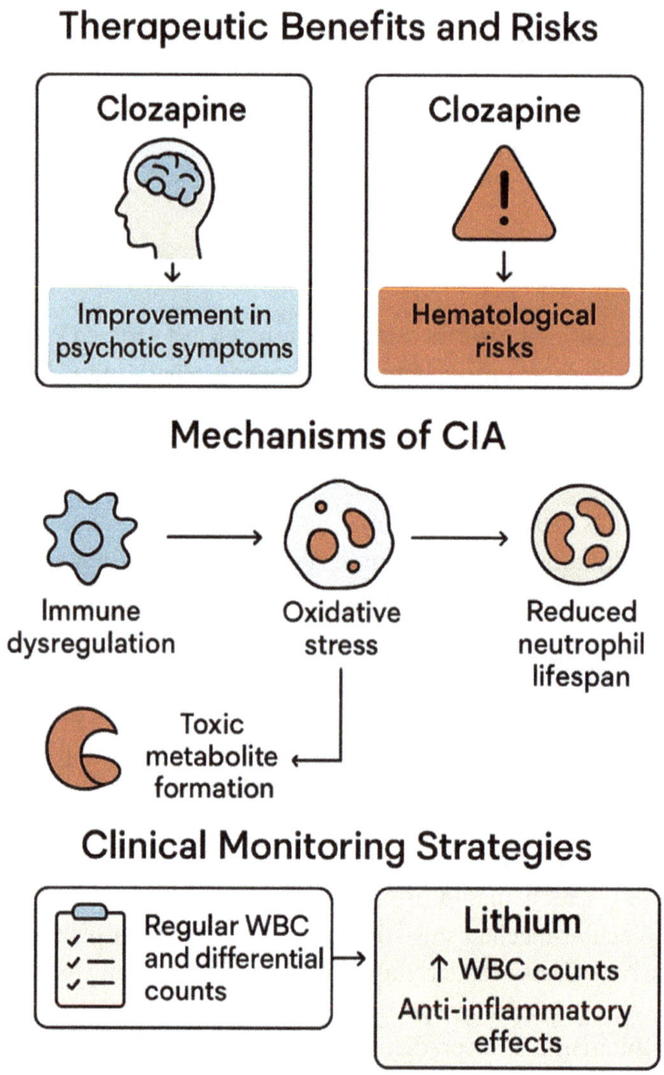

Table 1. Review of selected cases of patients with schizophrenia and Agranulocytosis

Article title	Reference	Results
Late-Onset Agranulocytosis in a Patient With Schizophrenia After 17 Months of Clozapine Treatment	Bhanji, N. H., Margolese, H. C., Chouinard, G., & Turnier, L. (2003). Late-onset agranulocytosis in a patient with schizophrenia after 17 months of clozapine treatment. *Journal of clinical psychopharmacology*, *23*(5), 522-523.	The article reported Late-Onset Agranulocytosis in a Patient With SCZ After 17 Months of Clozapine.
Clozapine-induced agranulocytosis in schizophrenic Caucasians: confirming clues for associations with human leukocyte class I and II antigens	Dettling, M., Cascorbi, I., Opgen-Rhein, C., & Schaub, R. (2007). Clozapine-induced agranulocytosis in schizophrenic Caucasians: confirming clues for associations with human leukocyte class I and II antigens. *The pharmacogenomics journal*, *7*(5), 325-332.	The intricate characteristics of Clozapine-triggered agranulocytosis suggest that a multitude of genes could be involved in its development.
Genetic risk factors for clozapine-induced neutropenia and agranulocytosis in a Dutch psychiatric population	Van Der Weide, K., Loovers, H., Pondman, K., Bogers, J., Van Der Straaten, T., Langemeijer, E., ... & Van Der Weide, J. (2017). Genetic risk factors for clozapine-induced neutropenia and agranulocytosis in a Dutch psychiatric population. *The Pharmacogenomics Journal*, *17*(5), 471-478.	Confirming whether combinations of the identified genetic risk factors possess greater predictive value warrants validation through a more extensive case-control study.
Incidence and risk for neutropenia/agranulocytosis among clozapine users: A retrospective cohort study	Ratanajamit, C., Musakopas, C., Vasiknanonte, S., & Reanmongkol, W. (2009). Incidence and risk for neutropenia/agranulocytosis among clozapine users: A retrospective cohort study. *International Journal of Psychiatry in Clinical Practice*, *14*(2), 109–115. https://doi.org/10.3109/13651500903402450	A single case of agranulocytosis was identified in the group not treated with clozapine.
Clozapine-induced agranulocytosis: A situation report up to August 1976	Anderman, B., & Griffith, R. W. (1977). Clozapine-induced agranulocytosis: a situation report up to August 1976. *European journal of clinical pharmacology*, *11*, 199-201.	With the exception of the notable "epidemic" observed in Finland, where the incidence rate was 21 times higher than in other nations, there is no indication that CIA is more prevalent than the disorder associated with phenothiazines.

Note: Review studies were excluded.
Abbreviations: SCZ, schizophrenia

Table 2. Lithium and agranulocytosis

Role of Lithium	Clinical Context	Typical Outcome
Therapeutic	Treatment of drug-induced agranulocytosis	Rapid recovery of ANC (often within 5–7 days).
Prophylactic	Clozapine initiation or rechallenge	Maintains WBC above the "red alert" threshold.
Diagnostic Risk	Masking effect	Can hide underlying marrow failure; risk of crash if Li is stopped.

Table 2 summarizes the multifaceted role of lithium in the context of agranulocytosis, particularly in patients receiving clozapine.

Table 3. Clozapine and Benefits

Category	Key Benefit	Detail and Clinical Significance
Gold Standard for Treatment Resistance	Superior Efficacy for Treatment-Resistant Schizophrenia (TRS)	It is the only FDA-approved medication for TRS (failure to respond to two prior antipsychotics). It leads to significant symptom reduction (positive and negative) in a substantial number of patients who were previously considered non-responders.
Suicide Prevention	Reduces the Risk of Recurrent Suicidal Behavior	It is the only antipsychotic with a specific FDA indication for reducing the risk of repeated suicidal behavior in patients with schizophrenia or schizoaffective disorder.
Movement Side Effects	Lowest Risk of Extrapyramidal Symptoms (EPS)	Due to its unique mechanism (weak D2 receptor binding), clozapine causes less Tardive Dyskinesia (TD), Parkinsonism, and Akathisia than most other antipsychotics, significantly improving quality of life.
Symptom Improvement	Reduces Negative Symptoms	Unlike many older antipsychotics that primarily target positive symptoms (hallucinations, delusions), clozapine is also effective at reducing negative symptoms (e.g., apathy, blunted affect).
Functional & Mortality Outcomes	Lower All-Cause Mortality	Patients treated with clozapine have been shown to have a lower risk of premature death compared to those on other antipsychotics, which may be related to decreased suicide rates and reduced relapse.
Other Refractory Conditions	Effective for Aggression/ Hostility and Psychosis in Parkinson's Disease	It is commonly used to manage severe aggression/ hostility that is refractory to other treatments and is often preferred for psychosis in Parkinson's disease due to its low EPS risk.

Table 3 outlines the benefits associated with clozapine and related treatments.

Table 4. Side effects of Clozapine

Category	Side Effect	Mechanism/Description	Monitoring Requirement
Life-Threatening/ Severe	Agranulocytosis	Severe drop in white blood cell count (specifically neutrophils), leading to a high risk of life-threatening infection.	Weekly blood count (ANC) monitoring for the first 6 months, then bi-weekly, then monthly, as mandated by REMS programs. Must be discontinued if ANC drops below a certain threshold.
	Myocarditis/Cardiomyopathy	Inflammation of the heart muscle, often presenting early in treatment with fever, fatigue, chest pain, and tachycardia. Can lead to heart failure.	Close monitoring of vital signs and cardiac symptoms (especially in the first month). Immediate discontinuation if suspected.
	Seizures	Clozapine significantly lowers the seizure threshold in a dose-dependent manner.	Start at a low dose and titrate slowly. Anti-epileptic medication may be needed in high-risk patients or at high clozapine doses.
Metabolic/Endocrine	Weight Gain	Significant and rapid weight gain (often exceeding 10 kg), contributing to metabolic syndrome.	Regular monitoring of BMI and weight. Lifestyle interventions.
	Type 2 Diabetes Mellitus	Insulin resistance and impaired glucose tolerance; risk is higher than with most other antipsychotics.	Baseline and regular monitoring of fasting glucose and HbA1c.
	Dyslipidemia	Increase in total cholesterol, LDL, and triglycerides.	Baseline and regular monitoring of lipid profile.
Common/Neurological	Sedation/Drowsiness	Extremely common, especially during initial titration and dose increases.	Often managed by taking the dose at night and slow titration.

continued on following page

Table 4. Continued

Category	Side Effect	Mechanism/Description	Monitoring Requirement
	Salivation (Sialorrhea)	Excessive drooling, particularly at night, which can cause skin irritation or aspiration risk.	Use of anticholinergic agents (e.g., benztropine or glycopyrrolate) at night.
	Dizziness/Orthostatic Hypotension	Drop in blood pressure upon standing, leading to risk of falls, particularly early in treatment.	Slow titration and advising patients to rise slowly. Monitoring blood pressure.
	Tremor/Other EPS	Less common than with typical antipsychotics, but still possible, especially at higher doses.	Dose reduction or use of anticholinergic medication.
Gastrointestinal	Constipation	Severe, potentially leading to ileus (bowel obstruction), which can be fatal. This is a common and serious complication.	Prophylactic laxatives/stool softeners are often prescribed routinely. Monitor bowel movements closely.

Table 4 presents a summary of the side effects associated with clozapine.

Table 5. Chronological Overview of Clozapine Development and Clinical Use

Year / Period	Milestone	Significance
1958–1959	Clozapine synthesized by Wander AG (Switzerland) (Hippius, 1999)	Development of the first atypical antipsychotic with a unique chemical structure
1960s	Early clinical testing in Europe	Demonstrated antipsychotic efficacy with minimal extrapyramidal side effects
1972	Introduced into clinical use in Europe	Widely adopted due to favorable neurological side-effect profile
1975	Reports of agranulocytosis in Finland	Temporary withdrawal in several countries following fatal cases
Late 1970s–1980s	Restricted use with hematological monitoring	Recognition that risks could be managed with regular blood testing
1988	Landmark US multicenter trial	Demonstrated superior efficacy in treatment-resistant schizophrenia
1989	FDA approval in the United States	Approved specifically for treatment-resistant schizophrenia with mandatory blood monitoring

continued on following page

Table 5. Continued

Year / Period	Milestone	Significance
1990s	Global reintroduction under monitoring programs	Establishment of national clozapine registries and safety protocols
2000s	Expanded indications and research	Evidence for reduced suicidality and benefits in refractory psychosis
2010s	Refinement of monitoring guidelines	Improved understanding of hematological, metabolic, and cardiac risks
2020s	Continued use as gold-standard for treatment resistance	Ongoing research into immunological effects, biomarkers, and optimization of safety

Table 5 provides a chronological overview of the development and clinical application of clozapine.

Table 6. Comparative Overview: Lithium vs. Clozapine

Feature	Lithium	Clozapine
Primary Indication	Bipolar Disorder (Mania & Maintenance)	Treatment-Resistant Schizophrenia
Effect on WBCs	Increase (Leukocytosis/Neutrophilia)	Potential Decrease (Risk of Agranulocytosis)
Systemic Risk	Renal & Thyroid Dysfunction	Metabolic Syndrome & Myocarditis
Neurological Risk	Tremor & Lithium Toxicity	Seizures & Sedation
Key Benefit	Anti-suicidal properties	Anti-suicidal properties

Table 6 presents a comparative overview of lithium and clozapine.

Table 7. Factors Influencing Clinical Success

Factor Category	Examples	Impact on Treatment Outcome
Demographics	Age, Gender, Ethnicity	Influences drug metabolism rates and susceptibility to side effects.
Lifestyle Habits	Smoking, Alcohol, Sleep patterns	Smoking can lower Clozapine levels; Alcohol increases sedation risks.
Comorbidities	Diabetes, Hypertension, Renal disease	Requires careful dosing (Lithium) or metabolic monitoring (Clozapine).
Adherence Tools	Mandatory Registries (REMS), Family support	Mandatory monitoring improves safety but may create barriers to access.

Table 7 outlines the factors that influence clinical success..

CONSENT FOR PUBLICATION

Written informed consent was obtained from the patients for publication of this case report. Consent obtained directly from patient.

COMPETING INTERESTS

The authors declare that they have no conflicts of interest to state.

AUTHOR CONTRIBUTIONS

The conceptualization and manuscript preparation were carried out by K.U. and S.U. Clinical data were collected by S.U. Both authors contributed to the revision and refinement of the final manuscript, and all authors provided approval for publication.

REFERENCES

Airainer, M., & Seifert, R. (2024). Lithium, the gold standard drug for bipolar disorder: Analysis of current clinical studies. *Naunyn-Schmiedeberg's Archives of Pharmacology*, *397*(12), 9723–9743. DOI: 10.1007/s00210-024-03210-8 PMID: 38916833

Alvir, J. M. J., Lieberman, J. A., Safferman, A. Z., Schwimmer, J. L., & Schaaf, J. A. (1993). Clozapine-induced agranulocytosis—Incidence and risk factors in the United States. *The New England Journal of Medicine*, *329*(3), 162–167. DOI: 10.1056/NEJM199307153290303 PMID: 8515788

Andrès, E., Zimmer, J., Mecili, M., Weitten, T., Alt, M., & Maloisel, F. (2011). Clinical presentation and management of drug-induced agranulocytosis. *Expert Review of Hematology*, *4*(2), 143–151. DOI: 10.1586/ehm.11.12 PMID: 21495924

Biso, L., Aringhieri, S., Carli, M., Scarselli, M., & Longoni, B. (2024). Therapeutic drug monitoring in psychiatry: Enhancing treatment precision and patient outcomes. *Pharmaceuticals (Basel, Switzerland)*, *17*(5), 642. DOI: 10.3390/ph17050642 PMID: 38794212

Blackman, G., Lisshammar, J. E. L., Zafar, R., Pollak, T. A., Pritchard, M., Cullen, A. E., Rogers, J., Carter, B., Griffiths, K., Nour, M., David, A. S., McGuire, P., Stewart, R., & MacCabe, J. (2021). Clozapine Response in Schizophrenia and Hematological Changes. *Journal of Clinical Psychopharmacology*, *41*(1), 19–24. DOI: 10.1097/JCP.0000000000001329 PMID: 33347018

Bleich, L., Grohmann, R., Greil, W., Dabbert, D., Erfurth, A., Toto, S., & Seifert, J. (2024). Clozapine-associated adverse drug reactions in 38,349 psychiatric inpatients: Drug surveillance data from the AMSP project between 1993 and 2016. *Journal of Neural Transmission (Vienna, Austria)*, *131*(9), 1117–1134. DOI: 10.1007/s00702-024-02818-7 PMID: 39136776

Bruijnzeel, D., Suryadevara, U., & Tandon, R. (2014). Antipsychotic treatment of schizophrenia: An update. *Asian Journal of Psychiatry*, *11*, 3–7. DOI: 10.1016/j.ajp.2014.08.002 PMID: 25216917

Cohen, D., Bogers, J. P., van Dijk, D., Bakker, B., & Schulte, P. F. (2012). Beyond white blood cell monitoring: Screening in the initial phase of clozapine therapy. *The Journal of Clinical Psychiatry*, *73*(10), 1887. DOI: 10.4088/JCP.11r06977 PMID: 23140648

Collares, S. F., de Ávila Júnior, A. M., Martins, T. C., Rezende, V. H. M., Romano-Silva, M. A., Santos, R. M. S., & de Miranda, D. M. (2025). Systematic review and meta-analysis of weight gain and metabolic changes in children and adolescents using second-generation antipsychotics. *Pharmacology, Biochemistry, and Behavior*, *251*, 174012. DOI: 10.1016/j.pbb.2025.174012 PMID: 40180054

De Berardis, D., Rapini, G., Olivieri, L., Di Nicola, D., Tomasetti, C., Valchera, A., & Di Nicola, M. (2018). Safety of antipsychotics for the treatment of schizophrenia: A focus on the adverse effects of clozapine. *Therapeutic Advances in Drug Safety*, *9*(5), 237–256. DOI: 10.1177/2042098618756261 PMID: 29796248

de Freitas, D. F., Patel, I., Kadra-Scalzo, G., Pritchard, M., Shetty, H., Broadbent, M., Patel, R., Downs, J., Segev, A., Khondoker, M., MacCabe, J. H., Bhui, K., & Hayes, R. D. (2022). Ethnic inequalities in clozapine use among people with treatment-resistant schizophrenia: A retrospective cohort study using data from electronic clinical records. *Social Psychiatry and Psychiatric Epidemiology*, *57*(7), 1341–1355. DOI: 10.1007/s00127-022-02257-3 PMID: 35246709

De Nayer, A., De Hert, M., Scheen, A., Van Gaal, L., Peuskens, J., De Nayer, A., De Hert, M., Scheen, A., Van Gaal, L., & Peuskens, J.on behalf of the Consensus Groupon behalf of the Consensus Group. (2005). Belgian consensus on metabolic problems associated with atypical antipsychotics. *International Journal of Psychiatry in Clinical Practice*, *9*(2), 130–137. DOI: 10.1080/13651500510018310 PMID: 24930795

Drzyzga, Ł., Obuchowicz, E., Marcinowska, A., & Herman, Z. S. (2006). Cytokines in schizophrenia and the effects of antipsychotic drugs. *Brain, Behavior, and Immunity*, *20*(6), 532–545. DOI: 10.1016/j.bbi.2006.02.002 PMID: 16580814

Ferensztajn-Rochowiak, E., & Rybakowski, J. K. (2023). Long-term lithium therapy: Side effects and interactions. *Pharmaceuticals (Basel, Switzerland)*, *16*(1), 74. DOI: 10.3390/ph16010074 PMID: 36678571

Goto, A., Yoshimi, A., Nagai, T., Ukigai, M., Mouri, A., Ozaki, N., & Noda, Y. (2017). Human neutrophils show decreased survival upon long-term exposure to clozapine. *Human Psychopharmacology*, *32*(6), e2629. DOI: 10.1002/hup.2629 PMID: 28913970

Hamina, A., Taipale, H., Lieslehto, J., Lähteenvuo, M., Tanskanen, A., Mittendorfer-Rutz, E., & Tiihonen, J. (2024). Comparative effectiveness of antipsychotics in patients with schizophrenia spectrum disorder. *JAMA Network Open*, *7*(10), e2438358–e2438358. DOI: 10.1001/jamanetworkopen.2024.38358 PMID: 39382894

Hippius, H. (1999). A historical perspective of clozapine. *The Journal of Clinical Psychiatry*, *60*(12), 22–23. PMID: 10372606

Islam, F., Hain, D., Lewis, D., Law, R., Brown, L. C., Tanner, J.-A., & Müller, D. J. (2022). Pharmacogenomics of Clozapine-induced agranulocytosis: A systematic review and meta-analysis. *The Pharmacogenomics Journal*, *22*(4), 230–240. DOI: 10.1038/s41397-022-00281-9 PMID: 35710824

Leucht, S., Arbter, D., Engel, R. R., Kissling, W., & Davis, J. M. (2009). How effective are second-generation antipsychotic drugs? A meta-analysis of placebo-controlled trials. *Molecular Psychiatry*, *14*(4), 429–447. DOI: 10.1038/sj.mp.4002136 PMID: 18180760

Li, X.-H., Zhong, X.-M., Lu, L., Zheng, W., Wang, S., Rao, W., Wang, S., Ng, C. H., Ungvari, G. S., Wang, G., & Xiang, Y.-T. (2020). The prevalence of agranulocytosis and related death in clozapine-treated patients: A comprehensive meta-analysis of observational studies. *Psychological Medicine*, *50*(4), 583–594. DOI: 10.1017/S0033291719000369 PMID: 30857568

Licht, R. W. (2012). Lithium: Still a major option in the management of bipolar disorder. *CNS Neuroscience & Therapeutics*, *18*(3), 219–226. DOI: 10.1111/j.1755-5949.2011.00260.x PMID: 22070642

Liu, J., Zhao, W., & Wang, Y. (2025). Lights and shadows of clozapine on the immune system in schizophrenia: A narrative literature review. *Metabolic Brain Disease*, *40*(2), 128. DOI: 10.1007/s11011-025-01558-1 PMID: 39954151

Malhi, G. S., Tanious, M., Das, P., Coulston, C. M., & Berk, M. (2013). Potential mechanisms of action of lithium in bipolar disorder: Current understanding. *CNS Drugs*, *27*(2), 135–153. DOI: 10.1007/s40263-013-0039-0 PMID: 23371914

McKnight, R. F., Adida, M., Budge, K., Stockton, S., Goodwin, G. M., & Geddes, J. R. (2012). Lithium toxicity profile: A systematic review and meta-analysis. *Lancet*, *379*(9817), 721–728. DOI: 10.1016/S0140-6736(11)61516-X PMID: 22265699

Moody, G., & Miller, B. J. (2018). Total and differential white blood cell counts and hemodynamic parameters in first-episode psychosis. *Psychiatry Research*, *260*, 307–312. DOI: 10.1016/j.psychres.2017.11.086 PMID: 29223800

Nassar, A., & Azab, A. N. (2014). Effects of lithium on inflammation. *ACS Chemical Neuroscience*, *5*(6), 451–458. DOI: 10.1021/cn500038f PMID: 24803181

Newman, W. J., & Newman, B. M. (2016). Rediscovering clozapine: After a turbulent history, current guidance on initiating and monitoring. *Current Psychiatry*, *15*(7), 42–46.

Novick, D., Montgomery, W., Treuer, T., Moneta, M. V., & Haro, J. M. (2017). Real-world Effectiveness of Antipsychotics for the Treatment of Negative Symptoms in Patients with Schizophrenia with Predominantly Negative Symptoms. *Pharmacopsychiatry, 50*(02), 56–63. DOI: 10.1055/s-0042-112818 PMID: 28208190

Oloyede, E., Nettey, V., Dzahini, O., Silva, E., Majkic, N., Montford, P., Secchi, A., Whiskey, E., & Taylor, D. (2025). Low awareness of clozapine-induced agranulocytosis in a mixed-method survey of 354 patients and carers. *Schizophrenia, 11*(1), 129. DOI: 10.1038/s41537-025-00639-5 PMID: 41168211

Opgen-Rhein, C., & Dettling, M. (2008). Clozapine-Induced Agranulocytosis and its Genetic Determinants. *Pharmacogenomics, 9*(8), 1101–1111. DOI: 10.2217/14622416.9.8.1101 PMID: 18681784

Pinioti, E., Glarou, E., Lappas, A. S., Fober, I., Helfer, B., Siafis, S., Christodoulou, N., Nikolakopoulou, A., Leucht, S., & Samara, M. (2025). Examining the safety profile of clozapine versus other antipsychotics: Systematic review and meta-analysis. *The British Journal of Psychiatry*, •••, 1–10. DOI: 10.1192/bjp.2025.10421 PMID: 41146456

Rattay, B., & Benndorf, R. A. (2021). Drug-Induced Idiosyncratic Agranulocytosis - Infrequent but Dangerous. *Frontiers in Pharmacology, 12*, 727717. Advance online publication. DOI: 10.3389/fphar.2021.727717 PMID: 34483939

Rubio, J. M., Kane, J. M., Tanskanen, A., Tiihonen, J., & Taipale, H. (2024). Long-term persistence of the risk of agranulocytosis with clozapine compared with other antipsychotics: A nationwide cohort and case–control study in Finland. *The Lancet. Psychiatry, 11*(6), 443–450. DOI: 10.1016/S2215-0366(24)00097-X PMID: 38697177

Schulte, P. F. J., Veerman, S. R. T., Bakker, B., Bogers, J. P. A. M., Jongkind, A., & Cohen, D. (2024). Risk of clozapine-associated agranulocytosis and mandatory white blood cell monitoring: Can the regulations be relaxed? *Schizophrenia Research, 268*, 74–81. DOI: 10.1016/j.schres.2023.09.024 PMID: 37770377

Shad, M. U. (2023). Pharmacogenomic screening for agranulocytosis and efficacy with clozapine. *Journal of Translational Genetics and Genomics, 7*(3), 141–165. DOI: 10.20517/jtgg.2023.11

Shao, L., Li, Y., Yuan, Z., Guo, X., Zeng, G., & Liu, J. (2024). The effect of clozapine on immune-related biomarkers in schizophrenia patients. *Brain Research Bulletin, 218*, 111104. DOI: 10.1016/j.brainresbull.2024.111104 PMID: 39424000

Siskind, D., Sharma, M., Pawar, M., Pearson, E., Wagner, E., Warren, N., & Kisely, S. (2021). Clozapine levels as a predictor for therapeutic response: A systematic review and meta-analysis. *Acta Psychiatrica Scandinavica, 144*(5), 422–432. DOI: 10.1111/acps.13361 PMID: 34374073

Tralongo, F., Konecki, C., Feliu, C., Kaladjian, A., & Djerada, Z. (2023). Association between clozapine plasma concentrations and treatment response: A systematic review, meta-analysis and individual participant data meta-analysis. *Clinical Pharmacokinetics, 62*(6), 807–818. DOI: 10.1007/s40262-023-01247-1 PMID: 37145296

Uludag, K. (2024a). Brain imaging studies on Tardive Dyskinesia in schizophrenia patients and animal models: A comprehensive review. *Future Neurology, 19*(1), 2433936. DOI: 10.1080/14796708.2024.2433936

Uludag, K. (2024b). Predicting Gender Based on Severity of Symptoms of Schizophrenia and Cognitive Parameters. In *Applications of Parallel Data Processing for Biomedical Imaging* (pp. 276–287). IGI Global. DOI: 10.4018/979-8-3693-2426-4.ch014

Uludag, K., & Kara, F. (2024). The impact of oxidative stress biomarkers on memory in individuals with schizophrenia and antioxidant use. In *Nutrition Controversies and Advances in Autoimmune Disease* (pp. 477–500). IGI Global. DOI: 10.4018/979-8-3693-5528-2.ch018

Uludag, K., Wang, D. M., Goodman, C., Wang, L., & Zhang, X. (2021). Prevalence, clinical correlates and risk factors associated with Tardive Dyskinesia in Chinese patients with schizophrenia. *Asian Journal of Psychiatry, 66*, 102877. DOI: 10.1016/j.ajp.2021.102877 PMID: 34638091

Ventura, A. M. B., Hayes, R. D., & Fonseca de Freitas, D. (2022). Ethnic disparities in clozapine prescription for service-users with schizophrenia-spectrum disorders: A systematic review. *Psychological Medicine, 52*(12), 2212–2223. DOI: 10.1017/S0033291722001878 PMID: 35787301

Wei, J., & Dong, T. (2025). The Effect of Clozapine on Immune-Related Biomarkers in Schizophrenia Patients. *Journal of Biochemical and Molecular Toxicology, 39*(9), e70503. DOI: 10.1002/jbt.70503 PMID: 40965598

Wheeler, A., Humberstone, V., & Robinson, G. (2009). Outcomes for schizophrenia patients with clozapine treatment: How good does it get? *Journal of Psychopharmacology (Oxford, England), 23*(8), 957–965. DOI: 10.1177/0269881108093588 PMID: 18635713

Willcocks, I. R., Legge, S. E., Nalmpanti, M., Mazzeo, L., King, A., Jansen, J., & Walters, J. T. (2021). Clozapine metabolism is associated with absolute neutrophil count in individuals with treatment-resistant schizophrenia. *Frontiers in Pharmacology, 12*, 658734. DOI: 10.3389/fphar.2021.658734 PMID: 33959025

Young, W. (2009). Review of Lithium Effects on Brain and Blood. *Cell Transplantation, 18*(9), 951–975. DOI: 10.3727/096368909X471251 PMID: 19523343

Yuan, X., Wang, S., Shi, Y., Yang, Y., Zhang, Y., Xia, L., Zhang, K., & Liu, H. (2022). Pro-inflammatory cytokine levels are elevated in female patients with schizophrenia treated with clozapine. *Psychopharmacology, 239*(3), 765–771. DOI: 10.1007/s00213-022-06067-y PMID: 35080634

Zhang, Y., Tao, S., Coid, J., Wei, W., Wang, Q., Yue, W., & Yang, G. (2024). The role of total white blood cell count in antipsychotic treatment for patients with schizophrenia. *Current Neuropharmacology, 22*(1), 159–167. DOI: 10.2174/1570159X21666230104090046 PMID: 36600620

Zhou, Y., Zheng, W., Guo, F., Wu, S., & Zhong, C. (2025). The anti-inflammation pharmacodynamics of lithium: Therapy of bipolar disorder. *Journal of Psychopharmacology (Oxford, England), 39*(6), 533–544. DOI: 10.1177/02698811251326942 PMID: 40138498

Chapter 2
Case Studies in Schizophrenia and Related Disorders

Jennifer Schulz
http://orcid.org/0009-0000-5822-4937
Ashland University, USA

EXECUTIVE SUMMARY

This chapter provides readers with a comprehensive overview of the "Schizophrenia Spectrum and Other Psychotic Disorders" chapter in the Diagnostic and Statistical Manual of Mental Disorders, Fifth edition, Text Revision (DSM-5-TR). It achieves this through the use of illustrative case studies, which provide real-life examples of psychotic disorders in clinical practice. The chapter provides background information on schizophrenia spectrum disorders, including their prevalence, symptoms, and evidence-based treatments, before detailing realistic case presentations.

INTRODUCTION

In the *Diagnostic and Statistical Manual of Mental Disorders, Fifth Edition, Text Revision* (*DSM-5-TR*), the chapter on "Schizophrenia Spectrum and Other Psychotic Disorders" contains a grouping of mental health conditions that involve unusual presentations of emotion, behavior, perception, and thought. Individuals with a disorder in this chapter show symptoms including odd behaviors, delusional beliefs, social withdrawal, and overall detachment from reality (American Psychiatric Association, 2022). For those employed in the behavioral health field, understanding the disorders in the schizophrenia spectrum chapter is essential. In the sections that follow, readers will learn about the prevalence of schizophrenia spectrum and other

DOI: 10.4018/979-8-3373-3084-6.ch002

psychotic disorders, the burdens associated with these conditions, and evidence-based treatment modalities. The chapter concludes with a collection of case studies that illustrate how these disorders may present in clinical practice, so current and future behavioral health professionals are prepared to identify patients with these disorders in clinical settings.

Chapter learning objectives are as follows:

1. Know the different disorders in the chapter on "Schizophrenia Spectrum and Other Psychotic Disorders" in the *DSM-5-TR*.
2. Recognize symptoms of schizophrenia-spectrum disorders in case presentations.
3. Understand how factors, such as marginalization and racism, can influence identification and treatment of psychotic disorders.
4. Identify patients with schizophrenia spectrum disorders in clinical settings.
5. Recognize when a patient requires treatment for a psychotic disorder.
6. Know effective treatment options for schizophrenia and related disorders.

KEY INFORMATION RELATED TO SCHIZOPHRENIA-SPECTRUM DISORDERS

Individuals working in behavioral health are likely to encounter patients living with symptoms of schizophrenia or a related psychotic disorder. According to a systematic review and meta-analysis that sought to determine the worldwide prevalence of this type of disorder, the median global prevalence of psychotic disorders in the general population is 5 per 1,000 people. Over the course of their lifetimes, an estimated 7.49 per 1,000 people will be diagnosed with a psychotic disorder (Moreno-Küstner et al., 2018).

The Disease Burden Associated with Psychotic Disorders

While the prevalence of schizophrenia and related disorders may seem low, it is essential for behavioral health providers to be cognizant of these conditions and competent in treating them, given the burdens associated with these diagnoses. Schizophrenia and other psychotic disorders are linked to indirect costs, such as unemployment, disability, premature death, and reliance on income assistance programs. These disorders are also associated with direct costs, including expenses linked to emergency room and inpatient treatment, as well as healthcare fees and the cost of rehabilitative services (Burns & Marder, 2023). Some groups are more at risk of dysfunction and disease burden from psychotic disorders than others. For instance, Black Americans, who are diagnosed with these disorders at over twice the rate as White Americans, show worse outcomes after diagnosis (Merritt et al., 2023).

The Benefits of Evidence-Based Treatments

Psychotic disorders can cause significant disability and impaired functioning. Fortunately, quality treatment can reduce the disease burden associated with schizophrenia and disorders similar to it. A recent systematic review revealed that second-generation antipsychotic medications, and especially long-acting injectables, improve quality of life for those living with schizophrenia and psychotic disorders (Sampogna et al., 2023). It is important to note, however, that research on pharmacological treatments for delusional disorder, which is included among the psychotic disorders, is limited (Le & Ruffalo, 2025; Muñoz-Negro & Cervilla, 2016).

Beyond medication, community psychiatric treatment can reduce disease burden by improving quality of life, wellbeing, and social connectedness, with psychosocial interventions including cognitive-behavioral therapy, psychoeducation, and social skills training being especially effective for these purposes (Černe Kolarič et al., 2024). While additional research is warranted, cognitive behavioral therapy and psychodynamic treatment may show promise for the treatment of delusional disorder, providing an alternative when medications are not effective (Le & Ruffalo, 2025).

Once effective interventions are established, keeping patients engaged in treatment is essential for maintaining long-term symptom reduction and improvement in quality of life. When patients stop taking medications, they are at risk of relapsing to a state in which symptoms such as hallucinations, delusions, and disorganized behavior become active again (Onitsuka et al., 2022). Relapse increases the risk of negative outcomes and societal costs including homelessness, unemployment, incarceration, and difficulties with sustaining independent living (Lin et al., 2021). To maintain sustained recovery and functioning, it is often necessary for patients to continue taking antipsychotic medications on a long-term basis. Furthermore, ongoing pharmacological management should be complemented by psychosocial treatments, such as psychotherapy and education provided by trained behavioral health professionals (Onitsuka et al., 2022). Given the burdens associated with schizophrenia and related psychotic disorders, as well as the consequences of relapse, behavioral health professionals must be prepared to identify these conditions in clinical practice and to provide evidence-based interventions, as well as referrals to appropriate treatments when warranted.

It is also essential that providers be prepared to offer culturally competent, antiracist care to marginalized populations. Compared to Whites, Black Americans with schizophrenia spectrum disorders experience worse neurocognitive functioning and higher levels of disorganized behavior. Black Americans may also experience distress related to racism, which worsens functioning (Merritt et al., 2023). Providers must consider these factors to ensure culturally competent care. Given their history of race-based trauma and mistreatment within both the criminal justice system and healthcare system, Black Americans may have mistrust toward White providers and thus may benefit from working with racially matched clinicians. At the very least, providers working with Black Americans must receive training in antiracist care and demonstrate awareness of the history of marginalization in this population (Faber et al., 2023).

IDENTIFYING SCHIZOPHRENIA AND RELATED DISORDERS IN CLINICAL PRACTICE

Given the disease burden associated with schizophrenia and related disorders, it is imperative that clinicians be able to identify these disorders so they can provide patients with evidence-based treatments. Identifying schizophrenia and related disorders begins with an understanding of diagnostic criteria, as delineated in the *DSM-5-TR*. Clinicians must also be skilled in differentiating among the different disorders in the chapter on schizophrenia and related psychotic conditions. A validated assessment tool, such as the CAT-Psychosis battery may be useful for professionals making a diagnosis (Guinart et al., 2021). The WERCAP Screen, which contains 16 questions that identify symptoms of psychotic and affective disorders and is available free of charge online, can also be beneficial for supporting a diagnosis (Mamah, 2011). Finally, the Positive and Negative Syndrome Scale (PANSS) can be used to support assessment and diagnosis. This scale measures general psychopathology, in addition to positive and negative symptoms of schizophrenia and related disorders. Negative symptoms include those like social withdrawal and blunted emotions, whereas positive symptoms include delusions, hallucinations, and strange thought content (Lim et al., 2021).

The aforementioned assessment tools each have their own strengths and weaknesses. The CAT-Psychosis demonstrates high diagnostic accuracy while requiring fewer items than traditional scales. It shows acceptable convergent validity and can reliably distinguish healthy controls from individuals in psychosis. Despite its efficiency, CAT-Psychosis requires access to technology and stable Internet systems, which may limit its use in low-resource or rural settings. It also relies on self-report, which may be unreliable in individuals with severe paranoia, cognitive impairment, or poor insight (Guinart et al., 2021). The WERCAP is cost-free and easily administered in community, primary care, and justice-involved settings. Mamah et al. (2014) found that the WERCAP showed good predictive validity for later psychotic disorders and strong internal consistency. It is especially useful for early detection, when symptoms may not yet meet full *DSM-5-TR* criteria. That being said, the WERCAP is a screening tool, not a diagnostic instrument. It may produce false positives and must be followed by structured clinical interviews (Mamah et al., 2014). Finally, the PANSS has strong reliability, validity, and sensitivity to symptom change. Kay et al. (1987) demonstrated that the PANSS reliably distinguishes positive, negative, and general psychopathology symptoms. It has long been considered a gold standard for symptom severity tracking in research and clinical trials. However, the PANSS is time-intensive, as administration tales 30–45 minutes. It is less practical for brief clinical settings and is not designed for early screening (Kay et al., 1987).

Assessment tools can be used to support a diagnosis and evaluate symptom severity, but clinicians should have an understanding of the signs that may point toward a diagnosis of schizophrenia or another psychotic disorder. This requires clinicians to have knowledge of symptoms, as well as the ability to use clinical judgment to identify symptoms in a specific individual. A patient who presents with evidence of delusional thinking, such as believing that they are performing a clandestine mission to support government activity, when there is no evidence of such, can point toward schizophrenia or another psychotic condition, such as delusional disorder. It is noted that paranoid delusions can be suggestive of a psychotic disorder, but in marginalized groups, paranoia may be a cultural manifestation of distrust rather than a clinical symptom, so paranoid delusions alone may not indicate psychosis (Gordon et al., 2023). Patients with a *DSM-5-TR* psychotic disorder may also experience hallucinations, which are sensory experiences that the patient perceives but are not actually physically present. For instance, a patient may report the presence of another individual in the room, who is not visible to the clinician or others; they may also endorse hearing voices that critique their activities or command them to take certain actions (American Psychiatric Association, 2022).

Delusions and hallucinations may be more obvious signs of psychotic disorders, but sometimes the indicators are subtler. While the presence of at least one symptom among hallucinations, delusions, or disorganized speech is required for a schizophrenia diagnosis (American Psychiatric Association, 2022), sometimes negative symptoms like lack of emotion, speech, or motivation are more prominent (Correll & Schooler, 2020). Classic psychotic symptoms like hallucinations and delusions can certainly point toward a diagnosis of schizophrenia or another psychotic disorder, but individuals with these conditions may display other warning signs. For instance, Sullivan et al. (2018) found that the following symptoms were linked to psychotic disorders among patients in primary care settings: bizarre behavior, suicidal thinking, lack of emotional expression, social withdrawal, manic symptoms, sleep disruption, depression, and difficulty with day-to-day functioning. Earlier research has identified suspiciousness, sleep disturbances, anger, disruptive behavior, and symptoms of anxiety and depression as being early warning signs for schizophrenia or a psychotic episode (Van Meijel et al., 2004). These symptoms may point toward a need to consider a schizophrenia-spectrum disorder when making a diagnosis.

Clinicians working in behavioral health settings, such as hospitals, outpatient clinics, or rehabilitation centers, must be prepared to identify patients showing signs of schizophrenia spectrum disorders and psychosis. Those who suspect a patient may be experiencing symptoms of one of these disorders must also remember that each patient will present uniquely. For instance, some patients may primarily show positive symptoms, such as hallucinations or delusional beliefs. On the other hand, negative symptoms like social and emotional withdrawal may predominate the clinical picture for other patients. Regardless of the specific symptom presentation, prompt identification and treatment are necessary to restore functioning and quality of life among individuals living with schizophrenia spectrum and other psychotic disorders.

Disorders on the Schizophrenia Spectrum

Assessment tools and awareness of psychotic symptoms can be useful for screening, but clinicians must also be aware of the different psychotic disorders to distinguish among them. There are multiple diagnoses in the *DSM-5-TR* chapter on "Schizophrenia Spectrum and Other Psychotic Disorders" (American Psychiatric Association, 2022). The purpose of the present chapter is not to describe the specific diagnostic criteria for each separate disorder, but rather to provide clinicians with background information to assist with the identification, assessment, and treatment of these disorders in clinical practice. This is achieved by the provision of this background information, alongside case studies to offer illustrative examples of the schizophrenia-spectrum disorders.

While it is beyond the scope of this chapter to describe the *DSM-5-TR* diagnostic criteria for all schizophrenia spectrum and related psychotic disorders in full detail, it is essential to have a baseline understanding of the main disorders in this category to assist with interpreting the case studies that follow. Consider the descriptions of the main disorders in this category below (American Psychiatric Association, 2022):

- **Brief psychotic disorder:** This diagnosis is reserved for people who show psychotic symptoms for at least one day but under one month.
- **Catatonia:** While not a standalone diagnosis, catatonia is recognized as a specifier for other disorders on the schizophrenia spectrum and involves psychomotor disturbances, such as stupor, limited verbal responses, grimacing, non-goal-directed movements, and mimicking of others' speech or movements.

- **Delusional disorder:** This disorder is diagnosed in individuals who subscribe to at least one delusion for a minimum of one month in the absence of other symptoms of schizophrenia.
- **Schizoaffective disorder:** This condition involves schizophrenia symptoms alongside major mood episodes, which can manifest as either mania or depression; to be diagnosed, there must be a period of at least two weeks during which a person shows evidence of hallucinations or delusions without any co-occurring mood episode symptoms.
- **Schizophrenia:** Diagnosed in people who show at least one symptom among hallucinations, delusions, and disorganized behavior, this disorder must involve a continued disturbance lasting at least six months, with at least one month of active symptoms (e.g. hallucinations, delusions, and disorganized behavior). Two symptoms must be present for diagnosis, and beyond the aforementioned active symptoms, a person might show disorganized/catatonic behavior or negative symptoms like blunted emotions.
- **Schizophreniform disorder:** This condition includes the same diagnostic criteria as schizophrenia, with the exception that symptoms last at least one month but under six months.

Beyond the specific diagnoses above, the *DSM-5-TR* includes conditions such as psychotic disorders induced by a substance/medication or a medical condition in the chapter on schizophrenia-spectrum disorders. There are also diagnostic codes for unspecified/other specified disorders that do not meet full criteria for another disorder in this category. Finally, the *DSM-5-TR* briefly addresses schizotypal personality disorder among the schizophrenia spectrum disorders, but it reserves the full description of this disorder for the chapter on personality disorders (American Psychiatric Association, 2022).

CLINICAL CASE STUDIES

Having background information about the various psychotic disorders is helpful, but clinical case studies enhance learning by offering real-world examples. As indicated in the aforementioned sections, there are varied presentations of psychotic disorders in clinical practice. The *DSM-5-TR* chapter outlining these disorders also contains a range of diagnoses, each with its own diagnostic criteria. Given these facts, it's helpful to review clinical case studies, which provide realistic examples of different symptom presentations that may be encountered in direct practice. The sections that follow provide real-world case examples of schizophrenia and various other related conditions. While these examples do not represent the actual, lived experiences of specific, identifiable patients, they are illustrative of commonly-encountered symptom presentations.

Schizophrenia Case Presentation

A 24-year-old male, James, is brought to the emergency department (ED) by local police after being found pacing outside a government office building late at night, loudly arguing with unseen individuals and attempting to enter restricted areas. Police report that James appeared frightened, confused, and unresponsive to verbal redirection. Upon arrival in the ED, James appears disheveled and poorly groomed. He is visibly agitated, scanning the room repeatedly and muttering under his breath. He intermittently covers his ears and appears startled by environmental noises that do not distress others. His speech is pressured and tangential, and when asked simple questions, his responses are loosely connected or even unrelated to the question that was asked.

When the clinical social worker assigned to James asks what brought him into the ED, James states, "They've been watching me for months. The cameras aren't just cameras; they transmit thoughts. I was chosen to stop them, but now they're trying to silence me." When asked who "they" are, James replies vaguely, "You know… the people running things. Government, satellites, corporations." The social worker asks James for more information about these beliefs, but James becomes increasingly distressed when questioned further. He does state that he hears voices telling him that he has messed up; he also reports that there are sometimes multiple voices who argue about him.

Throughout the assessment process, the social worker notices that James is oriented to person and place, but he is unable to sustain attention to the conversation. He reports feeling that he is justified in entering restricted government buildings, because he believes he has been commissioned by the government to perform specific tasks. James does not recognize that he is experiencing symptoms of mental illness. James paces around the hospital room during the assessment and oscillates between appearing fearful and displaying flat affect.

The social worker is able to contact James' mother, Cindy, to obtain collateral information. Cindy reports that James has not slept in several nights, and family members have been concerned because James has not been eating. Cindy states that James has been deteriorating over the last nine months. She indicates that James stopped showing up to his job and later was fired, and then he began isolating himself from friends and family. However, it has only been over the past two months that James has been fixated on his belief that he is conducting a mission alongside the government.

Ultimately, James is determined to lack decision-making capacity due to active psychosis and impaired reality testing. He is placed on an involuntary psychiatric hold for safety and stabilization and admitted to an inpatient psychiatric unit for initiation of antipsychotic treatment and comprehensive care.

Follow-Up Questions

The questions below are helpful for strengthening readers' understanding of James' case and of the diagnosis of schizophrenia:

- How does James meet diagnostic criteria for schizophrenia?
- Why does James not meet diagnostic criteria for a related condition, like schizophreniform disorder or brief psychotic disorder?
- What services should James' social worker refer him to upon discharge from the inpatient psychiatric unit?

These questions are designed to promote critical thinking and deeper engagement with the case study. Answering them may require utilizing additional resources outside of this chapter, such as the *DSM-5-TR* or books on evidence-based treatments for schizophrenia. Sample answers are provided in the appendix at the end of this chapter.

Schizoaffective Disorder Case Presentation

Marisol was referred for a psychiatric assessment by a local mental health court after multiple low-level legal violations related to behavioral disturbances in public spaces. Court records indicate that her behavior raised concerns about untreated serious mental illness, including periods of unresponsiveness, disorganized conduct, and inability to follow verbal commands. The court mandated a comprehensive psychiatric assessment to clarify diagnosis, treatment needs, and capacity for participation in outpatient treatment.

During her intake appointment, a longtime friend accompanies Marisol to offer support. Marisol appears motionless, seated upright in the waiting area for an extended period without speaking or shifting position. When approached, she does not respond verbally and maintains a fixed gaze. During the psychiatric interview, Marisol shows signs of a psychomotor disturbance, as she remains immobile for prolonged periods, before shifting into sudden, purposeless movements.

The psychologist conducting the intake appointment notes that Marisol is poorly groomed with mismatched clothing, poor hygiene, and unbrushed hair. Marisol also occasionally mimics the psychologist's movements without being instructed to do so. Marisol is mute for most of the evaluation, and when her friend prompts her to speak, Marisol's speech is slow, monotonic, and limited to two- and three-word responses. Marisol shows limited emotional reactivity but is able to verbalize that she hears voices commenting on her behavior and telling her she is contaminated.

Marisol's friend indicates that while Marisol appears flat and non-responsive during the assessment, she has recently had periods during which she shows risky behavior, such as going on spending sprees, driving recklessly, and engaging in sex with multiple new partners per day. During these periods, Marisol appears agitated, stays awake for days on end, and is convinced that she's invincible. Marisol has been chronically transient and is currently couch surfing; she has been staying on her friend's couch for the last month, because she has been unable to maintain stable employment or housing on her own.

Based on the presenting symptoms, the psychologist diagnoses Marisol with schizoaffective disorder, bipolar type, with catatonia. The psychologist will work with Marisol on an ongoing basis, providing cognitive-behavioral therapy and referrals to other needed services.

Follow-Up Questions

The questions below encourage critical thinking about Marisol's case; the answer key in the appendix of this chapter provides sample answers:

- Why does Marisol meet the criteria for schizoaffective disorder rather than schizophrenia?
- Why does the specifier "with catatonia" apply to Marisol's case?
- What services would be beneficial for Marisol?

Delusional Disorder Case Presentation

Her family doctor refers Elaine for psychiatric evaluation after Elaine has repeatedly contacted local authorities, her employer, and a homeowners' association to report that her neighbor is intentionally sabotaging her property and attempting to poison her through environmental exposure. Despite multiple investigations finding no evidence, Elaine remains convinced of malicious intent. During her assessment, Elaine states, "I'm not mentally ill. This is happening. No one is listening."

Elaine reports that approximately three years ago, she began noticing what she describes as "subtle attacks" from her neighbor, including strange odors that she believes are toxic chemicals and Internet outages she believes are the result of targeted interference. Elaine's beliefs remain consistent and unchanged over time. She has compiled lengthy written notes related to her observations, in addition to taking photographs, which she believes document the alleged persecution. Elaine insists that her beliefs are accurate, even when given reassurance and contradictory evidence.

While Elaine does become agitated when discussing the alleged poisoning from her neighbor, she is otherwise calm and cooperative, and her speech is coherent. She is well-groomed and neat in appearance, with no bizarre behaviors. Elaine is able to maintain stable employment and housing, and she has no history of hallucinations, hospitalizations, or pharmacological treatment for mental illness. Aside from her insistence that her neighbor is poisoning her, Elaine shows rational thinking patterns, and her mood is appropriate to the setting.

The clinical social worker working with Elaine diagnoses her with delusional disorder, persecutory type and begins treatment planning.

Follow-Up Questions

Consider the questions below to analyze Elaine's case further, and consult the answer key in the appendix for sample responses:

- Why is the given diagnosis appropriate for Elaine?
- Why does Elaine not meet criteria for schizophrenia?
- What should the social worker include on Elaine's treatment plan?

Schizotypal Personality Disorder Case Presentation

Schizotypal personality disorder is fully described in the *DSM-5-TR* chapter on personality disorders; however, it is briefly listed in the chapter on schizophrenia spectrum disorders because international manuals consider it to belong to this class of conditions. Individuals with schizotypal personality disorder may appear to show symptoms of psychosis, because they demonstrate distortions in cognition and perception, as well as strange, magical thinking patterns. They also present with unusual behavior, social anxiety, and a tendency to avoid close friendships or relationships. However, they do not meet criteria for a psychotic disorder like schizophrenia, because of the absence of periods of true psychosis, during which hallucinations or delusions are present (American Psychiatric Association, 2022). A case presentation for schizotypal personality disorder appears below, as some patients presenting for treatment may appear to have a disorder like schizophrenia, when a diagnosis of schizotypal personality disorder is actually more appropriate. The case study below illustrates schizotypal personality disorder, to allow readers to develop the ability to distinguish this personality disorder from schizophrenia and related disorders, such as brief psychotic disorder or delusional disorder:

Miguel is referred for a psychological evaluation at a community mental health clinic after his primary care physician becomes concerned about his mental status. During a routine appointment, Miguel, who has dangerously high blood pressure, states that he doesn't need to take medications, because he believes he is able to exert control over his blood pressure readings through a daily candle-lighting ritual. Miguel acknowledges that others likely find this to be hard to believe, but he is confident that he can manage his blood pressure without medical intervention, because his rituals are calming for him.

When Miguel presents to the community mental health clinic for his assessment with a licensed professional counselor, he reports that he has never really had close friendships. Starting in adolescence, Miguel distanced himself from peers, whom he says found him to be "odd." Miguel states that he just doesn't relate to many of his peers, so he spends most of his free time alone, reading about astrology. Miguel talks at length about "hidden patterns in the universe," which he finds to be fascinating. Miguel prefers to be alone, because he feels others cannot be trusted.

Miguel is able to maintain full-time employment in a shipping warehouse, which provides him with enough income to rent a studio apartment above a downtown business in the small town where he lives. He reports he shows up to work and completes his tasks but does not interact with colleagues. He has no desire to be promoted to a supervisory role, because he believes upper management would mock or judge him. This belief is based on Miguel's report that he senses "negative energy fields" from upper management.

The professional counselor notes that Miguel is dressed strangely for the weather; his assessment occurs on a hot, mid-summer day, but Miguel dresses in multiple layers, with bright, mismatched colors. He is cooperative with the assessment and able to engage in back-and-forth conversation, but his speech is tangential, and he has difficulty providing succinct responses to questions. He demonstrates thinking patterns that most people would find to be unusual, but his speech is coherent. Miguel's thinking patterns do not rise to the level of being delusional, and while Miguel reports a deep connection to the spiritual world, he does not endorse any hallucinations.

Based on symptom presentation, the counselor diagnoses Miguel with schizotypal personality disorder. Miguel agrees to participate in weekly counseling sessions. During sessions, the counselor emphasizes social skills training, which has shown benefits for patients with schizotypal personality disorder in existing research (Kirchner et al., 2018). Miguel views social skills training as meaningful, as he believes it can help him better understand his colleagues and peers.

Follow-Up Questions

Consider the questions below to further explore how Miguel's presentation differs from that associated with other schizophrenia-spectrum diagnoses; consult the appendix for example responses.

- How does Miguel meet the diagnostic criteria for a personality disorder?
- Why is schizotypal personality disorder a more appropriate diagnosis than schizophrenia?

CONCLUDING REMARKS

The case studies presented in this chapter highlight the diverse and often complex ways in which schizophrenia spectrum and other psychotic disorders may present in clinical practice. While these conditions share core features such as disturbances in perception, thought, and behavior, the case examples herein demonstrate that no two patients present identically. Differences in symptom profile, illness course, functional impact, and contextual factors, such as legal involvement, social support, and immediate safety concerns, require clinicians to approach each assessment with flexibility and sound clinical judgment.

Taken together, the cases of James, Marisol, Elaine, and Miguel illustrate the importance of careful differential diagnosis within the schizophrenia spectrum. James' presentation demonstrates a classic example of schizophrenia, as evidenced by positive symptoms, impaired functioning, and lack of insight into his illness. Marisol's case emphasizes the diagnostic distinction between schizophrenia and schizoaffective disorder, as well as the clinical significance of identifying specifiers such as catatonia, which are relevant when making a diagnosis. On the other hand, Elaine's presentation illustrates how delusional disorder may involve fixed, unfounded beliefs in the absence of hallucinations, disorganized speech, or deterioration in overall functioning, reminding behavioral health professionals that psychotic disorders exist along a spectrum of severity and impairment. Finally, Miguel's case reminds readers that a differential diagnosis, such as a personality disorder, may be more appropriate when patients present with strange beliefs in the absence of true psychosis.

These cases also reinforce the critical role of behavioral health professionals in early identification, comprehensive assessment, and coordination of evidence-based care for patients living with symptoms of schizophrenia or another psychotic disorder. Accurate diagnosis requires not only familiarity with *DSM-5-TR* criteria, but also the ability to use clinical judgment to make a diagnosis and refer patients to appropriate services to promote symptom reduction and restored functioning. The realistic case examples in this chapter aim to equip readers with the conceptual knowledge and applied skills necessary for identifying, assessing, and intervening with patients who live with schizophrenia and related disorders in real-world settings. Engaging with these patients and providing evidence-based services can play a central role in improving quality of life for individuals with these disorders, while also reducing significant costs to society, such as those arising from unemployment, disability, premature death, and healthcare expenditures (Burns & Marder, 2023; Černe Kolarič et al., 2024; Sampogna et al., 2023).

While evidence-based treatments for psychotic disorders have been established, future research must fill existing gaps, such as the lack of research exploring treatment of delusional disorder (Muñoz-Negro & Cervilla, 2016). Pharmacological treatments for delusional disorder remain limited; psychodynamic and cognitive-behavioral therapy may be beneficial, but additional research is warranted (Le & Ruffalo, 2025). Finally, researchers must continue to explore the effects of racism on functioning in those with schizophrenia and related disorders, to ensure marginalized populations can access effective, culturally competent care (Merritt et al., 2023).

REFERENCES

American Psychiatric Association. (2022). Personality disorders. In *Diagnostic and statistical manual of mental disorders* (5th ed., text rev.; pp. 629–684). https://doi .org/DOI: 10.1176/appi.books.9780890425787

American Psychiatric Association. (2022). Schizophrenia spectrum and other psychotic disorders. In *Diagnostic and statistical manual of mental disorders* (5th ed., text rev.; pp. 87–122). https://doi.org/DOI: 10.1176/appi.books.9780890425787

Burns, A. V., & Marder, S. (2023). Schizophrenia spectrum and other psychotic disorders. In IsHak, W. W. (Ed.), *Atlas of psychiatry* (pp. 469–492). Springer., DOI: 10.1007/978-3-031-15401-0_15

Černe Kolarič, J., Plemenitaš Ilješ, A., Kraner, D., Gönc, V., Lorber, M., Mlinar Reljić, N., Fekonja, Z., & Kmetec, S. (2024). Long-term impact of community psychiatric care on quality of life amongst people living with schizophrenia: A systematic review. *Health Care, 12*(17), 1750. DOI: 10.3390/healthcare12171750 PMID: 39273773

Correll, C. U., & Schooler, N. R. (2020). Negative symptoms in schizophrenia: A review and clinical guide for recognition, assessment, and treatment. *Neuropsychiatric Disease and Treatment, 16*, 519–534. DOI: 10.2147/NDT.S225643 PMID: 32110026

Faber, S. C., Roy, A. K., Michaels, T. I., & Williams, M. T. (2023). The weaponization of medicine: Early psychosis in the Black community and the need for racially informed mental healthcare. *Frontiers in Psychiatry, 14*, 1098292. DOI: 10.3389/fpsyt.2023.1098292 PMID: 36846217

González-Rodríguez, A., & Seeman, M. V. (2020). Addressing delusions in women and men with delusional disorder: Key points for clinical management. *International Journal of Environmental Research and Public Health, 17*(12), 4583. DOI: 10.3390/ijerph17124583 PMID: 32630566

Gordon, S., Mote, J., & Fulford, D. (2023). Qualitative analysis of paranoia reported in clinical interviews with Black and White adults with schizophrenia. *Psychiatric Services (Washington, D.C.), 74*(12), 1257–1264. DOI: 10.1176/appi.ps.20220089 PMID: 37254507

Guinart, D., de Filippis, R., Rosson, S., Patil, B., Prizgint, L., Talasazan, N., Meltzer, H., Kane, J. M., & Gibbons, R. D. (2021). Development and validation of a computerized adaptive assessment tool for discrimination and measurement of psychotic symptoms. *Schizophrenia Bulletin, 47*(3), 644–652. DOI: 10.1093/schbul/sbaa168 PMID: 33164091

Kay, S. R., Fiszbein, A., & Opler, L. A. (1987). The Positive and Negative Syndrome Scale (PANSS) for schizophrenia. *Schizophrenia Bulletin*, *13*(2), 261–276. DOI: 10.1093/schbul/13.2.261 PMID: 3616518

Kirchner, S. K., Roeh, A., Nolden, J., & Hasan, A. (2018). Diagnosis and treatment of schizotypal personality disorder: Evidence from a systematic review. *npj. Schizophrenia*, *4*(1), 20. DOI: 10.1038/s41537-018-0062-8 PMID: 30282970

Le, T., & Ruffalo, M. L. (2025). Psychotherapy for delusional disorder: Theoretical models and therapeutic techniques. *American Journal of Psychotherapy*, *78*(4), 251–255. DOI: 10.1176/appi.psychotherapy.20240061 PMID: 40495539

Lim, K., Peh, O.-H., Yang, Z., Rekhi, G., Rapisarda, A., See, Y.-M., Abdul Rashid, N. A., Ang, M.-S., Lee, S.-A., Sim, K., Huang, H., Lencz, T., Lee, J., & Lam, M. (2021). Large-scale evaluation of the Positive and Negative Syndrome Scale (PANSS) symptom architecture in schizophrenia. *Asian Journal of Psychiatry*, *62*, 102732. DOI: 10.1016/j.ajp.2021.102732 PMID: 34118560

Lin, D., Joshi, K., Keenan, A., Shepherd, J., Bailey, H., Berry, M., Wright, J., Meakin, S., Benson, C., & Kim, E. (2021). Associations between relapses and psychosocial outcomes in patients with schizophrenia in real-world settings in the United States. *Frontiers in Psychiatry*, *12*, 695672. DOI: 10.3389/fpsyt.2021.695672 PMID: 34764891

Mamah, D. (2011). *The Washington Early Recognition Center Affectivity and Psychosis (WERCAP) Screen*. Washington University School of Medicine in St. Louis. Retrieved from_https://werc.wustl.edu/Content/pdfs/WERCAP%20Screen%202022.pdf

Mamah, D., Owoso, A., Sheffield, J. M., & Bayer, C. (2014).

Merritt, C. C., Halverson, T. F., Elliott, T., Jarskog, L. F., Pedersen, C. A., & Penn, D. L. (2023). Racial disparities and predictors of functioning in schizophrenia. *The American Journal of Orthopsychiatry*, *93*(3), 177–187. DOI: 10.1037/ort0000661 PMID: 36931838

Moreno-Küstner, B., Martín, C., & Pastor, L. (2018). Prevalence of psychotic disorders and its association with methodological issues: A systematic review and meta-analyses. *PLoS One*, *13*(4), e0195687. DOI: 10.1371/journal.pone.0195687 PMID: 29649252

Muñoz-Negro, J. E., & Cervilla, J. A. (2016). A systematic review on the pharmacological treatment of delusional disorder. *Journal of Clinical Psychopharmacology*, *36*(6), 684–690. DOI: 10.1097/JCP.0000000000000595 PMID: 27811554

Onitsuka, T., Hirano, Y., Nakazawa, T., Ichihashi, K., Miura, K., Inada, K., Mitoma, R., Yasui-Furukori, N., & Hashimoto, R. (2022). Toward recovery in schizophrenia: Current concepts, findings, and future research directions. *Psychiatry and Clinical Neurosciences*, *76*(7), 282–291. DOI: 10.1111/pcn.13342 PMID: 35235256

Sampogna, G., Di Vincenzo, M., Giuliani, L., Menculini, G., Mancuso, E., Arsenio, E., Cipolla, S., Della Rocca, B., Martiadis, V., Signorelli, M. S., & Fiorillo, A. (2023). A systematic review on the effectiveness of antipsychotic drugs on the quality of life of patients with schizophrenia. *Brain Sciences*, *13*(11), 1577. DOI: 10.3390/brainsci13111577 PMID: 38002537

Sullivan, S. A., Hamilton, W., Tilling, K., Redaniel, T., Moran, P., & Lewis, G. (2018). Association of primary care consultation patterns with early signs and symptoms of psychosis. *JAMA Network Open*, *1*(7), e185174. DOI: 10.1001/jamanetworkopen.2018.5174 PMID: 30646393

The WERCAP Screen and the WERC Stress Screen: Psychometrics of self-rated i instruments for assessing bipolar and psychotic disorder risk and perceived stress burden. *Comprehensive Psychiatry*, *55*(7), 1757–1771. https://doi.org/DOI: 10.1016/j.comppsych.2014.07.004

Van Meijel, B., van der Gaag, M., Kahn, R. S., & Grypdonck, M. H. F. (2004). Recognition of early warning signs in patients with schizophrenia: A review of the literature. *International Journal of Mental Health Nursing*, *13*(2), 107–116. DOI: 10.1111/j.1440-0979.2004.00314.x PMID: 15318905

KEY TERMS AND DEFINITIONS

Active-Phase Symptoms: In schizophrenia spectrum disorders, those symptoms that fall under the category of hallucinations, delusions, or disorganized speech

Catatonia: A specifier applied when a person shows evidence of psychomotor disturbances, such as stupor, grimacing, or mimicking of others' speech or movements

Delusions: Fixed, false beliefs that a person maintains even when given evidenced that the beliefs are unfounded

Hallucinations: Sensory experiences that a person perceives, despite these experiences not actually being present in the environment or perceivable to others

Negative Symptoms: Those symptoms in schizophrenia spectrum and related disorders that involve disengagement and lack of speech, emotion, or motivation

Positive Symptoms: A term used to describe the addition of unexpected symptoms, such as hallucinations, delusions, and abnormal thinking patterns, in schizophrenia-spectrum disorders

Schizophrenia Spectrum and Other Psychotic Disorders: A group of mental health conditions that involves unusual presentations of emotion, behavior, perception, and thought

APPENDIX

Answer Key

Case Study 1: Schizophrenia (James)

- How does James meet diagnostic criteria for schizophrenia?

James meets diagnostic criteria for schizophrenia, because he shows evidence of delusions, based on his fixed belief that he is involved in some sort of government mission aimed at "stopping cameras." James also endorses hallucinations, as he hears voices arguing or telling him he has made mistakes. Additionally, James shows signs of disorganized speech, as evidenced by giving responses that are loosely related or unrelated to questions asked of him. Finally, James shows a flat affect during assessment, which aligns with the negative symptoms of schizophrenia. Based on these symptoms and the fact that James is no longer functioning in important life areas (e.g. work), he meets diagnostic criteria for schizophrenia (American Psychiatric Association, 2022).

- Why does James not meet diagnostic criteria for a related condition, like schizophreniform disorder or brief psychotic disorder?

The main feature that distinguishes schizophrenia from schizophreniform disorder or brief psychotic disorder is the duration of symptoms. In the case description, James has been experiencing a mental health disturbance for nine months, according to his mother. He has also been experiencing active symptoms (e.g. delusions) for two months. Given this symptom duration, James meets criteria for schizophrenia, which requires a disturbance to persist for at least six months, with active symptoms present for at least one month. Schizophreniform disorder would be an appropriate diagnosis if symptoms had been present for at least one month but under six months, whereas brief psychotic disorder would be diagnosed if symptoms were present for a minimum of a day but for under one month. Additionally, negative symptoms like emotional blunting are not part of the diagnostic criteria for brief psychotic disorder (American Psychiatric Association, 2022).

- What services should James' social worker refer him to upon discharge from the inpatient psychiatric unit?

Based on available evidence, James would benefit from a referral to a psychiatrist for ongoing medication management upon discharge. Ideally, James would be prescribed a second-generation antipsychotic during his hospitalization, and a psychiatrist would continue with this medication upon James' discharge. James should also be referred for psychosocial interventions, such as cognitive-behavioral therapy and/or a social skills group (Černe Kolarič et al., 2024; Sampogna et al., 2023).

Case Study 2: Schizoaffective Disorder (Marisol)

- Why does Marisol meet the criteria for schizoaffective disorder rather than schizophrenia?

Marisol meets the diagnostic criteria for schizoaffective disorder, bipolar type, because she shows evidence of manic behavior, consistent with a mood disorder, alongside symptoms of schizophrenia. If Marisol met diagnostic criteria for schizophrenia, she would not also experience mood disorder symptoms. It is also noted that because Marisol shows evidence of hallucinations in the absence of manic symptoms during the assessment, she meets the criterion of having hallucinations or delusions without the presence of mood symptoms for at least two weeks during the course of the illness (American Psychiatric Association, 2022).

- Why does the specifier "with catatonia" apply to Marisol's case?

The specifier "with catatonia" applies to Marisol's case, because she shows evidence consistent with catatonia, including lack of psychomotor activity (e.g. appearing motionless), mimicking the psychologist's movements, and limited verbal responses. The term catatonia is used to describe psychomotor disturbances (American Psychiatric Association, 2022).

- What services would be beneficial for Marisol?

In addition to participating in therapy, Marisol should be referred promptly to a psychiatrist for medication evaluation. A long-acting injectable antipsychotic would be beneficial, to encourage treatment adherence. Marisol would also benefit from psychoeducation to help her gain insight into her illness and understand the importance of medication adherence (Černe Kolarič et al., 2024; Sampogna et al., 2023). Case management services would be helpful for supporting Marisol within the community and linking her to needed resources, such as employment training and housing services.

Case Study 3: Delusional Disorder (Elaine)

- Why is the given diagnosis appropriate for Elaine?

Elaine meets criteria for delusional disorder because she has had a delusion for at least one month. She reports suspecting her neighbor of poisoning her, and this belief has persisted for several years. The belief meets the criteria for a delusion, because it is fixed and does not change when Elaine is provided with evidence to the contrary. More specifically, Elaine meets criteria for a delusional disorder, persecutory type, because she believes she is being subjected to poisoning (American Psychiatric Association, 2022).

- Why does Elaine not meet criteria for schizophrenia?

Elaine does not meet diagnostic criteria for schizophrenia, because the delusion is her only symptom, and she does not experience functional impairment. She is able to work and maintain housing, despite her insistence that her neighbor is poisoning her. Elaine doesn't show other signs of schizophrenia, such as hallucinations or disorganized speech (American Psychiatric Association, 2022).

- What should the social worker include on Elaine's treatment plan?

Compared to other schizophrenia spectrum disorders, there is a lack of research related to evidence-based treatments for delusional disorder; however, antipsychotic medications have been found to be effective for about one-third of patients (Muñoz-Negro & Cervilla, 2016). The social worker might refer Elaine to a psychiatrist to determine if medication would be beneficial for symptom management. The social worker should provide supportive psychotherapy to help Elaine cope with the anxiety associated with the delusions, while monitoring her for ongoing safety (González-Rodríguez & Seeman, 2020).

Case Study 4: Schizotypal Personality Disorder (Miguel)

- How does Miguel meet the diagnostic criteria for a personality disorder?

Personality disorders are described as involving enduring patterns that differ significantly from culturally normative behavior and thought processes (American Psychiatric Association, 2022). Miguel's presentation aligns with this definition, as he describes distancing himself from peers since adolescence. This suggests that his unusual behavior and social isolation represent a lasting pattern, which is characteristic of the personality disorders.

- Why is schizotypal personality disorder a more appropriate diagnosis than schizophrenia?

Miguel's symptoms do not align with a diagnosis of schizophrenia, because he does not demonstrate symptoms of true psychosis. While he does show peculiar thinking patterns and strange beliefs, they do not rise to the level of being delusional. Miguel has some insight into the fact that others perceive him to be unusual. He also does not experience hallucinations. In the absence of periods of psychosis, Miguel's presentation reflects personality features rather than disconnection from reality (American Psychiatric Association, 2022).

Chapter 3
Neurocognitive Disorders in the Elderly:
Delirium Dementia and Alzheimer's Disease

Samruddhi Datta Thube
http://orcid.org/0009-0002-0688-0830
SCES Indira College of Pharmacy, Tathawade, India

Pranoti Pramod Bendre
http://orcid.org/0009-0002-4130-8047
SCES Indira College of Pharmacy, Tathawade, India

Rohini Mahadev Chavan
http://orcid.org/0009-0005-8338-3338
SCES Indira College of Pharmacy, Tathawade, India

EXECUTIVE SUMMARY

Neurocognitive disorders, are becoming more common among older adults, which presents significant difficulties for individuals, those who care for them, and healthcare systems. This review emphasizes the significance of precise differentiation for effective care, highlighting the clinical features, diagnostic complexities, and treatment strategies of these conditions. While dementia and Alzheimer's involve progressive, irreversible neurodegeneration, delirium, which is frequently reversible, may indicate underlying cognitive decline. Improving patient outcomes necessitates personalized care, early diagnosis, caregiver support, and lifestyle interventions. The article also underscores the urgent need for continued research into disease-modifying therapies, early detection biomarkers, and health system improvements. To manage the growing burden of neurocognitive disorders and improve the qual-

DOI: 10.4018/979-8-3373-3084-6.ch003

ity of life for those who suffer from them, comprehensive strategies that integrate efforts at the policy, social, and clinical levels are essential as global populations age. (World Health Organization, 2021)

INTRODUCTION

As the world's population gets older, the number of neurocognitive disorders (NCDs) in older people has increased greatly, creating a significant public health problem. Aging raises the chances of facing mental issues such as delirium, dementia, and Alzheimer's disease, all of which greatly impact thinking skills and overall well-being. These conditions place a heavy burden not just on individuals and their support networks but also create complex issues for healthcare systems worldwide. (Inouye et al., 1990)

As life expectancy grows, the world's population is changing significantly. The World Health Organization (WHO) estimates that the number of people aged 60 and above will rise from 1 billion in 2020 to 1.4 billion by 2030 and 2.1 billion by 2050. This change poses one of the biggest public health challenges of this century. While living longer is a sign of medical and societal progress, it also leads to more age-related illnesses, particularly neurocognitive disorders (NCDs), including difficulties like delirium, dementia, and Alzheimer's disease. These disorders impact millions globally and place a heavy burden on families, caregivers, and health systems. (Petersen & Jack, 2009)

A drop in thinking skills—like memory, concentration, language, and problem-solving—that makes it difficult for someone to perform daily activities is the main sign of neurocognitive disorders. As people grow older, these disorders become more common. For instance, it is estimated that over 55 million people worldwide have dementia at any moment, with almost 10 million new cases diagnosed each year. Alzheimer's, the most common type of dementia, makes up 60-70% of all cases. Because the number of older adults is rising and access to early diagnosis and treatment is limited, the total number of people with dementia is expected to reach 139 million by 2050, with the largest increases anticipated in low- and middle-income countries. (Feldman & Gauthier, 2008)

Another serious but often missed neurocognitive issue, delirium, is especially common in older adults who have been hospitalized. Studies indicate that delirium affects about 15-30% of elderly patients admitted to hospitals, with even higher rates—up to 50%—in intensive care units and after surgeries. Unlike dementia and Alzheimer's disease, delirium begins suddenly and is often temporary, but it can signal more severe cognitive problems. It can complicate medical care for older patients and often indicates an underlying health issue or system problem. (Langa & Levine, 2014)

Delirium is a sudden condition characterized by changing levels of attention and awareness, often occurring due to illness or hospital stays. Although it usually goes away, it can worsen existing cognitive weaknesses and may signal the start of more cognitive decline. On the other hand, dementia is a long-term, gradual decline in cognitive abilities, with Alzheimer's disease being the most common type. Alzheimer's is marked by neurodegenerative changes like amyloid plaques and tau tangles, leading to slow memory loss and a drop in function. It is crucial to tell these conditions apart for effective treatment, as delirium, dementia, and Alzheimer's disease come from different reasons and need different management styles. Quick recognition and proper care are essential for reducing the chance of lasting cognitive difficulties and improving the quality of life for both patients and their caregivers. (Atri et al., 2024)

This aims to provide a short overview of the clinical features needed for diagnosis and treatment choices for these disorders. It highlights the importance of accurate diagnosis and personalized care and also points out the need for ongoing research to develop better treatment methods and caregiving strategies, especially with the growing older population. (World Health Organization, 2021)

BACKGROUND

Neurocognitive disorders (NCDs) have seen a significant rise in occurrence among elderly populations as the global demographic shifts towards an older age. The three most common conditions that negatively affect cognitive abilities in older individuals are delirium, dementia, and Alzheimer's disease. Each of these disorders poses notable challenges for patients, their families, and healthcare systems. Neurocognitive disorders are defined by a decline in cognitive functions that disrupts everyday living. The aging brain is particularly vulnerable to these conditions, especially when compounded by other health issues such as cardiovascular disease, diabetes, or stroke. Delirium which is a temporary state often triggered by illness or medication changes, manifests as fluctuating confusion and difficulties with attention. Although it can be reversed, delirium has the potential to exacerbate existing cognitive issues and complicate accurate diagnosis. Dementia, on the other hand, is characterized by a long-term decline in cognitive capabilities, with Alzheimer's disease being the most prevalent type. The gradual buildup of amyloid plaques and tau tangles is primarily responsible for the memory loss and brain degeneration commonly associated with Alzheimer's disease. The similarities in symptoms among delirium, dementia, and Alzheimer's complicate the process of distinguishing between them without comprehensive assessment. These disorders impose a significant burden on individuals, caregivers, and healthcare networks. For patients to achieve better outcomes and improved quality of life, accurate early diagnosis and focused treatment are essential. As the incidence of these disorders continues to increase, there is an urgent necessity for enhanced diagnostic methods, management approaches, and ongoing research to address this escalating public health issue. (American Psychiatric Association, 2013)

FOCUS OF THE ARTICLE

It looks closely at the increasing issue of neurocognitive disorders (NCDs) in older adults, focusing mainly on delirium, dementia, and Alzheimer's disease—three common and important cognitive problems affecting older people worldwide. Although these conditions have different beginnings, developments, and causes, they often share similar symptoms that can lead to wrong diagnoses, ineffective treatment, and unnecessary suffering for patients. The article aims to explain the signs, diagnostic difficulties, and treatment options related to each condition while also looking at their connections and effects on long-term brain health.

The article discusses several key points about mental health and aging by concentrating on these specific neurocognitive disorders:

1. Prevalence and Implications for Public Health: The review highlights the rising prevalence of NCDs in both rich and lower-income countries in line with global aging trends. The paper stresses the need for healthcare systems to adjust to this change by enhancing diagnosis and long-term care systems.
2. Clinical Characteristics and Diagnostic Nuances: One main goal is to differentiate between delirium, dementia, and Alzheimer's disease based on their clinical paths. Delirium is marked by sudden and changing issues with attention and awareness, often caused by outside factors like infections, medications, or surgeries. Dementia, including Alzheimer's disease, shows a gradual and irreversible decline in thinking ability that often leads to major challenges in daily tasks. It's important to tell these conditions apart because of the wide range of treatment options and serious results of a wrong diagnosis.
3. Relationships Between Conditions: The article examines how delirium and dementia interact in a complex way, especially how episodes of delirium can cause or worsen existing cognitive decline. People with dementia are particularly at risk of experiencing delirium during hospital stays or serious illnesses, and having delirium may speed up cognitive decline. Understanding these relationships

is crucial for doctors trying to use prevention methods and manage long-term results effectively.

4. Strategies for Treatment and Management: Another key focus is reviewing current non-drug and drug treatment options. The article looks at existing medications for dementia and Alzheimer's disease, like cholinesterase inhibitors and NMDA receptor antagonists, and also discusses the limits of current treatments in stopping disease progression. Important aspects of complete care, such as changes in the environment, cognitive exercises, and support for caregivers, are also mentioned.
5. Policy and Research Implications: The review aims to inform not just clinical practice but also health policies and future research. It highlights the need for early diagnosis, teamwork in care, and training for caregivers. Additionally, the article urges continued research into biomarkers, brain imaging tools, therapies to change the course of the disease, and methods to reduce inequalities in dementia care.

In simple terms, the aim of this article is to be a helpful guide for people in healthcare, researchers, and decision-makers who are dedicated to supporting and caring for older individuals. By combining current information on delirium, dementia, and Alzheimer's disease, it promotes better awareness, personalized treatment plans, and changes at the system level that can lead to an improved quality of life for millions of elderly people dealing with brain-related disorders. (Alzheimer's Association, 2023)

SOLUTIONS AND RECOMMENDATIONS

A comprehensive strategy is necessary to tackle neurocognitive disorders such as delirium, dementia, and Alzheimer's disease, which increasingly impact older adults. The following suggestions can enhance the diagnosis, treatment, and support for those affected by these conditions: (Inouye et al., 1990)

1.Early Diagnosis and Assessment- Conducting routine cognitive evaluations (e.g., MMSE, MoCA) for seniors can help identify early indicators of cognitive decline, allowing for prompt action. (Petersen & Jack, 2009) - Healthcare providers should employ a mixture of neuropsychological tests, patient history, brain imaging (MRI, CT), and biomarker analysis to differentiate between delirium, dementia, and Alzheimer's disease. An accurate diagnosis is essential for selecting the most effective treatment strategy. (Feldman & Gauthier, 2008)

2.Personalized and Holistic Care- When developing treatment strategies, it is important to consider each patient's specific needs, including the disease stage, any coexisting conditions, and caregiver involvement. Tailored plans can enhance symptom control and overall well-being. (Langa & Levine, 2014) - Engagement in cognitive stimulation therapy, physical activities, and social interactions has been demonstrated to boost cognitive abilities and slow the progression of certain types of dementia. Creating organized, supportive environments can diminish confusion and distress, especially for individuals with Alzheimer's. (Atri et al., 2024)

3. **Enhanced Delirium Prevention and Management**- Prompt identification and treatment of the root causes of delirium—such as infections, medications, or metabolic disturbances—are key to reducing its impact. (World Health Organization, 2021) - Ensuring a calm, familiar, and well-lit environment in hospitals and care settings can minimize the risk of delirium in older adults, especially those recovering from surgery or illness. (American Psychiatric Association, 2013) - To lessen the frequency and impact of delirium, healthcare professionals must be more aware of its symptoms and prevention strategies. (Alzheimer's Association, 2023)
4. **Caregiver Support and Education**- Caregivers of people with neurocognitive disorders should receive training on how to deal with challenging symptoms, manage behavioral changes, and offer emotional support. Caregiver burnout can be reduced and patient outcomes can be improved by this. (Inouye et al., 1990) - Caregivers can cope with the emotional and practical challenges of caring for loved ones with neurocognitive disorders by setting up local support groups and having access to resources. (Petersen & Jack, 2009)
5. **Medications and Treatments**- For Alzheimer's and other forms of dementia, medications like cholinesterase inhibitors (donepezil, rivastigmine) and glutamate regulators (memantine) can alleviate symptoms. However, they should be used judiciously, as they do not halt disease progression. (Feldman & Gauthier, 2008) - Antipsychotic medications may be necessary in managing severe agitation or psychosis, but they should be prescribed with caution due to the risk of adverse effects in elderly patients. (Langa & Levine, 2014)
6. **Research and Future Directions**- Advancing research into biomarkers for early detection and understanding the genetic underpinnings of Alzheimer's and other dementias could lead to more effective diagnostic tools and treatments. (Atri et al., 2024) - More research is needed to identify treatments that can slow or prevent the progression of Alzheimer's and other neurodegenerative diseases. The treatment of these disorders may change

in the future thanks to therapies that modify the disease. (World Health Organization, 2021) - Promoting healthy lifestyle choices (e.g., regular exercise, a balanced diet, and cognitive engagement) in midlife could reduce the risk of developing neurocognitive disorders in older age. (American Psychiatric Association, 2013)

7. **Policy and Healthcare System Improvements**- Governments and healthcare organizations should invest in expanding and improving long-term care facilities, ensuring they are well-equipped to handle the increasing number of patients with neurocognitive disorders. (Alzheimer's Association, 2023)
    - Increasing insurance coverage for long-term care and providing financial assistance to families of people with these conditions can lessen the financial strain on individuals and those who care for them. By addressing these key areas through a combination of early detection, personalized care, caregiver support, and continued research, the quality of life for patients with neurocognitive disorders can be improved, and the burden on families and healthcare systems can be reduced. (Inouye et al., 1990)

FUTURE RESEARCH DIRECTIONS

In order to improve diagnosis, treatment, and prevention for neurocognitive disorders, ongoing research is essential. Advances in our understanding and management of delirium, dementia, and Alzheimer's disease appear to be possible in several key areas of research: (Petersen & Jack, 2009)

1. Early Detection and Diagnostic Tools

Early diagnosis of brain disorders, especially Alzheimer's disease (AD), frontotemporal dementia (FTD), and dementia with Lewy bodies (DLB), is very important for improving patient care. (Feldman & Gauthier, 2008)

It allows for timely intervention, planning for future support, and encourages patient involvement in clinical trials for treatments that can change the disease. In the past, neurodegenerative illnesses were only diagnosed after noticeable cognitive decline began. However, with new diagnostic tools and technologies, it's now possible to find early stages of the disease before major symptoms appear. (Langa & Levine, 2014)

Early detection methods combine clinical evaluations, brain imaging, fluid markers, and genetic tests, which together give a better picture of disease processes before clear symptoms start to show. (Atri et al., 2024)

- **Biomarkers and Neuroimaging**
- Biomarkers are measurable signs of disease. For neurocognitive disorders, especially Alzheimer's disease, the National Institute on Aging–Alzheimer's Association (NIA-AA) has suggested a biological definition based on three main biomarkers: amyloid (A), tau (T), and neurodegeneration (N), referred to as the AT(N) framework. (World Health Organization, 2021)
- **Fluid Biomarkers**
  - Analyzing cerebrospinal fluid (CSF) is the best method for finding early signs of Alzheimer's disease. Lower levels of Aβ42 and higher levels of total tau (t-tau) and phosphorylated tau (p-tau) are signs of amyloid buildup and tau-related brain damage.
  - Recent developments in blood markers have shown hope as less invasive options:
  - The plasma Aβ42/40 ratio shows amyloid levels.
  - Levels of phosphorylated tau (p-tau181, p-tau217) in blood relate to tau damage in the brain and disease progression.
  - Neurofilament light chain (NFL) is a new marker for nerve damage and is increased in various neurodegenerative diseases.

These biomarkers are more frequently used in clinical trials and practice to enhance diagnosis, assess risk, and observe treatment responses. (American Psychiatric Association, 2013)

- **Neuroimaging Techniques**
  - Advanced brain imaging is crucial for spotting structural, metabolic, and molecular changes in the brain linked to neurodegenerative diseases. (Alzheimer's Association, 2023)
- **Positron Emission Tomography (PET)**
  - Amyloid PET imaging (such as florbetapir, florbetaben) shows the buildup of amyloid plaques in the brain.
  - Tau PET tracers (like flortaucipir) identify where and how much tau tangles are present.
  - FDG-PET examines brain glucose use, which often decreases in certain areas in Alzheimer's disease. (Inouye et al., 1990)
- **Magnetic Resonance Imaging (MRI)**
  - The shrinkage of the medial temporal lobe in Alzheimer's and the frontal lobe in FTD are two examples of brain shrinkage patterns detected by structural MRI. Volumetric MRI and cortical thickness mapping can monitor changes over time.

- Diffusion tensor imaging (DTI) and functional MRI (fMRI) provide insights into the health of white matter and changes in brain connectivity. (Petersen & Jack, 2009)

- **Artificial Intelligence and Machine Learning** are being used more and more in neuroimaging to improve early detection by spotting subtle patterns that traditional methods might miss. (Feldman & Gauthier, 2008)

2. Pathophysiology and Disease Mechanisms
    - Amyloid and Tau Research: In Alzheimer's research, the amyloid cascade hypothesis suggests that the build-up of beta-amyloid (Aβ) peptides in the brain starts a series of harmful events. (Langa & Levine, 2014)
    - These peptides aggregate to form external amyloid plaques, which hinder cell communication, cause inflammation, and cause nerve cell death. (Atri et al., 2024)
    - Enzymes (- and -secretases) cut Amyloid Precursor Protein (APP) to produce A.
    - The imbalance between how much Aβ is made and how much is removed causes its harmful build-up.
    - Although Aβ build-up is noticeable in the early stages of Alzheimer's, the link between plaque amount and cognitive decline is complicated. As a result, soluble oligomers rather than plaques may be the most hazardous forms. (World Health Organization, 2021)
    - At the same time, in Alzheimer's disease, tau proteins, which normally support nerve cell microtubules, become excessively phosphorylated. This causes the formation of intracellular neurofibrillary tangles (NFTs). Cell death is eventually brought on by these tangles, which prevent synaptic communication and disrupt signal transmission within cells. (American Psychiatric Association, 2013)
    - The spread of tau problems through connected brain areas closely matches the progress of the disease, indicating that tau plays a key role in cognitive decline. (Alzheimer's Association, 2023)
    - Neuroinflammation: There is mounting evidence that brain inflammation may play a significant role in the onset and progression of Alzheimer's disease and other forms of dementia. (Inouye et al., 1990)

- New anti-inflammatory treatments that slow the progression of the disease could be developed by comprehending the inflammatory processes involved. (Petersen & Jack, 2009)
- Synaptic Dysfunction and Neurodegeneration: Investigating the underlying causes of neurodegeneration and synaptic loss may lead to the discovery of novel therapeutic strategies for preserving and restoring brain neural connections. (Feldman & Gauthier, 2008)
- Neuroinflammation: There is mounting evidence that brain inflammation may play a significant role in the onset and progression of Alzheimer's disease and other forms of dementia. New anti-inflammatory treatments that slow the progression of the disease could be developed by comprehending the inflammatory processes involved. (Langa & Levine, 2014)
- Synaptic Dysfunction and Neurodegeneration: Investigating the underlying causes of neurodegeneration and synaptic loss may lead to the discovery of novel therapeutic strategies for preserving and restoring brain neural connections. (Atri et al., 2024)

3. Interventions that are both pharmacological and non-pharmacological

Effective treatment of neurocognitive disorders necessitates a comprehensive, multi-method strategy that incorporates both medication and non-medication options. There is a growing interest in disease-modifying therapies (DMTs), which aim to alter the underlying issues of Alzheimer's disease (AD) and other dementias. While current drug treatments alleviate symptoms, At the same time, non-drug methods, such as mental exercises, lifestyle improvements, and caregiver training, are vital for enhancing patient outcomes and quality of life. (World Health Organization, 2021)

- **Disease-Modifying Therapies (DMTs)**
  - Examples of current drug treatments that focus primarily on symptoms rather than the main causes of nerve damage include cholinesterase inhibitors like donepezil and rivastigmine and NMDA receptor blockers like memantine. On the other hand, new developments are concentrating on biological agents that solve problems specific to diseases. (American Psychiatric Association, 2013)
  - Treatments for Amyloid- The amyloid cascade theory suggests that the buildup of amyloid-beta (Aβ) peptides starts a series of nerve damage events. Monoclonal antibodies like aducanumab and lecanemab are made to bind to clumped A and assist in its removal from the brain. Despite the FDA's fast-track approval of aducanumab, mixed study

results raise questions about the drug's practicality. In contrast, lecanemab showed moderate slowing of cognitive decline in the CLARITY-AD trial and received standard FDA approval in 2023. (Alzheimer's Association, 2023)

- These treatments are not cures and can have risks like amyloid-related imaging abnormalities (ARIA), which shows the importance of careful patient selection and monitoring. (Inouye et al., 1990)
- Tau-Targeting Therapies-Unlike amyloid levels, tangled, hyperphosphorylated tau proteins are more closely linked to cognitive decline. Anti-tau antibodies, kinase inhibitors (for example, those that target GSK-3), and tau aggregation inhibitors are among the treatment options being explored. Many clinical trials are ongoing, but none have resulted in approved treatments yet. (Petersen & Jack, 2009)
- Neuroinflammation Modulation- Long-term neuroinflammation is a key feature of many neurodegenerative diseases. Researchers are looking into modulators of the innate immune system, such as agents that target cytokines and microglial activation inhibitors. Trials are taking place on tyrosine kinase inhibitors like masitinib and the anti-inflammatory antibiotic minocycline to see how they impact disease advancement. (Feldman & Gauthier, 2008)
- Cholinergic and Neurotransmitter-Based Therapies- Although not disease-modifying, improving neurotransmitter function (especially acetylcholine and glutamate) remains an important symptomatic strategy. Dual-acting agents that support neurotransmitters while also protecting nerve cells are one potential future approach. (Langa & Levine, 2014)
- Cognitive Enhancement and Neuroprotection-Besides modifying the disease, research is ongoing into ways to boost brain resilience and cognitive ability, especially in the early stages of decline. (Atri et al., 2024)
- Stem Cell Therapies -Mesenchymal stem cells (MSCs) and induced pluripotent stem cells (iPSCs) are being studied for their ability to turn into neurons, reduce inflammation, and repair damaged tissue. (World Health Organization, 2021)
- Early trials show promise for enhancing cognitive function and reducing neuroinflammation, despite the fact that long-term efficacy and safety have not been established. (American Psychiatric Association, 2013)
- **Neurotrophic Factors**-The survival of nerve cells and the ability for connections between them depend on nerve growth factor (NGF) and brain-derived neurotrophic factor (BDNF). Boosting natural levels or

using synthetic versions through gene therapy or infusion is under investigation. (Alzheimer's Association, 2023)

- Trials using NGF gene delivery with viral vectors or delivered by encapsulated cells have shown promise in stopping cognitive decline. (Inouye et al., 1990)
- **Gene Therapy**- The aim of targeted gene therapy is to manage the production of proteins that are important for disease, such as APP, tau, or APOE. Methods include editing with CRISPR/Cas9, sending corrective genes through viral vectors, and using antisense oligonucleotides (ASOs) to change protein production. (Petersen & Jack, 2009)

- **Cognitive Enhancing Compounds:**
  - Several experimental drugs focus on improving synaptic plasticity, encouraging new brain cell growth, or adjusting neurotransmitter systems to aid thinking. These include ampakines, nicotinic receptor activators, and histone deacetylase (HDAC) inhibitors. (Feldman & Gauthier, 2008)
- **Lifestyle Interventions:**
  - Non-drug strategies are key for preventive care and supportive treatment in brain disorders. There is increasing proof that changeable lifestyle factors can lower the chance of cognitive decline and delay its onset. (Langa & Levine, 2014)
  - Dietary Interventions: Diets high in antioxidants, polyphenols, and healthy fats—like the Mediterranean and MIND diets—are linked to slower cognitive decline. Nutrients such as vitamin D, B vitamins (especially folate and B12), and omega-3 fatty acids may protect brain health. (Atri et al., 2024)
  - Physical activity: Regular aerobic and strength training are linked to higher levels of neurotrophic factors (like BDNF), larger hippocampal volumes, and improved cognitive performance. Exercise may also help reduce vascular risk factors and improve sleep quality, both of which are important for preventing dementia. (World Health Organization, 2021)
  - Sleep and Circadian Health: The buildup of amyloid and cognitive decline is connected to poor sleep habits and sleep apnea. Maintaining a regular sleep schedule, treating sleep apnea, and practicing good sleep hygiene are all important for brain health. - Cognitive Training and Mental Stimulation: Cognitive stimulation therapy (CST), brain games, memory exercises, and ongoing education have been proven to slow cognitive decline, especially in mild cognitive impairment (MCI). People who engage in mental activities have greater cognitive reserves, according to long-term research. - Social Engagement and

Psychological Health: Changeable risk factors for dementia include depression and isolation. Taking part in community, social, and leisure activities improves mood and slows cognitive decline. Mindfulness-based stress reduction (MBSR) and therapy can enhance emotional health and cognitive abilities. (American Psychiatric Association, 2013)

4. Delirium and Its Relationship with Dementia

- Dementia and delirium are deeply intertwined conditions that frequently coexist with dementia in older adults, posing unique difficulties for diagnosis and treatment. Although delirium is an acute, fluctuating disturbance of attention and cognition, and dementia is a chronic, progressive decline in cognitive abilities, their overlapping features often lead to diagnostic overshadowing, where symptoms of delirium are mistakenly attributed to dementia progression. This misinterpretation can delay appropriate treatment and worsen patient outcomes. (Alzheimer's Association, 2023)
- Understanding the Relationship Between Delirium and Dementia Studies indicate that up to 60–80 percent of older adults with dementia experience delirium while in the hospital. Delirium is very common in people with dementia. Moreover, patients with pre-existing dementia are more vulnerable to developing delirium due to diminished cognitive reserve, making even minor physiological or environmental stressors capable of triggering acute confusion. (Inouye et al., 1990)
- Delirium is not only a comorbid condition but also a potential accelerant of neurodegenerative processes, according to recent research. A delirious episode may result in persistent cognitive decline, accelerating the progression from mild cognitive impairment (MCI) to dementia or increasing the severity of existing dementia, according to clinical studies. In patients who experienced delirium, structural neuroimaging revealed increased cortical atrophy and decreased hippocampal volume, indicating a neurotoxic effect. Multiple pathophysiological mechanisms have been proposed to explain how delirium contributes to long-term cognitive decline, including: (Petersen & Jack, 2009)
- Neuroinflammation: Delirium triggers acute systemic and central nervous system inflammation. In patients with dementia, chronic neuroinflammation is already present, and superimposed inflammatory episodes can exacerbate neuronal damage. (Feldman & Gauthier, 2008)
- Cholinergic Hypothesis: Impaired cholinergic neurotransmission is linked to both delirium and Alzheimer's disease. Acute-on-chronic failure of this system may be reflected in delirium, particularly in dementia patients. Through oxidative stress, mitochondrial dysfunction, and

excitotoxicity, delirium may accelerate the disconnection of synapses and the loss of neurons. Disruption of Brain Network Connectivity: Functional MRI studies suggest that delirium leads to sustained alterations in large-scale brain networks (such as the default mode and salience networks), which are crucial for attention, memory, and awareness. (Langa & Levine, 2014)

5. Quality of Life and Support from Caregivers

- The progression of neurocognitive disorders like dementia, Alzheimer's disease, and delirium has a significant impact not only on the affected individuals but also on the people who take care of them. As the disease advances, patients often require continuous assistance with daily activities, medical care, and emotional support. This dependency places a considerable physical, emotional, and financial burden on caregivers, often leading to caregiver stress, depression, and burnout. Therefore, improving the quality of life for both patients and caregivers is a vital area of clinical practice and research. (Atri et al., 2024)
- Interventions by Caregivers Caregivers, often family members, form the backbone of long-term care for older adults with neurocognitive disorders. However, they frequently lack the necessary preparation and support, which contributes to significant psychological distress and lowers the quality of care. Targeted caregiver interventions are essential for enhancing patient outcomes and sustaining the caregiver's well-being. (World Health Organization, 2021)
- Key strategies and findings in this domain include:
- Education and Training Programs: Providing caregivers with structured training about the nature of dementia and delirium, symptom management, behavioral challenges, and communication techniques has been shown to reduce stress and increase confidence. Studies such as the REACH II trial (Resources for Enhancing Alzheimer's Caregiver Health) demonstrated that tailored education combined with skills training can substantially reduce caregiver burden and depression. (American Psychiatric Association, 2013)
- Psychosocial and Emotional Support: Emotional well-being is central to caregiver resilience. Interventions such as support groups, individual counseling, and mindfulness-based stress reduction programs have proven effective in alleviating symptoms of anxiety and depression among caregivers. Additionally, these facilitate peer support networks, reducing caregivers' sense of isolation. Respite Care Services: Short-term relief options, including adult day care programs, in-home respite services, and temporary institutional placements, give caregivers the

chance to rest and recover. Access to respite care has been associated with lower caregiver burnout and can even delay the institutionalization of the care recipient. (Alzheimer's Association, 2023)

- Impact on Patient Outcomes: Importantly, caregiver support interventions are not only beneficial for the caregiver but also improve outcomes for individuals with neurocognitive disorders. Better-informed and emotionally supported caregivers are more capable of managing behavioral disturbances, adhering to care plans, and promoting a stable environment, which can delay cognitive decline and reduce hospitalization rates. (Inouye et al., 1990)
- Cultural Considerations: Interventions must take into account family structures, beliefs, and cultural norms. Research indicates that caregiving experiences and challenges differ by ethnicity, affecting how support should be tailored for diverse populations. (Petersen & Jack, 2009)
- Technology and Caregiving
- The integration of digital health tools is transforming how care is delivered to individuals with neurocognitive disorders and how caregivers access support. As the population ages and the need for care grows, technology offers creative and scalable solutions to the problems of providing care. Some notable advancements in technology include: Telemedicine and remote consultations: Patients and caregivers can access healthcare providers without having to leave their homes through virtual medical visits, which is especially helpful for those who struggle with mobility or live in rural areas. Telehealth can facilitate early diagnosis, regular monitoring, medication adjustments, and behavioral assessments with reduced logistical burdens. (Feldman & Gauthier, 2008)
- Digital Monitoring Systems: In-home sensors, GPS trackers, fall detectors, and wearable health monitors can alert caregivers to safety concerns, wandering behavior, or medical emergencies. These tools promote patient autonomy while providing caregivers with peace of mind. (Langa & Levine, 2014)
- Cognitive Training Applications: There is growing interest in the use of apps and software platforms that offer brain-training exercises, memory games, and mental stimulation activities. Some studies suggest that these tools may slow cognitive decline and encourage engagement in people with early-stage dementia, although the evidence for their effectiveness varies. Virtual Reality (VR) and Augmented Reality (AR): New research is looking into whether dementia patients' agitation, anxiety, and depression can be reduced in VR environments. VR can also be used in caregiver training modules to simulate real-life scenarios and

teach best practices for communication and care delivery. (Atri et al., 2024)

- Predictive Analytics and Artificial Intelligence (AI): AI-driven platforms are being developed to analyze patient data and predict changes in behavior or health status, providing caregivers and clinicians with preemptive alerts. These systems may help reduce emergency visits and improve chronic disease management. (World Health Organization, 2021)
- Resources and Online Support Networks: Through digital platforms, caregivers can connect with forums, educational materials, webinars, and coaching services. A convenient and adaptable method for acquiring knowledge and receiving emotional support is provided by these online communities. Future Directions for Improving the Well-Being and Support of Caregivers Looking forward, research should prioritize: (American Psychiatric Association, 2013)
- Longitudinal studies that track how different interventions influence caregiver health, patient outcomes, and long-term healthcare utilization. (Alzheimer's Association, 2023)
- models of integrated care that combine psychological, social, and medical support for patients and caregivers with interdisciplinary teams Analyses of cost-effectiveness to help policymakers make decisions about how to fund caregiver interventions and tech-based solutions. Personalized interventions based on the stage of disease, caregiver experience, cultural background, and specific stressors. (Inouye et al., 1990)

6. Disparities in health care across the globe

- Access to diagnosis, treatment, and long-term care for neurocognitive disorders varies greatly across regions, particularly between high-income countries and low- and middle-income countries (LMICs). A complex web of cultural, socioeconomic, infrastructure, and policy-related factors contribute to these disparities. To ensure that all older adults, regardless of where they live, receive timely and effective care, these disparities must be addressed. Factors from culture and society at large Perceptions of aging, cognitive decline, and mental illness are significantly influenced by cultural beliefs and social norms. In many societies, dementia symptoms may be misattributed to "normal aging" or even to supernatural causes, which leads to delayed help-seeking behaviors and underdiagnosis. Families are even less likely to use healthcare options because of the stigma associated with mental and cognitive disorders. The treatment of neurocognitive disorders is directly influenced by socioeconomic factors like income, education, and access to healthcare resources. For instance: Limited health literacy often results in late-stage diagnosis and inadequate understanding of treatment plans. (Petersen & Jack, 2009)

- Long-term care is out of reach for many people, especially in nations with weak public health systems, due to inadequate insurance coverage or a lack of financial resources. Urban-rural healthcare divides lead to unequal access to neurologists, diagnostic imaging, and specialized dementia care units. (Feldman & Gauthier, 2008)
- As a result, research must concentrate on how these factors influence patient outcomes and should direct interventions that are culturally appropriate and financially viable. Aging Populations in Low- and Middle-Income Countries (LMICs)
- While the majority of dementia research is conducted in high-income nations, LMICs have the fastest-growing older population. Unique obstacles exist in these regions, including: a lack of geriatricians, neurologists, and mental health professionals in underfunded health systems. There is no formal caregiving infrastructure, so a lot of people have to rely on family members who might not have the training or support they need. Due to high prices and a lack of availability, advanced treatments and diagnostic tools are difficult to obtain. Given that LMICs will account for more than 70% of people with dementia by 2050 (World Alzheimer Report), it is critical to develop low-cost, scalable solutions tailored to the infrastructure and cultural contexts of these regions. This includes public awareness campaigns, mobile health technologies, training for community health workers, and simplified screening tools. (Langa & Levine, 2014)

7. Policy and Health Care Research

- The rising burden of neurocognitive disorders calls for robust, evidence-based health system responses. Research into the economic impact, care delivery models, and resource allocation required to support people living with cognitive decline must serve as the foundation for effective policies. Policy on Healthcare Cost-Efficiency Neurocognitive disorders place an immense financial strain on individuals, families, and health systems due to costs associated with: (Atri et al., 2024)
- Residence-based long-term care medical treatments and hospitalizations
- Informal caregiving (which often leads to income loss)
- Behavioral symptom management
- Global dementia costs are expected to double by 2030, according to a report from Alzheimer's Disease International. In 2020, they are pro-

jected to exceed $1.3 trillion. These projections emphasize the urgent requirement for cost-effectiveness analyses to direct the development of sustainable policies. In terms of delaying institutionalization, improving patient outcomes, and supporting caregivers, research must determine which interventions provide the best value for money. Integration of Care Models (World Health Organization, 2021)

- A multidisciplinary approach known as an integrated care model incorporates social, psychological, and medical support to provide patients with ongoing, coordinated care. There is evidence that these models can: Improve patient and caregiver satisfaction (American Psychiatric Association, 2013)
- Reduce hospital readmissions
- Promote early intervention and continuity of care
- The following are essential aspects of successful integration: Care that is team-based and involves mental health professionals, nurses, social workers, and doctors. shared electronic health records for improved provider communication Systems for case management that monitor the progression of diseases and adjust care plans Pilot programs in Europe and North America, such as the Innovative Care for Chronic Conditions Framework by the WHO, demonstrate the potential of integrated models to improve dementia outcomes, especially when customized to local contexts. Further research is needed to evaluate their adaptability and effectiveness in different regions, especially LMICs. (Alzheimer's Association, 2023)

8. **Future Outlook and Research Priorities**

- Neurocognitive disorders will emerge as one of the most pressing public health issues of the 21st century as the world's population ages. Multidisciplinary and collaborative research is essential to meet this challenge through: (Inouye et al., 1990)
- utilizing readily available biomarkers and imaging technologies to improve early diagnosis Deepening understanding of disease mechanisms, including neuroinflammation, genetic factors, and environmental risks (Petersen & Jack, 2009)
- Advancing therapeutic development, from disease-modifying drugs to regenerative medicine and neuroprotective agents
- Expanding non-pharmacological interventions, such as cognitive training, lifestyle modifications, and caregiver education (Feldman & Gauthier, 2008)
- Leveraging digital health technologies, including telemedicine, AI-driven care planning, and remote monitoring

- Promoting equitable global health, ensuring all individuals—regardless of geography or income—have access to quality dementia care (Langa & Levine, 2014)
- To turn research findings into interventions that can be implemented in the real world, it is essential to work together across fields, countries, and disciplines. Policy changes informed by science, community engagement, and international cooperation will be necessary to reduce the burden of neurocognitive disorders and to foster resilience among patients, caregivers, and healthcare systems. (Atri et al., 2024)

9. Research on Health Systems and Policy

- Cost-Effectiveness and Healthcare Policy: Healthcare policies will be informed by research into the economic impact of neurocognitive disorders, such as the cost of care, insurance coverage, and long-term care facilities. As the world's aging population grows, cost-effective interventions that strike a balance between providing high-quality care and being financially feasible will be crucial. (World Health Organization, 2021)
- Integration of Care Models: Research into integrated care models, which combine medical, social, and psychological support for patients with neurocognitive disorders, could improve care coordination and outcomes. The efficacy of these models ought to be evaluated across a variety of healthcare settings. (American Psychiatric Association, 2013)
- Enhancing early diagnosis, comprehending disease mechanisms, developing effective treatments, and assisting caregivers are the future of neurocognitive disorder research. A combination of advanced technologies, pharmacological interventions, lifestyle changes, and healthcare system improvements will be essential in addressing the growing challenge of delirium, dementia, and Alzheimer's disease as the global population ages. We can develop novel solutions that enhance the lives of people with neurocognitive disorders and their families by concentrating on these essential area (Alzheimer's Association, 2023)

CONCLUSION

One of the most significant and difficult health issues affecting the aging population worldwide is neurocognitive disorders, particularly delirium, dementia, and Alzheimer's disease. The prevalence of these disorders is sharply rising, with profound effects on individuals, families, healthcare systems, and economies as a result of rising life expectancy and demographic shifts that increase the number of elderly people. In the case of delirium, these conditions are characterized by acute confusion and inattention that frequently go unnoticed, progressive cognitive decline, and impairments in memory, judgment, and functional independence. As their clinical presentations may overlap, early and accurate differentiation between delirium, dementia, and Alzheimer's disease is essential. However, they require distinct diagnostic approaches and tailored management strategies. Inappropriate treatments, faster functional deterioration, and an increased burden on caregivers can result from delayed or inaccurate diagnosis. Despite advancements in symptom management, most existing pharmacological treatments provide only temporary or partial relief. Disease-modifying treatments that can alter the underlying processes of neurodegeneration are still desperately needed. Promising areas of ongoing research include anti-amyloid and anti-tau therapies, neuroinflammation modulation, synaptic repair, and the use of regenerative strategies such as stem cell therapy and gene editing. Similarly, the integration of biomarkers and advanced neuroimaging technologies offers potential for earlier diagnosis—possibly even in preclinical stages—thus opening new windows for intervention. (Inouye et al., 1990)

Non-pharmacological strategies also play a pivotal role in managing neurocognitive disorders. Physical activity, cognitive stimulation, healthy eating, and social engagement are all examples of lifestyle interventions that have the potential to delay disease onset and reduce symptoms. Equally critical is the need to address the psychosocial aspects of care, particularly the well-being of caregivers, who often face significant emotional, physical, and financial stress. A holistic care model must include interventions that provide psychological support, respite care, and caregiver education. These disorders have a global impact that is not evenly distributed. Access to healthcare, diagnostic capabilities, and long-term care infrastructure disparities are major obstacles, particularly in low- and middle-income nations. These disparities emphasize the significance of developing care models that are scalable, cost-effective, and culturally appropriate. To ensure that research findings and best practices are translated into effective and equitable care for diverse populations and healthcare systems, global collaboration is essential. At the health policy level, long-term planning and investment in dementia-capable systems of care are crucial. This entails developing public health strategies that place a priority on brain health across the lifespan, integrating care across disciplines, and building workforce capacity. Policymakers must consider the economic implications of neurocognitive disorders and implement funding mechanisms to support research, care delivery, and caregiver assistance. (Petersen & Jack, 2009)

Interdisciplinary endeavors that integrate neuroscience, gerontology, public health, technology, and health policy are likely to produce the most significant advancements in the future. Based on genetics, biomarkers, and individual risk profiles, the shift toward personalized and precision medicine holds great promise for these conditions' prevention and individualized treatment. In conclusion, a multifaceted and globally coordinated response is required to combat the growing problem of neurocognitive disorders. By aligning scientific innovation, public policy, and compassionate caregiving, we can not only improve diagnostic and treatment outcomes but also significantly enhance the quality of life for millions of older adults worldwide. To address this pressing public health issue going forward, a strong commitment to research, healthcare equity, and supportive infrastructure will be essential. (Feldman & Gauthier, 2008)

REFERENCES

Alzheimer’s Association. (2023). 2023 Alzheimer’s Disease Facts and Figures. Alzheimer's & Dementia, 19(4), 1-50. doi:.DOI: 10.1002/alz.13177

American Psychiatric Association. (2013). Diagnostic and Statistical Manual of Mental Disorders (DSM-5). 5th Edition. Arlington, VA: American Psychiatric Publishing.

Atri, A., Dickerson, B. C., Clevenger, C., Karlawish, J., Knopman, D., Lin, P., Norman, M., Onyike, C., Sano, M., Scanland, S., & Carrillo, M. (2024). Alzheimer’s Association clinical practice guideline for the Diagnostic Evaluation, Testing, Counseling, and Disclosure of Suspected Alzheimer’s Disease and Related Disorders (DETeCD-ADRD): Executive summary of recommendations for primary care. Alzheimer’s & Dementia, alz.14333. DOI: 10.1002/alz.14333

Ellis, G., & Sevda Lis, N. (2019). Understanding and improving multidisciplinary team working in geriatric medicine. Age and Ageing, 48(4), 498–505. DOI: 10.1093/ageing/afz021

Feldman, H. H., & Gauthier, S. (2008). Management of Alzheimer's Disease: Practical Insights and Emerging Therapies. Journal of Clinical Psychiatry, 69(11), 1704-1711. DOI: 10.4088/JCP.v69n1104

Inouye, S. K., van Dyck, C. H., Alessi, C. A., Balkin, S., Siegal, A. P., & Horwitz, R. I. (1990). The delirium syndrome: The incidence, mortality, and long-term consequences of delirium in hospitalized elderly patients. Journal of the American Geriatrics Society, 38(12), 1425-1432. doi:. 1990.tb01758.xDOI: 10.1111/j.1532-5415

Langa, K. M., & Levine, D. A. (2014). The Diagnosis and Management of Mild Cognitive Impairment: A Review. JAMA, 312(23), 2551-2561. doi:DOI: 10.1001/jama.2014.15204

Petersen, R. C., & Jack, C. R. (2009). Alzheimer’s Disease and Dementia: The Future of Early Detection and Intervention. The Lancet Neurology, 8(7), 563-572. doi:DOI: 10.1016/S1474-4422(09)70142-7

World Health Organization (WHO). (2021). Dementia. [WHO Fact Sheet]. Retrieved from https://www.who.int/news-room/fact-sheets/detail/dementia

KEY TERMS AND DEFINITIONS

Alzheimer's Disease: It is a type of dementia, it is characterized by a gradual decline in cognitive functioning, especially memory loss, along with changes in behavior and thought processes. This condition is associated with neuronal damage resulting from the build: up of amyloid plaques and tau tangles in the brain. (Atri et al., 2024)

BPSD (Behavioral and Psychological Symptoms of Dementia): These are non: cognitive symptoms experienced by individuals with dementia, such as agitation, sadness, anxiety, aggression, and hallucinations. Such symptoms considerably impact the quality of life for both patients and their caregivers. (Alzheimer's Association, 2023)

Cognitive Stimulation Therapy (CST): A non: drug intervention designed to enhance cognitive abilities in individuals with dementia through activities that foster thinking, memory, and problem: solving skills. CST has demonstrated positive effects on cognitive and emotional health. (Inouye et al., 1990)

Delirium: A rapid emergence of confusion and an altered mental state, often initiated by medical issues such as infections, side effects of medications, or dehydration. (Feldman & Gauthier, 2008)

Dementia: A general term denoting a notable decline in cognitive functions that disrupts everyday life. It encompasses Alzheimer's disease, vascular dementia, and frontotemporal dementia, all of which involve a progressive loss of memory, poor decision: making, and changes in personality. (Langa & Levine, 2014)

Disorder of the Brain (NCD): This is an extensive category of conditions marked by a deterioration in cognitive abilities. Examples of NCDs that generally impact older individuals include dementia, Alzheimer's disease, and delirium. This decline can affect various cognitive functions, such as memory, attention, reasoning, language, and executive functions. (Petersen & Jack, 2009)

Mild Cognitive Impairment (MCI): A condition marked by noticeable cognitive or memory issues that are not severe enough to disrupt daily activities but may heighten the risk of developing dementia, including Alzheimer's disease. (American Psychiatric Association, 2013)

Molecular Imaging: This refers to advanced imaging methods, such as PET scans, utilized to identify abnormalities associated with Alzheimer's disease and other dementias, including the accumulation of amyloid plaques, tau tangles, and neuroinflammation. (Petersen & Jack, 2009)

Neuroinflammation: a brain based immune response that is becoming more and more recognized as a factor in the pathophysiology of neurodegenerative diseases. Chronic inflammation may exacerbate neuronal damage and is considered a potential therapeutic target for slowing disease progression in dementia and Alzheimer’s. (Feldman & Gauthier, 2008)

Synaptic Dysfunction: Disruption in the communication between neurons at synapses, often preceding visible neurodegeneration. This dysfunction plays a role in the cognitive symptoms of Alzheimer's disease and other dementias and is one of the main areas of focus when developing treatments to keep or restore cognitive function. (Langa & Levine, 2014)

Vascular Dementia: This type of dementia arises from diminished blood flow to the brain, often due to strokes or other vascular problems. Symptoms commonly include confusion, memory lapses, and challenges with planning and making decisions. (World Health Organization, 2021)

Chapter 4

Understanding and Managing Anxiety, Schizophrenia, Depression, and Bipolar Disorder in Children:

Our Children's Care – Key to Sustainable Inclusion

Wasswa Shafik
http://orcid.org/0000-0002-9320-3186
Dig Connectivity Research Laboratory (DCRLab), Uganda

EXECUTIVE SUMMARY

Understanding and managing anxiety, schizophrenia, depression, and bipolar disorder in children is critical for promoting their mental health and well-being. These conditions can manifest differently in younger populations, requiring tailored approaches to diagnosis and treatment. Anxiety in children often presents as excessive worry or fear, while schizophrenia may involve delusions, hallucinations, and impaired social functioning. Depression in children can lead to mood disturbances, irritability, and withdrawal from activities, while bipolar disorder is characterized by extreme mood swings, ranging from manic episodes to deep depression. Early identification and intervention, including therapy, medication, and support from caregivers, are essential to managing these disorders effectively. A comprehensive approach that includes medical, psychological, and educational strategies can help children cope with and manage these conditions, improving their overall quality of life.

DOI: 10.4018/979-8-3373-3084-6.ch004

1 INTRODUCTION

Mental health can affect daily functioning from school to play, from managing behavior challenges at home to having the ability to sit for meals, from stress levels to the ability to facilitate and maintain efficient learning, and from coping with a mild cold to managing a chronic illness. Even the common conditions previously mentioned can have an ultimate impact on a child's health and functioning, and many times, they are not visible. They are not the cause (Schneider et al., 2023). Our perception, treatment, and understanding of chronic physical health problems in children have undergone radical changes over the last decade. What did you want to become when you were a child? An astronaut, a firefighter, possibly a teacher, or a pop star? Both children and adults have different life and occupational objectives that may sound noble or trivial, visionary or too practical, depending on personal interests and circumstances. However, the way to become fulfilled in the future is not necessarily easier in adulthood, and each phase of human life is a challenge that requires strength and determination (Wilson et al., 2022). In fact, the evolution of children exposed to stress during their development is quite complex because anxiety may precede or follow poor quality of life or represent an inherited vulnerability. In addition, when the problem is real and not trivial, feelings of worry, fears, and the severity of anxiety can increase with age, and other serious mental health disorders such as schizophrenia, depression, and bipolar disorder can be expressed or triggered by anxiety attacks, poor school performance, putting academic plans at risk (Bozzatello et al., 2021).

In a recent study related to the social isolation experienced by parents during COVID-19, a significant increase in the frequency of new-onset and exacerbation of psychiatric conditions such as major depressive disorder, anxiety disorder, and endorsement of psychotic-like experiences in children and their first-degree relatives was found (Abubakari, 2021). In conclusion, serious emotional and behavioral problems are relatively common in children and adolescents, affecting approximately 12–21% of young people within the first year of life. These problems tend to emerge early, with symptoms typically reaching their highest levels between ages 2–3 years in girls and 4–5 years in boys. Compared to children who do not experience such difficulties, affected individuals often show lower levels of cooperation, increased oppositional behavior, and reduced ability to cope with frustration. Over time, these early challenges can have long-term consequences, increasing the risk of developing mood, anxiety, and behavioral disorders during adolescence and adulthood. Additionally, these individuals are more vulnerable to serious outcomes, including suicidal thoughts and attempts later in life. For this reason, childhood mental health is a major public health concern and represents a major challenge, with many factors contributing to the onset and maintenance of these childhood expressions of anxiety and distress (Shafik, 2024d). It is essential to recognize the most appropriate and indicated diagnostic and treatment paths and engage individuals in effective prevention, treatment, and management programs.

1.1 Overview of Anxiety Disorders in Children

Anxiety disorders are the most common mental health problem for children and adolescents, affecting as many as one in ten each year. The usual childhood fears and worries change as a child grows and develops; the barrage of "what if" questions that linger in younger children's minds diminish. More complex ones replace unsophisticated but socially acceptable fears and rituals, take longer to generate, and lack an element of social acceptability. Childhood anxiety disorders unfold at different ages, in different settings, and with low to high intensity (Schneider et al., 2023). The development of anxiety disorders is a function of the child's traits and behaviors, such as the ability to inhibit, to control emotions, and to receive negative feedback. Predisposing characteristics of these children do not have as strong an effect as the immediate determinants, such as daily stress events, family environment, and friends, in terms of the anxiety and phobias shown. Based on characteristics and new criteria in the Diagnostic and Statistical Manual of Mental Disorders, these disorders are organized into four modality types: generalized anxiety disorders, phobic disorders, separation anxiety disorders, and panic disorders. Any of these disorders, even their severest forms, can be treated effectively once a professional accurately diagnoses the problem (Bozzatello et al., 2021).

1.2 Understanding Schizophrenia in the Pediatric Population

Childhood schizophrenia is a rare psychiatric disorder that typically first appears during the preteen or adolescent years. Before puberty, the condition occurs at similar rates in boys and girls; however, following puberty, it becomes more prevalent in boys than in girls. Because schizophrenia is a rare condition and because the symptoms are similar to other childhood mental illnesses, it is often difficult to make as specific a diagnosis as the situation requires. People who develop schizophrenia as adults report an insidious onset that is yearlong, but for children, the onset is difficult to pinpoint and seems to have had a more chaotic and rapid acceleration (Shafik, 2025). For children, the more typical incipient symptoms of odd or passive behavior are not necessarily related to schizophrenia, developmental disorders, personality disorders, or PTSD. Symptoms vary in presentation, the primary difference being that children can lose a lot of developmental ground and fall very disorganized. Because of these variations in onset and not all children suffer from the same difficulty and have very different types of reasoning for why they are so disabled, it is helpful to describe the children in terms of symptoms and disorganization rather than attaching a specific criterion to relate it to the adult manifestation of schizophrenia (Wilson et al., 2022). Lifetime suicide rates are higher in schizophrenia, and neurotransmitter dysfunction is believed to be the reason for psychosis. Treatments with other neurotransmitter dysfunctions, such as depression and anxiety, to control these illnesses are now being researched. For improvement, please consider providing publications focused on the needs of children of parents with mental illness, humanoid hallucination, management of severe public issues, as well as the management of anxiety, ODD, and bipolar disorder.

1.3 Depression in Children: Causes and Symptoms

Children and pre-adolescents also suffer from depression, but signs of these disorders are often not recognized and treated. Some children might be under emotional and psychological strain because of the onset of puberty, changing family or school settings, or the difficulties that relate to starting to become individuals with their responsibilities and concerns. The child suffering from depression assumes the rest of the world feels as she does—unrelieved despair—and further assumes that help and understanding are unattainable (Merrill, 2022). The child's depression demonstrates the importance that early intervention and treatment have for depressive illnesses. It was once thought that children could not suffer from clinical depression. That belief is now known to be wrong. Although adult and child depression alone is not likely to lead to serious acting-out behaviors, if unresolved, the long-term implications are more severe for the child suffering from depression. The pre-adolescent or adolescent struggling with an episode of depression is not seeking attention, nor is they likely to respond to problem-solving advice that might have worked in the past. Mentally ill children—including the child who periodically experience severe emotional disturbances that might include depression or manic-depressive illness—are not likely to seek help. They are, in fact, without the insight and often the encouragement of peers (Richards et al., 2019). Most adolescents in need are not receiving some of the support and encouragement of peers.

1.4 Bipolar Disorder in Childhood

Childhood-onset bipolar disorder (BD) is a severe form of BD, which is usually preceded by depression and often has a chronic course in adulthood. The cardinal symptoms of BD, like mania, hypomania, depression, or irritability, can be observed in childhood as well as in adolescence. Using the same diagnostic criteria for BD in adults for children has been a controversial topic for many years. While many researchers and clinicians believe that applying the adult diagnostic criteria is adequate for the diagnosis of BD in children and adolescents, others are hesitant to do so (Dubey et al., 2021). After an episode of major depressive disorder (MDD) occurs in more than 80% of pediatric BD patients, the average patient goes on to have an estimated nine episodes throughout their lifetime. The average duration of an episode is barely an estimated nine months, and nearly 50% of developing patients with childhood-onset BD will have frequent episodes. Early-onset bipolar disorder is also more predominantly characterized by a continuous presentation; as a result, nearly half of the children's functioning has been rated as “only fair” or “poor” (Ashdown-Franks et al., 2020).

1.5 Signs and Symptoms

The expression of the factors in early childhood behavior and social interactions that are probably characteristics of normal development; the relationship of fearful-anxious behavior in children to later depression; the impact of each identified risk factor on developmental pathways that are relevant to adrenarche changes between puberty and early adulthood; and implications for children with specific disorders seen as related to pathways of increased risk for later severe depression (Duffy et al., 2019). It can be hard for parents to know whether their child may have bipolar disorder or whether recurring mood and behavior changes are due to other childhood or even growth-related issues. Symptoms can resemble and often be misdiagnosed as other conditions. These include attention deficit hyperactivity disorder, oppositional defiant disorder, or conduct disorder. Those conditions are more common than bipolar disorder, and they can also occur along with mood episodes. Therefore, when diagnosing bipolar disorder in a child, it is important to form a broad picture of the child's behavior and recent history (Ashdown-Franks et al., 2020). There are a number of warning signs that may indicate a child is at health risk for bipolar disorder. In most cases, the symptoms in childhood are not the same as those in adults suffering from episodes of mania or depression. Children and young adolescents with bipolar disorder, particularly those without supportive, nurturing, and loving care, go through extremely rapid mood changes within a day. These symptoms are magnified in the presence of sleep problems. As the illness progresses, episodes of mood states may swing back and forth with or without long periods of stability between episodes. Symptoms also vary by the developmental stage (Richards et al., 2019).

2 SCHIZOPHRENIA IN CHILDREN

Schizophrenia is a mental illness characterized by major disturbances in thought, perception, and emotion, as well as paranoia or an exaggerated feeling of self-importance. It is considered an extremely serious illness, and most individuals who develop this disorder suffer silently for a long time. Childhood-onset schizophrenia is distinct from other psychiatric disorders because it is characterized by a sudden onset of symptoms, often including hallucinations, delusions, and severe disturbances in thinking and behavior. Although they may have already had disturbances of some kind and may not have been thought of as a "happy-go-lucky" child, the emergence of the full constellation of psychotic symptoms associated with this disorder is what sets childhood-onset schizophrenia apart from other child psychiatric disorders (Shafik, 2024c). The child's journey to this illness, however, is not different from that of any other psychiatric disorder. The onset of childhood-onset schizophrenia occurs before the age of 13. The symptoms are like those observed in the adult form of the illness, but show some particularities. In children younger than age 6, symptoms may be less obvious and can manifest themselves through two or more of the following: delusions, hallucinations, language disorders, difficulty expressing emotion, and a flat affect that other people notice. Schizophrenia in young children is a very severe disorder. Even as the children grow older, schizophrenia grows with them (Paron, 2024). Unlike other disorders, young children with schizophrenia not only become incapable of functioning at a relatively young age, but their ability to take care of themselves and feed themselves never develops.

2.1 DEFINITION AND CHARACTERISTICS OF SCHIZOPHRENIA

Schizophrenia is a complex disorder involving three main categories of symptoms: the so-called positive symptoms, such as delusions and hallucinations; negative symptoms, such as withdrawal and social isolation; and disturbances of thought, such as illogical thinking or loss of normal thought processes. Schizophrenia is relatively uncommon in childhood, but it probably has the most devastating and long-term effects if it is present in children (Liu, 2024). Because of this, there has been quite a bit of research on the treatment of childhood schizophrenia, and it has also captured much professional attention. Schizophrenia has an estimated prevalence of approximately 1 in 10,000 people, and its onset in children younger than 11 years of age is extremely rare. Several types of schizophrenia have been described, and children are thought to disproportionately fall into a category that is rapid in its onset and either severe or very slow and more insidious as the full illness develops, but it is less disabling than in adults if the child receives the appropriate treatment and services (Simon et al., 2020).

2.2 Prevalence and Incidence

Although there is a great deal of interest in and attention paid to childhood and adolescent anxiety, schizophrenia, depression, and bipolar disorder, the general lack of prevalence and incidence data for these diagnoses is noteworthy. Similarly, though studies to estimate the prevalence rates of psychological disorders in adults utilize a combination of diagnostic assessment interviews, medical claims, medical records, or the reports of healthcare professionals, the few studies that have attempted to estimate the prevalence and incidence rates of anxiety, schizophrenia, depression, and bipolar disorders in children have typically relied exclusively on information provided by only one or a small number of these sources (Gahona-Villegas et al., 2023). The use of parent or self-reports is clearly insufficient to provide accurate incidence and prevalence estimates for many anxiety, schizophrenia, depression, and bipolar disorder diagnoses. Indeed, by failing to capture the physical health service use of children and adolescents provided by family physicians or pediatricians and the mental health service use provided through hospital or clinic contacts, substantial undercounts in the actual prevalence of emotional or behavioral disorders in children and adolescents may result. Regarding the use of diagnostic interviews to assess rates of psychological disorders, several other issues and concerns motivate this review of the epidemiologic evidence on the childhood and adolescent incidence and prevalence of psychological disorders, adult and child depression, and child bipolar disorder, in particular (Davis et al., 2019).

2.3 Causes and Risk Factors

To better understand anxiety, schizophrenia, depression, and bipolar disorder, and to manage them effectively, it is important to examine their underlying causes and the factors that may increase a child's risk of developing one or more of these conditions. When these disorders are not properly recognized and treated, they can lead to significant emotional distress and long-term impairment in a child's functioning and quality of life. Understanding how these conditions arise or are exacerbated can help primary care providers and youth-serving professionals work with children, their families, and educators to provide the support, resources, and services they may require (Shahid et al., 2021). Research has not identified a single cause for anxiety, schizophrenia, depression, or bipolar disorder. Each of these disorders likely arises from a mix of genetic, biological, psychological, and environmental factors. Although the origins of these conditions can be complex and difficult to tease apart, the search for these origins can also provide critical insights when prevention, detection, or treatment is concerned. Such research is powered by findings drawn from studies interested in risk and protective factors for these conditions. Such studies identify characteristics that tend to differentiate children with these conditions from children who do not yet have them (Hannaway, 2024). This can help provide important keys to effective prevention and treatment.

2.4 Symptoms and Diagnostic Criteria

Anxiety in children may be associated with excessive fear, excessive worrying, or fear in response to a traumatic event. The child may assume life experiences will turn out badly and may feel helpless, panicked, or out of control. Physical symptoms may include a pounding heart, sweating, a knotted stomach, rapid or shallow breathing, or headaches. A child may refuse to eat or sleep and experience nightmares, bedwetting, screaming, or other symptoms of distress. The child may also become tense, irritable, demanding, or have temper tantrums and freeze or become clumsy (Zhang & Liu, 2023). Performance or productivity may suffer. A diagnosis of anxiety is made when the child finds it hard to control the worry or fear and when the symptoms interfere with the boy's or girl's functioning at school, home, or with friends. Sometimes, it is also important to know if a past or current traumatic event has harmed the child. Symptoms must last at least six months. If the symptoms last fewer than six months, the diagnosis is made that the child has "not otherwise specified anxiety disorder." In this case, the symptoms may be fairly severe. It is important to know that anxiety is common in children, who may once or twice refuse to go to school or have symptoms similar to stomach flu, but false alarms are not the fault of the child, and treatment should be sought, especially when dangerous activities are contemplated (Madej, 2024).

2.5 Treatment Approaches

There are currently a variety of common treatments for anxiety in children and adolescents, including psychological treatments, psychopharmacological agents, structured school programs, and individualized behavior plans. Psychological treatments include cognitive-behavioral therapies, exposure therapies, play therapy, and family or parent involvement. Social skills training and applied relaxation therapies that teach children to relax during fearful situations have both demonstrated reductions in anxiety. In addition to affective disorders such as GAD and depression, anxiety or somatic disorders are frequent coexisting conditions in comorbid clinical populations (Saliba et al., 2023). Panic disorder is treated similarly to anxiety disorders. Agoraphobia is also treated with exposure and social skills training while continuing school. Medications that are commonly effective during the initial stages of treatment include beta-blockers, selective serotonin reuptake inhibitors (SSRIs), and benzodiazepines. Desensitization is an exposure-based treatment often used in treating school phobia. Treatment should be kept at a pace that the child is comfortable with and should begin by addressing school skills at home. School visits are best not to make until the child is comfortable with traveling around the block. Cognitive-behavioral therapy is not recommended until the child is comfortable being in their school or on their bus. Approximate returns to school are made unless the child has experienced a precipitous event, such as a parental or peer death or standing up to the bully (Morris, 2014). Then, cognitive-behavioral therapy for panic attacks is appropriate.

3 ASSESSMENT AND DIAGNOSIS OF MENTAL HEALTH DISORDERS IN CHILDREN

Assessment is a general term that refers to the entire process through which knowledge is obtained regarding a child's emotional or mental health. A diagnosis is a specific classification based on this knowledge. Diagnoses are generally organized into taxonomies or classifications. These are schemes that group diagnoses into categories according to common characteristics. The best-known diagnostic taxonomies in the mental health field are the DSM and the ICD (Jung et al., 2021). The DSM is the most commonly used diagnostic system by mental health professionals in the United States. When properly conducted, the assessment should systematically evaluate all potential causes leading to a child's difficulties. The mental health professional's final diagnosis should include all conditions that apply, distinguishing primary from secondary conditions. Primary conditions are the child's most central or immediate concerns. These generally cause the greatest distress and impairment and are most in need of treatment. Secondary conditions are other significant concerns that may influence or maintain the primary conditions. These may need to be addressed as well. Proper assessment results in symptoms being properly classified and organized and thus effectively addressed. For example, a child who is persistently moody, irritable, prone to excessive worrying or fears, easily upset, and often found in a weepy state may meet the diagnostic criteria for an anxiety disorder (Stein et al., 2024). However, the child's problems might actually be secondary to an unrecognized or previously treated mood disorder such as depression, with anxiety serving only as a symptom of the depression. In this case, the child might be unnecessarily treated for the anxiety with coping and relaxation skills only. The child's underlying depression is missed, and the child remains untreated for the correct disorder, which, if treated, might relieve all other concerns. Conversely, the recognition that the child is primarily depressed would focus treatment away from anxiety coping strategies to properly address the root disorder of the child's symptoms of both mood and anxiety (Ng et al., 2024). Once symptoms and behaviors are observed in children, they should be assessed and diagnosed. Early recognition and treatment of mental health problems usually make the problems more manageable, reduce their intensity and duration, and diminish their interference with the child's development. Parents, caregivers, other professional staff, and the child should contribute to an accurate diagnosis. Evaluation by professionals typically includes the following components: parental interview, child observation, child interview, psychological testing, neurological examination, and laboratory tests. For reliable and valid results, psychologists need information from multiple sources (Opie et al., 2024). Examples include teachers, peers, other family members, and significant others in the child's life. If the child is very young, the psychologist may need to observe the child while engaged in different tasks, as they may not be capable of expressing how they feel. If the child is school-age or older, they usually will be interviewed. Although the psychologist will spend the greatest amount of time with the parent or primary caregivers, the child will also probably be seen at least once to provide impressions about behavior and to give input about feelings and the current situation. After diagnostic assessment, and in conjunction with the child and caregivers, the professional develops a treatment plan, which should be tailored to the individual and should consider specific needs and preferences (Gurtner et al., 2022; Ng et al., 2024; Stein et al., 2024).

3.1 Screening Tools and Techniques

Pediatricians have many screening tools available to them that can be used at different stages of child development infant, child, and adolescent—to screen for risks of mental illness within the developmental context. These tools can be helpful for identifying potential concerns before they become significant problems, leading to better care for children and their families during the early stages of mental illness. By understanding the symptoms found within various mental illnesses and knowing the specific signs and symptoms to look for in different developmental stages, pediatricians can help keep risk in perspective (Merrill, 2022). In addition, by understanding when, how, and with whom to use these tools, pediatricians can help prevent the one-size-fits-all mentality from being applied to childhood development. Each child brings a variety of assets and liabilities to the developmental stage. The capacity of a child's environment to support their emotional and physical well-being is a major factor in how a diagnosis will progress over time (Richards et al., 2019). This pediatric emphasis on both the individual and their environment sets up a positive model for preventive care throughout a lifetime, regardless of illness.

3.2 Diagnostic Criteria and Assessment Procedures

Before determining whether or not a child meets the criteria for a disorder, the clinician must become familiar with the clinical description of the disorder. However, because children are still growing up, many of the symptoms that are listed in the criteria for adult disorders do not apply to children. A separate set of diagnostic criteria has, therefore, been developed. Once a clear definition of a disorder is in place, the next step in assessment is identification. Quantitative methods of assessment begin with collecting information, usually in the form of self-reports, reports from parents, and observations (Dubey et al., 2021). Commonly prescribed interviews are used. Classrooms and summer camps may also be considered suitable reference groups for children and adolescents, provided the prevalence of psychiatric disorders is not known to differ from that in the general community or the clinicians have sufficient knowledge of the properties of the scales they are using. Cognitive assessment is often an important part of the assessment for anxiety, schizophrenia, depression, and bipolar disorder (Merrill, 2022).

However, because children with depressive and hypomanic disorders may be at increased risk for school-based problems, such as peer rejection and academic difficulties, assessment instruments should identify individuals with these comorbid conditions, preferably in a reliable manner. To assess medication management or psychosocial treatment response, self-report measures of symptoms, disability, or mood state are essential. Two commonly used rating scales contain overlapping symptoms. According to a child behavior checklist, four syndromes are likely to contain subscales that assess mood: anxious/depressed, withdrawn, somatic complaints, and thought problems; moreover, the dimensions of externalizing and cognitive problems are likely to contain elements that assess impulsivity and inappropriate behavior (Duffy et al., 2019). At the same time, the prospective assessment of suicidal thoughts or acts is one of the most important responsibilities of the clinician. In the depression literature, there is no consistent agreement on what specifically is being measured by the self-reports and informant reports for young children. Self-report instruments may be used as a tool to aid in data-gathering when working with children. There are no specific neuropsychological tests available that do not contain confounding factors that also occur in other endogenous disorders when evaluating a suspected child with depression (Hofmann et al., 2012).

4 EVIDENCE-BASED TREATMENTS FOR CHILDHOOD MENTAL HEALTH DISORDERS

The development of effective treatments for mental health disorders is not a recent phenomenon. Decades of research have begun to uncover the specific characteristics of several disorders, including anxiety, depression, and conduct disorder. Through this body of work, many treatments have been developed and tested. This constitutes the standard of care for treating youth with mental health concerns (Shafik, 2024a). These evidence-based treatments should be made widely available to all youth. Unfortunately, many do not receive these effective treatments. In many communities, over two-thirds of children with mental health disorders remain untreated. Common reasons are a lack of knowledge about effective treatments by educators and parents and limited professionals to conduct treatments. To facilitate access, evidence-based treatments can be disseminated through various implementation strategies (Merrill, 2022).

One treatment that has been developed and tested over the past fifty years is family-based exposure therapy for treating anxiety. Exposure therapy is effective across a range of anxiety-related problems and is currently the gold standard when treating childhood anxiety disorders. Additional treatments demonstrating strong empirical support are sertraline and fluoxetine. These are especially effective for children of preschool age diagnosed with social phobia (Chung & Teo, 2022). The availability of proven treatments and the fact that childhood anxiety often predicts mood and substance abuse disorders in adulthood suggests that all clinicians evaluate for anxiety disorders when assessing youth with emotional and behavioral problems. Moreover, ever-increasing prevention interventions are being developed and tested for youth at risk for sudden anxiety disorders. Two interventional strategies come in the form of cognitive-behavioral therapy and the family check-up program. The development of effective treatments for mental health disorders will take a coordinated effort by government, research, philanthropy, and providers. However, prevention and early intervention hold the greatest hope for reducing the enormous burden of illness among children (Bozzatello et al., 2021).

4.1 Cognitive-Behavioral Therapy (CBT)

The efficacy of CBT in treating symptoms associated with anxiety and mood disorders has been demonstrated in many studies. There are primarily three types of CBT aimed at reducing anxiety symptoms: 1) psychoeducation, which empowers families by providing information and teaching them concrete strategies for dealing with anxiety that their child may exhibit; 2) cognitive therapy, which focuses on helping children change their maladaptive beliefs, distorted thoughts, and perceived threats; and 3) exposure/response prevention, in which children learn the techniques for increasing tolerance of anxiety by repeatedly exposing them to thoughts, situations, and other stimuli that cause fear or anxiety (Wilson et al., 2022). In a pilot group CBT trial for children aged eight to twelve with bipolar disorder, various assessment scales decreased significantly over nine months, and the improvement scale improved for a significant percentage of subjects. In a large open trial of anxious youth, overall response rates were high for primary anxiety disorders, and a majority had at least some response to treatment (Bostock et al., 2017). The majority had experienced anxiety disorders for an average of 57 months or more.

4.2 Pharmacological Interventions

Research studies are finding that children respond to psychoactive medications in the same way as adults and are similarly susceptible to their side effects. The medications that are effective with adults are generally similar for children. These include tricyclic antidepressants, selective serotonin reuptake inhibitors for depression, benzodiazepines for panic attacks and generalized anxiety, lithium for mania, and beta-blockers for aggression and akathisia. Unlike adults, the routine use of antipsychotics is avoided because of their numerous severe side effects (Duffy et al., 2019). Overall, about half of children with anxiety or depression respond reasonably well to an adequate trial of an SSRI. For those children who do not, the typical response is little to no improvement. Various individual cases of schizoaffective episodes resembling those seen in adults often respond to lithium salts already in use; moreover, in clinical practice, lithium is often used in situations in which boys have been initially overtreated with neuroleptics by psychiatrists unfamiliar with the very rare onset of mania in adolescence. When psychopharmacological treatments with children are introduced in combination with their families and the rapid dissemination of information on its general and specific effects, the children often respond better and provide quicker recovery than they do without such combinations of treatments (Dubey et al., 2021).

4.3 Family-Based Interventions

Treatments that are based within a family context are effective in addressing various behavioral, emotional, and social issues with children and are tools that are currently underutilized by parents. Yet, examples are available. Communication skills, conflict resolution skills, problem-solving skills, anger management skills, and coping skills (to name a few) are areas of intervention. All of these can be seen as skills to be identified, cultivated, and encouraged by the parents, who can act as 'behavior managers', 'social skills trainers', and 'emotional coaches' for their children

(Schneider et al., 2023). With the help of friends, family, mental health professionals, schools, and communities, parents can be even more effective. The present chapter outlines, discusses, or suggests family-based interventions for depression, mania, schizophrenia, generalized anxiety, specific anxiety, social anxiety, school anxiety, performance anxiety, separation anxiety, and associated features in development (Bozzatello et al., 2021).

Consideration of the family in assessing and treating the disorders of the child and youth can serve to counterbalance the prevailing tendency toward individualist methodology in the field. It should be recognized that identifying behaviors and thoughts that modify symptoms and identifying nonmodifiable features are always key tasks. The presence of symptoms in a child can change the entire family environment and require attention to various family factors (Wan et al., 2023). The challenge for clinicians and researchers is to recognize and validate family problems and to provide parents, children, and siblings with the attention and interventions appropriate for these concerns. This approach is consistent with the policy of educating parents to manage their children effectively and with the movement toward multimodal treatments. Those who work with the family will typically start their intervention planning with a question such as, "What caused the problem or issue?" Family-based approaches are allowing for a more comprehensive understanding of mental illness and are becoming increasingly important in child and family interventions (Chung & Teo, 2022).

5 PREVENTIVE STRATEGIES AND EARLY INTERVENTION

Preventive strategies promote good sleep, exercise, diet, and positive behaviors. Early intervention is also critical. There are interventions that can help parents and children reduce risk by changing negative thinking. Challenge negative thinking – look for evidence and find alternative views. Halt that thought – if it's not helpful or true, stop, stamp, and swap it for a better thought. Tell yourself a good thought. React differently – stay calm and relax or make a plan and do something brave and smart (Ashdown-Franks et al., 2020)! Patterns of activity using cognitive behavioral therapy can help reduce trauma for children in high-risk family environments by introducing trauma-focused approaches and by helping parents add skills to cope with stress and family demands, such as good communication and parenting, and time for themselves. The aim is to encourage positive family togetherness rather than over-perfection, over-scheduling, rigidity, and criticism that contribute to the development of anxiety in children. Such programs provide the chance for parents to develop new skills for managing concerns and for children to learn tools and approaches for managing stress or worry when they experience it (Schneider et al.,

2023). In this way, programs help reduce the risk of anxiety and related symptoms and patterns from becoming a problem for kids and increase the possibility of happy, balanced, and satisfying family lives.

5.1 Promoting Resilience in Children

We have identified a number of strategies for promoting resilience in children. As well as addressing factors such as abuse and neglect, the provision of opportunities for children to develop social relationships and enhance their self-esteem is important. Parents also need to be encouraged to implement such social interventions. The fact that some interventions are willingly implemented even when there is a waiting list for other highly desirable treatments, with the outcome of beneficial effects on children, emphasizes the potential value of these procedures (Bozzatello et al., 2021)social factors have been shown to be protective: multiple support systems for children who face difficulties, effective schools that can have powerful effects as protective factors, low alienation from the school, a high sense of connectedness, and an effective community providing protective resources and opportunities such as recreational facilities. Thus, it is clear that some psychiatric disorders can be prevented or reduced by simple measures, promoting optimal development through infancy, utilizing the existing strength of families to keep children from falling through the growing cracks in the social safety network, and promoting personal and social competencies in children. The data indicate that this approach works, even with high-risk groups (Deng & He, 2023). To help children cope and succeed, it makes a great deal of sense to stop dithering and start doing.

5.2 School-Based Mental Health Programs

There are some sampled instances of school-based mental health programs, as briefly presented.

5.2.1 Referral Services

Awareness must also be developed about the availability of mental health services within the community. Cost, transportation, and access can be obstacles to accessing available services. Developing referral services for the school or neighborhood and cost-effective opening of mental health clinics or centers would be beneficial.

5.2.2 Health Educators as Liaisons

Health educators in the school setting can be used to stimulate program planning and execution. They can function as liaisons between the school system and health and social agencies within the community. Health educators can aid in curriculum-based mental health programs. Prevention activities by health educators will reduce the service costs of the community in dealing with larger mental health problems (Merrill, 2022).

5.2.3 Developing Student-Awareness Programs

When developing prevention programs, student feedback can be invaluable. By integrating individual problems or areas of concern, as indicated by the student body, into the curriculum, related knowledge and coping skills can be developed. Although it is not a formal part of the school service system, self-referral or peer referral procedures should be an option for children. A school counselor or mental health professional may be employed to conduct informational meetings, discussions, or speaking engagements based on the individual needs of children (Richards et al., 2019).

6 SPECIAL CONSIDERATIONS IN TREATMENT AND MANAGEMENT

This article has reviewed four major types of severe emotional and behavioral disorders: anxiety, schizophrenia, depression, and bipolar disorder in children. We have presented a framework to assist clinicians in conceptualizing and, we hope, resolving the considerable challenge that these disorders pose. Clearly, most general pediatric clinicians are not prepared to manage these children and their families. They require a context of cooperation and consultation with mental health professionals (Dubey et al., 2021). Therefore, any strategies that facilitate giving these children fundamental respect and helping and supporting their families in what may be a long and difficult set of steps deserve full exploration and fruition.

Suppose the general pediatric clinician is going to be asked to recognize children who are vulnerable to such severe mental health disorders as prepsychotic children or anxious and depressed children, as well as facilitate the ongoing care of these children and their families. In that case, some focus on providing context-adapted services for these young people is called for. There are special considerations to keep in mind. And they are not quite just about the children either (Richards et al., 2019). Rather, the focus needs to be wider: the child in their family and clinical context.

6.1 Comorbidity and Dual Diagnosis

Comorbidity and dual diagnosis refer to individuals who experience more than one type of psychological disturbance at the same time. A classic example of this concern is children who experience both anxiety and depression simultaneously. Individuals with comorbid disorders are often at considerably higher risk for more negative outcomes than individuals diagnosed with just a single disorder. Depression is often a part of many childhood disorders. Since individuals with depression often talk about such symptoms as saying they are no good, sad, or anxious, it is not earth-shattering to realize that anxiety is another aspect of depression (Chung & Teo, 2022). Just because these symptoms are present, this does not mean that your child actually has a diagnosis of depression. To fit this category, your child would also have to experience a loss of interest or pleasure in things they are usually interested in. Some complex comorbidity implies children who have some form of altered sensory processing, attention disorders, and anxiety. From time to time, children present a pattern of very intense and agitated symptoms of Attention deficit hyperactivity disorder (ADHD), anxiety, motor tics, and a vocal tic. Researchers are now looking for a possible link between physical and neurological imbalances in the brain and the sudden onset of obsessive-compulsive disorder and tic symptoms (Wilson et al., 2022). Children of this nature do not fit a traditional diagnosis easily. Other forms of comorbidity include the relationship of germ phobia, an obsessive-compulsive disorder in which the person has to perform hand washing rituals before each meal to avoid unpleasant consequences, anxiety, anorexia, or the relation between depression and panic disorder. An interesting duplication of symptoms occurs in children with both Tourette's syndrome and obsessive-compulsive disorder (Akaishi et al., 2023). These children have been shown to have deficits in information processing that are limited to selecting and focusing on relevant stimuli.

6.2 Cultural and Societal Factors

Among the several factors, this section presents some cultural and social concerns as presented below.

6.2.1 Stigmatization

Families also face much of the stigmatization faced by adults with mental illness with children who have a mental illness. Feelings of fear, anger, and misunderstanding prevail when adults and children meet and look different from the rest of society. Mental illness in children causes stress from reduced income due to parental absence from work, the financial burden of medical bills, and costly social services. Although the child's behavior is the effect, the parent often feels blamed, thereby increasing feelings of guilt, shame, and the need for avoidance (Ashdown-Franks et al., 2020).

6.2.2 Ethnic Factors

While sharing the same symptoms as the general population, ethnic children with severe emotional disturbances are less likely to receive care than white children. With helpless available for ethnic children, their problems are likely to get worse before treatment is received. The longstanding interest in healing and compassion for those who sense disparagement has undoubtedly shaped the psychiatric service system's approach to people with emotional disturbances (Chung & Teo, 2022). On the other hand, ethnic cultures may view emotional disturbances as signs of divine possession, which can be cured through exorcism. Many cultures isolate family members with extreme emotional conduct to avoid exposure to shame and to protect the sick from evil spirits. In the case of Mexican culture, however, the reverse is true, and psychiatric care may be criticized as overly alienating and scientific. There is also discrimination within a number of diverse ethnic and cultural groups (Schneider et al., 2023). Dominant white individuals tend to receive superior mental health services over minorities.

6.2.3 Societal Factors

The familial and social structure and culture of society also affect the treatment plan, contributing to the emotional disturbances of a child as well as to the recovery of the child and, eventually, the adult. Three of the most significant sociocultural groups characteristically face issues in the mental health treatment of their children: social classes, those from lower-income families, and citizens who are causal reasons for mental health being subcultural. Major disparity identifies the mentally ill who are institutionalized. Many people in our society believe that the mentally ill belong in institutions. Their appearances frighten people, beliefs about mental illness frighten people, and the notion of suffering through care frightens people. Many people do not want to do more than their fair share, so they vote to spend as little of their money as possible (Deng & He, 2023). Fear also drives law-abiding citizens to resist educating their children in institutions rumored to care for the unruly and potentially violent. Finally, the realization that other people in institutions constitute the group of our society that is most at risk generates fear and resistance to change.

7 SUPPORTING PARENTS AND CAREGIVERS

Parents and caregivers serve as the front-line advocates for the mental health needs of their children. However, when this responsibility is combined with managing their children's emotional and behavioral difficulties, parenting can be overwhelming, exhausting, and demoralizing. This situation may be especially true for caregivers of children with serious emotional disturbances such as anxiety disorders, mood disorders, and psychotic disorders (Chung & Teo, 2022). As a result, it is easy to understand why parental stress and depression are serious risks for the parents of these children and that the risk is even greater for families living in poverty or where multiple stressors, such as residing in an unsafe neighborhood or having an unsupportive or overtaxed social network are present. Consequently, clinicians who work with these children need to have a good working knowledge of the family-based interventions that have been developed to promote positive mental health within these families (Duffy et al., 2019). These programs have developed resource materials, provided training for other organizations in adaptations, and initiated several support groups. Materials include manuals for parent empowerment and disaster preparation activity workbooks for children and families. Leaders have been invited to speak at local, state, and national conferences, organizational meetings, focus groups, and other forums to promote the concept of supporting family members involved in the advocacy for mental healthcare services (Merrill, 2022).

7.1 Parental Education and Training Programs

Parents of children who have anxiety disorders and social anxiety disorder often have trouble understanding their child's symptoms. When parents do understand their child's symptoms, they may respond in a way that inadvertently reinforces the child's worry symptoms or prevents the child from learning to cope. Thus, parents need to learn important principles about anxiety and its treatment, including knowing when and how to help the child practice facing different anxiety-provoking situations and challenging negative automatic thoughts (Akaishi et al., 2023). Unfortunately, no well-designed, large-scale studies have yet been conducted on the efficacy of a brief parental education program to help children with anxiety or their parents. Thus, the majority of literature is based on the content and importance of parental education rather than the benefits of specific programs. In the Youth FAST, the parent group incorporates information on learning to detect and challenge children's avoidant thinking, assisting children with developing problem-solving skills and developing self-efficacy through reinforcement, modeling, and appropriate support. Noting the potential benefits of teaching fathers of anxious children, a video was also developed aimed at providing fathers with an easy-to-use, self-paced, structured format for acquiring basic skills in positive parenting techniques (Ashdown-Franks et al., 2020).

7.2 Community Resources and Support Groups

Parents can often benefit from talking with other people who have had similar experiences. Many communities have parent support groups that provide support, education, and advocacy for people and families dealing with serious mental illness. Local telephone books or other parents likely will have information about the various support groups in the area. In addition to parent support groups, many communities have groups for ill children and adolescents. Ask doctors, therapists, or psychologists where to find these groups. Many mental health practitioners can tell parents what is being offered in the community and suggest therapists or other professionals who may be able to help (Akaishi et al., 2023). To locate mental health professionals in the community, contact the mental health association, the hospital outpatient department, university medical school departments, and other parents who have children with emotional disorders. Universities often have grant programs, and many students are being trained to work with children and adolescents with serious emotional disorders. Religious leaders, pediatricians, and family practice physicians can be helpful, as well as child advocacy organizations, therapy programs, respite care services, and the local school. These are often excellent resources for parents who are just learning about the various treatment options available in the community (Richards et al., 2019).

8 LEGAL AND ETHICAL ISSUES IN CHILDHOOD MENTAL HEALTH CARE

A compelling legal and ethical question revolves around the ability of parents to refuse treatment for their mentally ill children. In most situations, parents have the authority and the responsibility to decide whether their children should receive medical care, including care for mental illnesses. The decisions of the parents are binding unless the state intervenes on behalf of the best interest of the child. In life-threatening emergencies, physicians may need to act without consent or consultation to avert severe harm. Potential solutions are not simple. Parents certainly have a responsibility for their children's distress (Wan et al., 2023). However, parents cannot be expected to accept every physician's recommendation at face value, nor can parents be expected to have an in-depth understanding of the risks, benefits, and alternatives of a particular treatment or calculation of proportionality of drug benefit against long-term side effects or cost. The denial of medical treatment must be based on a thorough understanding of the therapeutic options, the potential effects of the illness on the child's education, peer relationships, family dynamics, and broader family well-being and functioning, as well as other potential implications for life adaptation and adjustment (Ashdown-Franks et al., 2020). In addition, the consequences of the care, or lack thereof, for expensive public, child welfare, and mental health systems must also be considered.

8.1 Confidentiality and Informed Consent

Many of the ethical issues in child psychotherapy parallel issues that arise in working with adults, such as privacy, confidentiality, and rules about informed consent. However, working with relatives and teachers, consent laws, the duty to protect, and the client's developmental capacity greatly affect how psychotherapists handle ethical dilemmas with children, adolescents, and their families. Psychotherapists confront considerable struggles involving the expression of trust and behavior among all parties in treatment. Furthermore, psychotherapists managing the care of minors require well-constructed policies, procedures, and clinical standards for the recognition and release of confidential data (Dubey et al., 2021; Shafik, 2024b). Developing a clinically high-quality, ethically sound relationship with a child or adolescent often requires a container of trust, which means always respecting the child's or adolescent's confidential information unless it is necessary and beneficial to reveal that person's confidences to the parents and ensure that doing so is not harmful to the client. The trust container should encompass a child's or adolescent's conversations that portray a mature sophistication in identifying and addressing their difficulties. A seemingly involuntary challenge of the therapist is always legitimate, complex, and often frightening as an unanticipated consequence of the trust that the child has sparked and may subsume (Shafik et al., 2024). This involves the therapist skillfully managing the therapeutic alliance with the chronologically young child while still providing care that allows for the preservation of the adolescent's welfare.

8.2 Child Advocacy and Rights

Although we are all in favor of protecting the rights of children, provisions for child advocacy and rights also contain the seeds for considerable confusion and disarray. In general, legal child advocates claim the power of providing legal counsel to children outside of family influence, for the purpose either of representing the child in family matters or of assisting such cases to be brought on the child's behalf. At the same time, many professional advocates for children function in a legislative or advisory capacity, where they may offer expert insights about specific issues (Sharma et al., 2021). Schools, as well as the child's peer group, may provide important resources for advocacy, in some cases representing children in an educational system that frequently has its own identity and autonomy separate from that of the family. Limited child advocates may be attributed to other professions that come into contact with children, such as lawyers, probation officers, and social workers. Also, certified pediatric or child psychiatrists may claim the role of being child advocates, but their primary responsibilities are to the adults in the case. The adult professions may not allow special problems that are attendant in play or to the premises of child advocacy, such as privacy in the doctor-patient relationship, enforceable confidentiality on the part of the child, and clearly defined responsibility for offsetting the vulnerability of children (Schneider et al., 2023).

9 FUTURE DIRECTIONS IN RESEARCH AND PRACTICE

Progress, while significant in a number of areas, is slow in the scientific inquiry into the understanding and management of anxiety, schizophrenia, depression, and bipolar disorder in infants, children, and adolescents. Research in such areas as genetics, gender-based development, cross-cultural dimensions at the time of onset, specific biomarkers, precise brain identity for the onset of pediatric psychiatric disease, and identification of environmental, temperament, and contextual triggering factors has been delayed or less systematically examined. Longitudinal studies, some initiated in childhood or adolescence with follow-up into midlife, the most common timing of onset of schizophrenia, produce unique datasets with unparalleled potential for studies of the pathogenesis of psychiatric disorders (Wan et al., 2023). In summary, the overlap of psychiatric symptoms in these childhood-onset disorders, the natural history of these disorders, their transitory instability, and similarities by gender and symptoms raise the question of whether the disorder is, in fact, one or multiple disorders, the sensory and response capacities of very young children to assess and respond to treatment, the significant issues of long-term medication exposure in young age groups, and the common variability we see during typical and atypical development, suggest a significant research effort to define these important childhood-onset disorders more clearly (Akaishi et al., 2023).

9.1 Innovations in Pediatric Mental Health Care

Though parenting is hard, it does not have to be needlessly harrowing when a child has a mental disorder. Research in the early detection and treatment of emotional and behavioral disorders has advanced rapidly in the past several years, especially in the area of emotional disorders such as anxiety and depression. These advances demonstrate the viability of involving pediatric primary care practitioners, school personnel, and mental health workers in making use of this new knowledge, helping create a comprehensive community-based system of mental health care with the least stigma possible (Hofmann et al., 2012). Such a public health approach to mental health should be able to diagnose and contain children's mental disorders early on, limiting the disadvantage these disorders place on individuals and reducing the ripple effect of suffering they create in the families, schools, and communities where children live (Shafik, 2024e). Imagine a place where pediatric citizens combine a healthful immunity to stress with a considerable capacity for trust and affection, resilience in the face of the unknown, hope in the coping capacity of themselves and others, and a creative sense of what it means to be alive. In homes, schools, neighborhoods, and playgrounds everywhere, adults guide the children with a savvy blend of realism, flexibility, and, most of all, love. Developmental tasks are met with reasonable success and humor (Richards et al., 2019). These children neither dissolve under pressure easily nor unravel permanently. All children have their sad times, their apprehensions, and their irrational moments, but these children tolerate the slings and arrows of childhood with a measure of grace. What is this place? It is a community dedicated to understanding the nature of mental health, just as we now understand the nature of physical health. All adults and institutions that touch the lives of these children know how to replenish these mental health resources with care. Integrated strategies thrive in this community even for children who are ill; they, too, can recover their balance (Merrill, 2022). Preventive efforts constantly renew the productive health of young minds.

9.2 Emerging Therapeutic Approaches

A number of new approaches for addressing pediatric mental illness are currently under development. These include sleep therapies for depression, wellness programs to prevent pediatric bipolar disorder and depression, and school-based cognitive-behavioral trauma therapy. Also being studied are the effects of antidepressants, schizophrenia, sleep function, and new treatments to restore sleep in bipolar illness. One of the most exciting new advances is the recent dramatic increase in the early detection and prevention of major psychiatric illnesses (Schneider et al., 2023). Adolescent and Child Bipolar Services is embarking on a community-based prevention research project for adolescents at very high risk for developing bipolar illness because of family history. Just as the willingness to include young children in treatment research with an eye toward prevention and early intervention marks a significant pivot point in our development as a society, there are many more innovative treatments on the horizon, reaching toward a brighter and healthier future for our children. The upcoming years will see the reorganization and reshaping of services to both adults and children based on a dramatically improved understanding of disease processes, plus the development of a range of novel therapies (Bozzatello et al., 2021).

10 CONCLUSION

Recognizing that cultural and societal factors need to be considered in understanding and addressing the emotional problems of young people is important. All societies have experienced children displaying early symptoms of the mental disorders discussed. Within specific contexts, early symptoms are understood and tolerated, while later symptoms may or may not be. Commonly, the biomedical model of mental disorders is supported by an apparent progression of symptoms toward poor function. Culture, society, language, and genetic makeup interact to form sets of beliefs about the significance of unusual emotional and behavioral symptoms, in turn shaping the expectations communicated to young people about behaviors that may only sometimes fit scientific definitions of mental disorders. These expectations shape the emotional experiences and self-concepts of those affected. The idea that mental health conditions in children will get worse if they aren't treated is just one reason why it's important for parents to recognize mental health concerns in their children and to engage with healthcare professionals to ensure their children's mental health is being taken care of. Parents are the best advocates their children have, and they must communicate openly and freely with their children. Children with better mental health will grow into adults with better mental health. While not every case of anxiety, depression, or conduct problems goes away without treatment, many interventions help children get better. Evaluating all four of the children and adolescents in your life requires observing how they function in different settings with different people at different points throughout the day. Finally, there are things that all of us can do to foster resilience and protect children from the problems that lead to poor mental health. Children with good mental health don't just appear out of nowhere – they have people looking after them who take the time and trouble to help them.

REFERENCES

Abubakari, M. S. (2021). The Internet of Things (IoT) as an Emerging Technological Solution for the Covid-19 Pandemic Mitigation: An Overview. In M. Khairudin, R. Asnawi, I. W. Djatmiko, P. Sudira, S. Hadi, & F. Arifin (Eds.), *Journal of Physics: Conference Series* (Vol. 1737, Issue 1). IOP Publishing Ltd. DOI: 10.1088/1742-6596/1737/1/012003

Akaishi, T., Tarasawa, K., Fushimi, K., Hamada, H., Saito, M., Kobayashi, N., Kikuchi, S., Tomita, H., Ishii, T., Fujimori, K., & Yaegashi, N. (2023). Risk Factors Associated with Peripartum Suicide Attempts in Japan. *JAMA Network Open*, *6*(1), e2250661. Advance online publication. DOI: 10.1001/jamanetworkopen.2022.50661 PMID: 36633845

Ashdown-Franks, G., Firth, J., Carney, R., Carvalho, A. F., Hallgren, M., Koyanagi, A., Rosenbaum, S., Schuch, F. B., Smith, L., Solmi, M., Vancampfort, D., & Stubbs, B. (2020). Exercise as Medicine for Mental and Substance Use Disorders: A Meta-review of the Benefits for Neuropsychiatric and Cognitive Outcomes. In *Sports Medicine* (Vol. 50, Issue 1). DOI: 10.1007/s40279-019-01187-6

Bostock, E. C. S., Kirkby, K. C., & Taylor, B. V. M. (2017). The current status of the ketogenic diet in psychiatry. In *Frontiers in Psychiatry* (Vol. 8). Issue MAR., DOI: 10.3389/fpsyt.2017.00043

Bozzatello, P., Blua, C., Rocca, P., & Bellino, S. (2021). Mental health in childhood and adolescence: The role of polyunsaturated fatty acids. *Biomedicines*, *9*(8), 850. Advance online publication. DOI: 10.3390/biomedicines9080850 PMID: 34440053

Chung, J., & Teo, J. (2022). Mental Health Prediction Using Machine Learning: Taxonomy, Applications, and Challenges. In *Applied Computational Intelligence and Soft Computing* (Vol. 2022). DOI: 10.1155/2022/9970363

Davis, N., Harris, L., & Cunningham, U. (2019). Professional ecologies shaping technology adoption in early childhood education with multilingual children. *British Journal of Educational Technology*, *50*(3), 1320–1339. Advance online publication. DOI: 10.1111/bjet.12774

Deng, Y., & He, J. (2023). A Comparison between before and during the Pandemic in Nonsuicidal Self-Injury Behaviors of Bipolar Disorder. *The Journal of Nervous and Mental Disease*, *211*(12), 896–901. Advance online publication. DOI: 10.1097/NMD.0000000000001572 PMID: 36044661

Dubey, P., Thakur, B., Rodriguez, S., Cox, J., Sanchez, S., Fonseca, A., Reddy, S., Clegg, D., & Dwivedi, A. K. (2021). A systematic review and meta-analysis of the association between maternal polycystic ovary syndrome and neuropsychiatric disorders in children. In *Translational Psychiatry* (Vol. 11, Issue 1). DOI: 10.1038/s41398-021-01699-8

Duffy, A., Goodday, S., Keown-Stoneman, C., & Grof, P. (2019). The emergent course of bipolar disorder: Observations over two decades from the Canadian high-risk offspring cohort. *The American Journal of Psychiatry*, *176*(9), 720–729. Advance online publication. DOI: 10.1176/appi.ajp.2018.18040461 PMID: 30525908

Gahona-Villegas, J. R., Reyes-Jurado, P., & Ríos-Méndez, R. E. (2023). Renovascular arterial hypertension in children. Three case report. *Acta Pediátrica de México*, *44*(3). Advance online publication. DOI: 10.18233/apm.v44i3.2264

Gurtner, M., Smith, M., Gage, R., Howey-Brown, A., Wang, X., Latavao, T., Deng, J. D., Zwanenburg, S. P., Stanley, J., & Signal, L. (2022). Objective Assessment of the Nature and Extent of Children's Internet-Based World: Protocol for the Kids Online Aotearoa Study. *JMIR Research Protocols*, *11*(10), e39017. Advance online publication. DOI: 10.2196/39017 PMID: 36129809

Hannaway, D. (2024). Digital learning in childhood: Possibilities for pedagogical transformation in South Africa. *South African Journal of Childhood Education*, *14*(1). Advance online publication. DOI: 10.4102/sajce.v14i1.1422

Hofmann, S. G., Asnaani, A., Vonk, I. J. J., Sawyer, A. T., & Fang, A. (2012). The efficacy of cognitive behavioral therapy: A review of meta-analyses. In *Cognitive Therapy and Research* (Vol. 36, Issue 5). DOI: 10.1007/s10608-012-9476-1

Jung, M., Lim, C., Lee, C., Kim, S., & Kim, J. (2021). Human dietitians vs. Artificial intelligence: Which diet design do you prefer for your children? *The Journal of Allergy and Clinical Immunology*, *147*(2), AB117. Advance online publication. DOI: 10.1016/j.jaci.2020.12.430

Liu, X. (2024). Ethical research on the artificial intelligence training system for preschoolers under the guidance of child-centered theory. *Applied and Computational Engineering*, *32*(1), 171–176. Advance online publication. DOI: 10.54254/2755-2721/32/20230206

Madej, K. (2024). Representation of Disability in Children's Video Games. In *Representation of Disability in Children's Video Games*. DOI: 10.4324/9781003430445

Merrill, R. M. (2022). Mental Health Conditions According to Stress and Sleep Disorders. *International Journal of Environmental Research and Public Health, 19*(13), 7957. Advance online publication. DOI: 10.3390/ijerph19137957 PMID: 35805615

Morris, N. (2014). Silenced in Childhood: A Survivor of Abuse Finds her Voice through Group Dramatherapy. *Dramatherapy : the Journal of the British Association of Dramatherapy, 36*(1), 3–17. Advance online publication. DOI: 10.1080/02630672.2014.926958

Ng, D. C. E., Liew, C. H., Tan, K. K., Awang, E. H., Nazri, F. N. A., Maran, A. K. T., Mohan, V. A. C., Ramachandran, D., Chok, M., Teh, C. H., Mohamad Nor, A., Baharuddin, S., & Khoo, E. J. (2024). Clinical comparison of HMPV and RSV infections in hospitalised Malaysian children: A propensity score matched study. *The Clinical Respiratory Journal, 18*(3), e13747. Advance online publication. DOI: 10.1111/crj.13747 PMID: 38529669

Opie, J. E., Esler, T. B., Clancy, E. M., Wright, B., Painter, F., Vuong, A., Booth, A. T., Newman, L., Johns-Hayden, A., Hameed, M., Hooker, L., Olsson, C., & McIntosh, J. E. (2024). Universal Digital Programs for Promoting Mental and Relational Health for Parents of Young Children: A Systematic Review and Meta-Analysis. In *Clinical Child and Family Psychology Review* (Vol. 27, Issue 1). DOI: 10.1007/s10567-023-00457-0

Paron, K. (2024). Exploring Child-Patient Autonomy: Findings from an Ethnographic Study of Clinic Visits by Children. *Child Indicators Research, 17*(1), 99–121. Advance online publication. DOI: 10.1007/s12187-023-10077-3

Richards, A., Horwood, J., Boden, J., Kennedy, M., Sellers, R., Riglin, L., Mistry, S., Jones, H., Smith, D. J., Zammit, S., Owen, M., O'Donovan, M. C., & Harold, G. T. (2019). Associations between schizophrenia genetic risk, anxiety disorders and manic/hypomanic episode in a longitudinal population cohort study. *The British Journal of Psychiatry, 214*(2), 96–102. Advance online publication. DOI: 10.1192/bjp.2018.227 PMID: 30472973

Saliba, M., Drapeau, N., Skime, M., Hu, X., Accardi, C. J., Athreya, A. P., Kolacz, J., Shekunov, J., Jones, D. P., Croarkin, P. E., & Romanowicz, M. (2023). PISTACHIo (PreemptIon of diSrupTive behAvior in CHIldren): Real-time monitoring of sleep and behavior of children 3–7 years old receiving parent–child interaction therapy augment with artificial intelligence — the study protocol, pilot study. *Pilot and Feasibility Studies, 9*(1), 23. Advance online publication. DOI: 10.1186/s40814-023-01254-w PMID: 36759915

Schneider, A., Zeiler, M., Kopp, K., Wagner, G., & Karwautz, A. (2023). The Therapeutic Potential of Prebiotics and Probiotics in Child and Adolescent Psychiatric Disorders. In *Zeitschrift fur Kinder- und Jugendpsychiatrie und Psychotherapie* (Vol. 51, Issue 6). DOI: 10.1024/1422-4917/a000930

Shafik, W. (2024a). Connected healthcare—the impact of Internet of Things on medical services. In *Artificial Intelligence and Internet of Things based Augmented Trends for Data Driven Systems* (pp. 181–217). CRC Press., DOI: 10.1201/9781003497318-10

Shafik, W. (2024b). Deep Learning Impacts in the Field of Artificial Intelligence. In *Deep Learning Concepts in Operations Research* (pp. 9–26). Auerbach Publications., DOI: 10.1201/9781003433309-2

Shafik, W. (2024c). Generative AI for Social Good and Sustainable Development. In *Generative AI: Current Trends and Applications* (pp. 185–217). Springer. DOI: 10.1007/978-981-97-8460-8_10

Shafik, W. (2024d). Science of Emotional Intelligence. In *Enhancing and Predicting Digital Consumer Behavior with AI* (pp. 284–310). IGI Global. DOI: 10.4018/979-8-3693-4453-8.ch015

Shafik, W. (2024e). Towards Trustworthy and Explainable AI Educational Systems. In *Explainable AI for Education: Recent Trends and Challenges* (pp. 17–41). Springer. DOI: 10.1007/978-3-031-72410-7_2

Shafik, W. (2025). Human-Computer Interaction (HCI) Technologies in Socially-Enabled Artificial Intelligence. In *Future of Digital Technology and AI in Social Sectors* (pp. 121–150). IGI Global.

Shafik, W., Kalinaki, K., Fahim, K. E., & Adam, M. (2024). Safeguarding Data Privacy and Security in Federated Learning Systems. In *Federated Deep Learning for Healthcare* (pp. 170–190). CRC Press., DOI: 10.1201/9781032694870-13

Shahid, S., Mubin, O., Al Mahmud, A., Iftikhar, Z., & Arshad, R. (2021). Child-Computer Interaction in the Global South: Designing for Children on the Margins. *Proceedings of Interaction Design and Children, IDC, 2021*, 655–657. Advance online publication. DOI: 10.1145/3459990.3460518

Sharma, P., Jain, S., Gupta, S., & Chamola, V. (2021). Role of machine learning and deep learning in securing 5G-driven industrial IoT applications. *Ad Hoc Networks, 123*, 102685. Advance online publication. DOI: 10.1016/j.adhoc.2021.102685

Simon, J., Luetzow, A., & Conte, J. R. (2020). Thirty years of the convention on the rights of the child: Developments in child sexual abuse and exploitation. *Child Abuse & Neglect, 110*, 104399. Advance online publication. DOI: 10.1016/j.chiabu.2020.104399 PMID: 32122640

Stein, R., Garay, M., & Nguyen, A. (2024). It Matters: Early Childhood Mental Health, Educator Stress, and Burnout. *Early Childhood Education Journal, 52*(2), 333–344. Advance online publication. DOI: 10.1007/s10643-022-01438-8 PMID: 36619683

Wan, J., Shin, D. B., Syed, M. N., Abuabara, K., Lemeshow, A. R., & Gelfand, J. M. (2023). Atopic dermatitis and risk of major neuropsychiatric disorders in children: A population-based cohort study. *Journal of the European Academy of Dermatology and Venereology, 37*(1), 114–122. Advance online publication. DOI: 10.1111/jdv.18564 PMID: 36018560

Wilson, C. A., Newham, J., Rankin, J., Ismail, K., Simonoff, E., Reynolds, R. M., Stoll, N., & Howard, L. M. (2022). Systematic review and meta-analysis of risk of gestational diabetes in women with preconception mental disorders. In *Journal of Psychiatric Research* (Vol. 149). DOI: 10.1016/j.jpsychires.2022.03.013

Zhang, W., & Liu, Q. (2023). Investigation and analysis of digital demand for children's books. *Nurture, 17*(4), 653–663. Advance online publication. DOI: 10.55951/nurture.v17i4.450

Chapter 5
Cardiopulmonary Rehabilitation in Patients With Bipolar Disorder

Irem Huzmeli
http://orcid.org/0000-0003-3400-6016
Hatay Mustafa Kemal University, Turkey

Sabiha Bezgin
Hatay Mustafa Kemal University, Turkey

EXECUTIVE SUMMARY

The cardiorespiratory effects in mental illnesses have recently received much attention. However, the cardiovascular and respiratory effects in patients with bipolar disorder and the corresponding rehabilitation strategies have not been clearly demonstrated. This chapter aims to demonstrate exercise capacity, respiratory strength, pulmonary function, dyspnea, physical activity level and rehabilitation strategies in patient with bipolar disorder (BD). The patients had dyspnea, expiratory muscle weakness, small airway dysfunction, obesity, smoking, reduced exercise capacity and physical inactivity. Eight-week cardiopulmonary rehabilitation program were recommended to BD patient that consist of lifestyle modification training, expiratory muscle training, aerobic and resistance training.

CLINICAL PRESENTATION

A 38-year-old female patient, employed as a teacher, has a height of 164 cm, a body weight of 90 kg, and a body mass index (BMI) of 33.5 kg/m^2, indicating

DOI: 10.4018/979-8-3373-3084-6.ch005

class II obesity. The patient has been under follow-up for the past eight years by the Department of Psychiatry with a diagnosis of bipolar disorder.

The patient has no additional comorbidities; however, there is a family history of cardiovascular disease. She reports experiencing dyspnea during vigorous activities, with a Modified Borg Scale (MBS) score of 4. Additionally, she has complaints of nocturnal dyspnea, which intensifies at night. The patient complaint from exertional dyspnea, received sleep support, had a Modified Medical Research Council (MMRC) dyspnea score of 2. While hospitalized in the psychiatric service, she was referred to for cardiopulmonary rehabilitation.

The patient's dyspnea was assessed using the Modified Borg Scale and the MMRC dyspnea scale. Respiratory muscle strength Maximal inspiratory pressure (MIP), Maximal Expiratory Pressure (MEP) was evaluated by mouth pressure measurement device (MicroRPM,) while pulmonary function was assessed using spirometry (MIR). Physical activity levels were determined with the short form International Physical Activity Questionnaire (IPAQ), and exercise capacity was evaluated by 6-minute walk test (6-MWT).

INTRODUCTION

Individuals with severe mental disorders are at an increased risk for comorbid conditions and premature mortality, and these disorders contribute significantly to economic burden. This situation results from a combination of factors, including genetic predisposition, illness-related and treatment-associated complications, unhealthy lifestyle behaviors, social discrimination, and barriers to accessing preventive health services. Additionally, alterations in the transport or concentration of neurochemical substances that mediate intercellular communication in the brain may disrupt neural signaling, thereby impairing the regulation of cognition, memory, learning, and mood (Launders et al., 2022; Manji et al., 2003).

Bipolar disorders, including bipolar I and bipolar II, are chronic psychiatric conditions characterized by the occurrence of acute mood episodes—manic, hypomanic, depressive, or mixed—and the presence of either absent or subsyndromal symptoms during inter-episode periods. The lifetime prevalence is estimated to range from 0.4% to 1.1% (Oliva et al., 2025). According to the Global Burden of Disease Report (2019), the global prevalence of bipolar disorders has remained relatively stable, comparable to that of schizophrenia, suggesting a strong genetic component underlying these conditions (GBD 2019 Mental Disease Collaborators, 2022; Oliva et al., 2025).

The Diagnostic and Statistical Manual of Mental Disorders, Fifth Edition (DSM-5), and the International Classification of Diseases (ICD) provide standardized criteria for the diagnosis of bipolar disorders. Bipolar I disorder is defined by the occurrence of at least one manic episode; while major depressive episodes are frequently observed, they are not necessary for diagnosis. In contrast, the diagnosis of bipolar II disorder requires the presence of at least one hypomanic episode and one major depressive episode (First et al., 2023).

The manic phase of bipolar disorder is characterized by an abnormally elevated or irritable mood accompanied by heightened energy and enthusiasm. During this period, individuals may exhibit grandiosity, inflated self-esteem, or unrealistic beliefs about their abilities or plans. Common symptoms include racing thoughts, reduced need for sleep (often with denial of fatigue), excessive involvement in pleasurable or risky activities without consideration of potential consequences (e.g., excessive spending, reckless driving), and heightened goal-directed behavior. In contrast, the depressive phase represents a marked shift toward low mood and diminished interest or pleasure in previously enjoyable activities. Symptoms may include feelings of sadness, hopelessness, pessimism, low self-esteem, excessive guilt or regret, loss of appetite, insomnia or hypersomnia, fatigue, psychomotor changes, recurrent thoughts of death or suicide, and somatic complaints without a clear medical cause. Stressful or traumatic life events—such as the loss of a loved one, job loss, childbirth, or relocation—can precipitate the onset or recurrence of mood episodes in individuals with bipolar disorder (First et al., 2023).

The underlying causes of premature mortality in individuals with bipolar disorder (BD) remain under investigation. However, there is consistent evidence linking BD to an elevated risk of cardiovascular mortality compared to the general population. The disorder presents with a range of physiological symptoms—such as fatigue, exhaustion, and tachycardia—that some theories attribute to dysfunctions in the cardiovascular, thermoregulatory, and hematopoietic systems. These systemic disturbances may contribute to increased mortality among hospitalized patients (Weiner et al., 2011). Despite accumulating data supporting the association between BD and cardiovascular morbidity, critical questions remain. For instance, the temporal and causal relationships between mood episodes and cardiovascular comorbidity are not fully understood, and it is unclear which specific symptoms, if any, mediate this connection (Weiner et al., 2011).

In addition to cardiovascular concerns, individuals with BD also face a significantly increased risk of mortality due to respiratory diseases. Studies have shown that respiratory-related deaths occur at disproportionately higher rates among people with BD compared to the general population, with mortality risk estimated to be nearly threefold higher than that associated with cardiovascular causes (Hayes et al., 2015). This elevated risk carries profound personal, societal, and economic consequences, similar to those seen with other medical comorbidities (Laguna-Muñoz et al., 2025). Multiple contributing factors have been identified, including genetic vulnerability, characteristics of the psychiatric illness and its pharmacological management, adverse health behaviors, social stigma, and limited access to preventive and timely medical care. Despite the severity of this issue, respiratory health in individuals with BD has received comparatively less attention than cardiovascular and metabolic health, underscoring the urgent need for targeted prevention and intervention strategies (Swartz & Swanson, 2014).

Physical health is increasingly recognized as a significant determinant of neurocognitive functioning in both psychiatric and non-psychiatric populations. Elevated body mass index (BMI) has been associated with poorer cognitive performance and reduced gray matter volume in healthy individuals (Elias et al., 2017; Masouleh et al., 2016). Consequently, preventive interventions play a critical role in the management of bipolar disorder (BD). Although there is no definitive cure for BD, individualized treatment plans are essential. These typically include pharmacological therapy alongside psychosocial and lifestyle modifications. Effective management strategies involve establishing structured daily routines, avoiding unhealthy dietary habits and the use of alcohol or illicit substances, fostering positive cognitive and behavioral skills, learning stress management techniques, and gaining comprehensive knowledge of the illness course (Oliva et al., 2025).

While the presence of mental disorders cannot be denied, the availability and effectiveness of therapeutic interventions in the modern era are equally undeniable. In addition to pharmacotherapy and psychotherapy—which remain the cornerstone treatments—physical activity is widely recognized as a beneficial adjunct intervention for various psychiatric conditions (Bay & Yilmaz, 2020). In individuals with BD, regular exercise has been shown to improve mood and quality of life, as well as reduce the risk of physical comorbidities, such as obesity and cardiovascular disease (Bay & Yilmaz, 2020). Furthermore, increased cardiovascular fitness has been linked to enhanced cognitive function and increased brain volume in individuals with schizophrenia (Kimhy et al., 2015; Firth et al., 2018). Although evidence regarding the impact of exercise on brain structure and function in individuals with mood disorders remains inconsistent, studies have demonstrated a significant positive association between physical activity and cognitive function in individuals with depression (Stubbs et al., 2016; Firth et al., 2018).

There is growing interest in the potential role of physical activity in preventing the onset of bipolar disorder in at-risk individuals and in enhancing coping strategies among those already affected (Stubbs et al., 2018). While physical activity has been widely studied and recommended in the context of depression (Thomson et al., 2015), the manic symptoms of bipolar disorder represent a clinical presentation that contrasts significantly with depressive features. Research consistently shows that individuals with bipolar disorder are generally less physically active than the general population (Vancampfort et al., 2017; Pereira et al., 2019). However, physical activity levels vary substantially depending on the current mood state: individuals experiencing manic or hypomanic episodes typically display higher activity levels, whereas those in depressive episodes exhibit markedly reduced activity (Sylvia et al., 2013; Kang et al., 2018). Moreover, some evidence suggests that intense physical exercise may potentially act as a trigger for manic episodes in susceptible individuals (Sylvia et al., 2013). Physical fitness may also play a mediating role in physical activity engagement, although this relationship requires further investigation (Svensson et al., 2022).

In addition to its well-established cardioprotective effects, a growing body of research indicates that various exercise regimens contribute significantly to improvements in brain function. Although the precise underlying mechanisms remain to be fully elucidated, accumulating evidence supports the neuroprotective effects of physical activity in both human and animal studies. These benefits have been observed across multiple domains, including mental health, neurodegenerative diseases, and acquired brain injuries, highlighting the therapeutic potential of exercise in promoting brain resilience and function (Liu et al., 2019).

In addition to physical activity, breathing exercises have gained increasing attention as complementary interventions in the treatment of mental health disorders. One such technique, deep breathing—also referred to as diaphragmatic breathing—involves voluntary, controlled respiration that engages the diaphragm muscle more actively during inhalation (Neves, 2011). Deep breathing is a simple yet effective relaxation method that, with sufficient training, can be easily learned and implemented by individuals. These exercises influence key anatomical structures and neural pathways involved in the regulation of emotion, attention, perception, and problem-solving (Brown et al., 2013). Notably, deep breathing enhances activation of the parasympathetic branch of the autonomic nervous system, which promotes neural flexibility, alters information processing, and contributes to the treatment of psychological disorders by alleviating symptoms such as anxiety and insomnia (Bentley et al., 2023).

A range of physiological and psychological benefits have been attributed to deep breathing, including stabilization of the autonomic nervous system, increased heart rate variability, reduced blood pressure, improved pulmonary and immune function, enhanced circulation of blood and lymph, improved digestion, and better sleep quality. These changes collectively contribute to greater biopsychosocial well-being and overall quality of life (Van Dixhoorn, 2007). In individuals with bipolar disorder (BD), research has shown elevated sympathetic nervous system activity and reduced parasympathetic activity (Göçen & Özden, 2024). Given that deep breathing is known to enhance parasympathetic activation, it is proposed as a potential adjunctive therapy in the management of BD (Serafim et al., 2019).

Respiratory muscle training (RMT), a form of respiratory exercise, has increasingly been incorporated into non-pharmacological treatment programs in recent years. Respiratory muscle dysfunction—resulting from various etiological factors—can lead to both inspiratory and expiratory muscle weakness. Inspiratory muscle weakness is often associated with exertional dyspnea, orthopnea (dyspnea when lying supine), bending-related dyspnea, and shortness of breath while standing. Expiratory muscle weakness, on the other hand, is commonly linked to ineffective coughing and secretion clearance, which may lead to recurrent respiratory infections. Additionally, respiratory muscle dysfunction can contribute to nocturnal hypoventilation, which is characterized by symptoms such as morning headaches, daytime sleepiness, impaired concentration, and disrupted sleep patterns (Hüzmeli & Katayıfçı, 2022).

Beyond these symptoms, clinical manifestations may include tachypnea, followed by central bradypnea, reduced respiratory rate, and eventually dyspnea (Hüzmeli & Katayıfçı, 2022). Respiratory muscle strength is also closely related to vital capacity (VC), success in weaning from mechanical ventilation in intensive care settings, the severity of dyspnea, exercise tolerance, and overall mortality risk (Bissett et al., 2020). Assessment of respiratory muscle function is typically performed using measurements of respiratory pressures and lung volumes. Spirometric parameters such as VC and forced vital capacity (FVC) help identify muscle weakness. Other relevant indicators include total lung capacity (TLC), residual volume (RV), and functional residual capacity (FRC), which provide insight into the mechanical performance of the respiratory system.

In cases of respiratory muscle weakness, reduced lung compliance and elasticity are common, often leading to decreased lung volumes, including TLC. However, maximum inspiratory pressure (MIP) and maximum expiratory pressure (MEP)—measured via mouth pressure techniques—are frequently preferred over VC and FVC due to their cost-effectiveness, minimal requirement for additional maneuvers, high reproducibility, and availability of well-established normative values. A reduction of 30% or more in VC in the supine position compared to standing is considered a strong indicator of significant respiratory muscle weakness. RMT and the assessment of respiratory muscle strength are particularly relevant in patients with neuromuscular diseases, postural abnormalities, cardiovascular or respiratory conditions, postoperative dyspnea (following thoracic or abdominal surgery), corticosteroid-induced weakness, mental health-related dyspnea, and in patients experiencing difficulty weaning from mechanical ventilation (McConnell, 2013).

Respiratory muscle training (RMT) encompasses various modalities, including respiratory muscle endurance training, respiratory muscle strength training, and functional respiratory muscle training. Common techniques include inspiratory muscle training (IMT), expiratory muscle training (EMT), and sniff pressure (Psniff) training (McConnell, 2013). IMT primarily targets the strengthening of inspiratory muscles, notably the diaphragm, as well as accessory muscles such as the external intercostals, scalenes, and sternocleidomastoid. This intervention is applicable across clinical populations, athletes, and healthy individuals.

Clinically, IMT has demonstrated efficacy in managing respiratory system pathologies characterized by muscle weakness, altered lung volumes, and expiratory flow limitation. Such improvements translate to enhanced clinical status, increased exercise capacity, and better quality of life (Shei et al., 2022). EMT is particularly utilized in patient populations experiencing respiratory failure, aiming to augment expiratory muscle strength and respiratory function. This is especially relevant in conditions such as Parkinson's disease, obstructive and restrictive lung diseases. EMT enables patients to overcome positive airway pressure, generate sufficient expiratory force, and initiate effective expiration. Training typically involves the use of a threshold loading device and mouthpiece, with a workload calibrated between 30–75% of maximum expiratory pressure (MEP), independent of patient positioning (McConnell, 2013; Shei et al., 2022). For meaningful structural and biochemical adaptations in respiratory muscles, these training regimens should be sustained for a minimum of six weeks (McConnell, 2013; Hüzmeli & Katayıfçı, 2022).

Evidence suggests that while IMT alone improves dyspnea, functional exercise capacity, and quality of life, combined respiratory muscle training (IMT + EMT) produces superior outcomes compared to IMT alone (Gosselink et al., 2011). Although EMT is less frequently applied in chronic obstructive pulmonary disease (COPD) patients, studies have reported increases in expiratory muscle strength alongside improvements in resting dyspnea and health-related quality of life (Mota et al., 2007). EMT is widely employed in managing swallowing disorders, dysphagia, multiple sclerosis, Parkinson's disease, and other neuromuscular conditions, typically involving five sets of five repetitions at 75% MEP intensity. Darling-White and Huber (2017) demonstrated that eight weeks of EMT at 75% MEP in Parkinson's patients significantly increased MEP and induced favorable changes in lung volumes. Furthermore, in a recent study examining the effects of high- and low-intensity expiratory muscle strength training (EMST) in obstructive sleep apnea syndrome (OSAS), a 12-week home-based program (25 breaths per session, once daily, seven days per week) significantly reduced systemic inflammation and oxidative stress while enhancing expiratory muscle strength in male patients with moderate OSAS (Ertürk et al., 2024).

In conclusion people with bipolar disorder have an increased risk of premature death, with a higher respiratory tract mortality rate compared to the general population. This leads to significant personal, societal, and economic costs (Laguna-Muñoz et al., 2025). Various factors contribute to this result, including genetic predisposition, aspects related to mental illness and its treatment, health behaviors, social discrimination, and limited access to preventive healthcare, timely diagnosis, and appropriate treatment. The risk of death from respiratory diseases is nearly three times higher in individuals with BD, surpassing that of cardiovascular events (Hayes et al., 2015). However, respiratory issues have received less attention compared to cardiovascular and metabolic conditions, highlighting the urgent need for prevention. This case report aimed to demonstrate the changes in cardiovascular and respiratory parameters with cardiopulmonary rehabilitation program in patient with BD.

ASSESSMENTS

Disease Status: The patient was diagnosed with Bipolar Type 2 disorder, currently in a depressive episode.

Charlson Comorbidity Index: This index is utilized to grade and define the comorbidity status of patients. Comorbid conditions are scored according to their severity. The comorbidity level is categorized as follows: a score of 0 indicates mild, 1-2 points denote moderate, 3-4 points signify severe, and a score of ≥5 reflects very severe comorbidity. A Charlson Comorbidity Index score of 0 indicated that the patient had no comorbidities.

Surgery History: None

Family History: The patient's mother had a diagnosis of hypertension

Smoking Status: 26 pack-year smoking exposure and current smoker

Drinking Status: Yes

Physical Activity Status: Inactive

The Coronary Artery Risk Score (Table 1) was used to evaluate the patient's risk of developing coronary artery disease (CAD).

Table 1. Coronary Artery Disease Risk Factors

Risk Factor	Present	Absent
Advanced Age (Men >45 years, Women >55 years)		X
Hypertension (HT)		X
Diabetes Mellitus (DM)		X
Hypercholesterolemia		X
Family History of CAD	X	
Smoking History	X	

The patient has two risk factors for CAD: Family history of CAD and Smoking history. These factors contribute to an increased risk for developing coronary artery disease over time.

CLINICAL IMPLICATIONS & RECOMMENDATIONS

- **Lifestyle modifications**: Smoking cessation, regular exercise, and a heart-healthy diet should be encouraged.
- **Regular screening**: Monitoring **lipid profile, blood pressure, and glucose levels** is essential to detect early metabolic changes.
- **Further risk assessment**: If necessary, additional cardiovascular risk scoring (e.g., **Framingham Risk Score** or **ASCVD Risk Calculator**) may provide a more comprehensive risk evaluation.
- Medication was shown in table 2. Antiepileptic (mood stabilizer), antidepressant (SNRI), beta-blocker, anxiolytic (Benzodiazepine), antipsychotic (Atypical) drug were the mediation.

Table 2. Medication

Drug	**Dose**	**Frequency**	**Mechanism of Action**
Depakine	500 mg	3 times/day	Antiepileptic (mood stabilizer)
Efexor	40 mg	Once daily	Antidepressant (SNRI)
Diaderal	75 mg	Once daily	Beta-blocker
Xanax	5 mg	Once daily	Anxiolytic (Benzodiazepine)
Rixper	1 mg	Once daily	Antipsychotic (Atypical)
Gyrex	300 mg	Once daily	Antipsychotic (Atypical)
Abilify Maintena	-	Once monthly	Antipsychotic (Long acting)

Subjective Assessments

- **Dyspnea:** Yes
- **Resting Dyspnea:** Present
    - o **Severity:** 2 points (Modified Borg Scale)
- **Exertional Dyspnea:** Present
    - o **Severity:**4 points (Modified Borg Scale)
    - o **Triggers:** Climbing stairs, walking uphill
- **Orthopnea:** Absent
- **Paroxysmal Nocturnal Dyspnea:** Absent
- **Cough:** Present
- **Sputum Production:** Absent
- **Hemoptysis:** Absent

- **Wheezing:** Absent
- **Chest Pain:** Absent
- **Fever:** Absent
- **Peripheral Edema:** Absent

Objective assessments

a. Chest Examination

Inspection: Visual inspection of the thorax revealed no deformities, asymmetries, or abnormal respiratory patterns.

Palpation:

Tracheal position: Midline, without deviation.

Thoracic expansion: Symmetrical involvement of both hemithoraces during spontaneous respiration. Systematic palpation was performed:

- *Upper thorax:* Normal symmetrical expansion with full aeration.
- *Epigastric/subcostal regions:* Symmetrical expansion but with mildly reduced aeration, suggesting possible diaphragmatic or lower airway involvement.

Percussion:

Comparative percussion (anterior/posterior, apical to basal) yielded normal resonant tones bilaterally, with no dullness or hyperresonance detected.

Auscultation:

- *Bronchial sounds:* Physiologically present over the trachea and main bronchi.
- *Bronchovesicular sounds:* Normal at the sternal borders (1st–2nd intercostal spaces).
- *Vesicular sounds:* Significantly diminished in bilateral basal lobes (posterior lower zones), though no adventitious sounds (crackles, wheezes, or rhonchi) were noted. This finding may indicate subclinical atelectasis, early restrictive pathology, or reduced diaphragmatic excursion.

Table 3 shows the pulmonary function test results.

Table 3. Pulmonary Function Test Results

	Lt	%
FEV_1	2.48	78
FVC	2.89	79
FEV_1/ FVC	78	
PEF	5.80	75
$FEF_{25\text{-}75}$	2.79	69

FEV1: forced expiratory volume in 1 s; FVC: forced vital capacity; PEF: peak expiratory flow; FEF%25–75 (%): forced expiratory flow at 25–75% of the pulmonary volume, MIP: maximal inspiratory pressure; MEP: maximal expiratory pressure, %: Percent, Lt: Liter

Interpretation:

1. Forced Expiratory Volume in 1 Second (FEV_1): 2.48 L (78%)
   - FEV_1 represents the amount of air exhaled forcefully in the first second.
   - A value of 78% of the predicted indicates mild airflow limitation but is still within the lower normal range.
2. Forced Vital Capacity (FVC): 2.89 L (79%)
   - FVC represents the total volume of air exhaled after a full inspiration.
   - A value of 79% of predicted suggests mild restriction but does not meet the threshold for a restrictive lung disease diagnosis (<70%).
3. FEV_1/FVC Ratio: 78%
   - This ratio is critical in differentiating obstructive vs. restrictive lung diseases.
   - A normal or slightly reduced FEV_1/FVC (≥70%) suggests a possible restrictive pattern or mild airflow obstruction.
   - In obstructive diseases (e.g., COPD, asthma), this ratio is usually <70%.
4. Peak Expiratory Flow (PEF): 5.80 L/s (75%)
   - Indicates moderate reduction in expiratory flow, suggesting possible small airway involvement.
5. Forced Expiratory Flow at 25-75% (FEF_{25-75}%): 2.79 L/s (69%)
   - FEF_{25-75}% reflects small airway function.
   - A reduced value (<70%) suggests mild small airway obstruction, which can be seen in early obstructive airway diseases such as asthma or chronic bronchitis.

No definitive obstruction or restriction, but borderline FVC suggests possible mild restrictive lung involvement (could be due to obesity). Correlation with clinical symptoms, history, and additional tests (e.g., lung volumes, diffusion capacity) is necessary for a definitive diagnosis. Spirometry revealed decreased FEF25-75%, consistent with small airways disease. This pattern is clinically associated with obesity-related respiratory compromise and/or tobacco-induced bronchial inflammation.

b. Respiratory Muscle Strength Assessment

The inspiratory and expiratory muscle strength (Table 4) was measured using a mouth pressure device (Micro Medical MicroRPM, UK) following ATS/ERS guidelines (Laveneziana et al., 2019).

Table 4. **Respiratory Muscle Strength Results**

Parameter	Measured Value (cmH_2O)	Cut-off Value for Weakness (Females)	Interpretation
MIP (Maximal Inspiratory Pressure)	110	62	Normal
MEP (Maximal Expiratory Pressure)	69	81	Weak

The patient's MIP value (110 cmH_2O) is above the threshold for respiratory muscle weakness, indicating normal inspiratory muscle strength. The patient's MEP value (69 cmH_2O) is below the cut-off (81 cmH_2O), suggesting expiratory muscle weakness.

Clinical Implications & Recommendations

- Expiratory muscle weakness may contribute to reduced cough efficiency, increasing the risk of mucus retention and respiratory infections.
- Respiratory muscle training (RMT), particularly expiratory muscle strengthening exercises, could be beneficial to improve respiratory function.
- Regular monitoring of respiratory muscle strength is recommended to assess progression and response to intervention.

Cut-off points for respiratory muscle weakness based on T-scores ≥2.5 SD below the peak mean value achieved at a young age were: 62 and 83cmH_2O for PImax and 81 and 109cmH_2O for PEmax in females and males, respectively (Lista-Paz et al., 2023).

Quantitative assessment revealed reduced expiratory muscle strength in this bipolar disorder patient (MEP: [69] cmH_2O), potentially contributing to the observed small airway dysfunction.

c. Exercise Capacity Assessment

Exercise capacity was evaluated using the Six-Minute Walk Test (6MWT, Table 5) in accordance with ATS/ERS guidelines (ATS Committee on Proficiency Standards for Clinical Pulmonary Function Laboratories, 2002). The following physiological parameters were recorded:

Table 5. **Six-Minute Walk Test Results**

Parameters	At Rest	Post-Test	1st Min Recovery
Heart Rate (bpm)	89	100	91
SpO_2 (%)	96	94	96
Blood Pressure (mmHg)	90/80	100/85	95/83
Respiratory Rate (breaths/min)	12	16	14
Dyspnea (Modified Borg Scale, 0-10)	0	4	1
Fatigue (Modified Borg Scale, 0-10)	0	4	1
Leg Fatigue (Modified Borg Scale, 0-10)	0	5	2
Distance Walked (m)	480	-	-
Distance (% of Predicted)	67.88%	-	-

bpm: Beats per minute, SpO2: Peripheral oxygen saturation, mmHg: Millimeters of mercury, m: Meters

- Heart rate was monitored using a heart rate monitor (Polar FT I00, China).
- Blood pressure was measured with a sphygmomanometer.
- Respiratory rate was determined by counting breaths per minute.
- Peripheral oxygen saturation (SpO_2) was assessed using a portable pulse oximeter (Choicemed MD300C15D, Germany).
- Fatigue and dyspnea perception were evaluated using the Modified Borg Scale.

At Rest: The patient's systolic blood pressure was reduced, while other vital signs were within normal limits.

Post-Test: The patient reached 54.94% of the predicted maximal heart rate (220 - age), indicating a submaximal effort. There was no significant oxygen desaturation (SpO_2 reduction <4%). The increase in blood pressure was within the expected physiological range. No excessive respiratory distress was observed (respiratory rate remained <40 breaths/min). According to the Modified Borg Scale, the patient experienced moderate dyspnea, generalized fatigue, and leg fatigue.

Walking Distance: The patient walked 480 meters during the test. The distance covered was 67.88% of the predicted value, which was below 80% of the expected distance. This result indicated a reduced exercise capacity. The predicted 6MWT distance was calculated using the formula from Gibbons et al., 2001:

Predicted 6MWT Distance=868.8−(Age×2.99)−(Gender: Male=0,Female=1×74.7

Recovery: The patient's heart rate recovery at 1 minute was 9 bpm, which is considered suboptimal as it was <12 bpm. According to the Modified Borg Scale, the patient continued to experience mild to moderate dyspnea, fatigue, and leg fatigue during the recovery phase.

- The submaximal nature of the test and the absence of oxygen desaturation suggest that cardiopulmonary function was preserved to some extent.
- However, the reduced 6MWT distance (<80% of predicted) and suboptimal heart rate recovery indicate impaired functional exercise capacity, which may be related to deconditioning, obesity, or underlying respiratory/cardiovascular factors.
- Further evaluation and cardiopulmonary rehabilitation are recommended to improve exercise tolerance and functional capacity.

d. Modified Medical Research Council (MMRC) Dyspnea Scale

- The MMRC Dyspnea Scale was used to evaluate breathlessness during daily activities (Mahler and Wells, 1988).
- The patient’s MMRC score was 2, indicating that dyspnea occurs during brisk walking on level ground or when walking uphill.

e. Short form-International Physical Activity Questionnaire (IPAQ)

- The short form of the International Physical Activity Questionnaire (IPAQ) was used to assess physical activity level (Table 6).
- According to the total physical activity score (<600 MET-min/week), the patient is classified as physically inactive.
- The high sitting time (4410 minutes per week) further supports a sedentary lifestyle, which may contribute to reduced exercise capacity and dyspnea symptoms.

- Encouraging structured physical activity and reducing sedentary time may be beneficial for improving functional capacity and overall health status(Craig et al., 2003; Sağlam et al., 2010).

Table 6. **Patient's IPAQ Results**

Activity Type	**MET-min/week**
Vigorous Physical Activity	0
Moderate Physical Activity	160
Walking	346.50
Total Physical Activity	506.50
Sitting Time (min/week)	4410

MET: Metabolic Equivalent of Task, min: Minutes

PROBLEM LIST

1. Dyspnea
2. Expiratory muscle weakness
3. Small airway dysfunction
4. Obesity
5. Smoking
6. Reduced exercise capacity
7. Physical inactivity

Management Targets

Short-Term Goals (0-4 weeks):

1. Respiratory symptom control:
    a. Instruction in breathing control techniques
    b. Education on dyspnea-relieving positions (e.g., forward lean, tripod positioning)
2. Symptom mitigation:
    a. Reduction in perceived breathlessness
3. Energy conservation strategies:
    a. Activity pacing techniques
    b. Work simplification methods

4. Pulmonary rehabilitation:
    a. Improvement in lung aeration through incentive spirometry/diaphragmatic breathing

Long-Term Goals (>4 weeks):

1. Muscle strength enhancement:
    a. Progressive respiratory muscle training (expiratory)
    b. Peripheral muscle strengthening program
2. Functional improvement:
    a. Graduated increase in exercise capacity (6MWT target: [708]m)
    b. Enhanced physical activity level (target: [7500-10000] steps/day)
3. Lifestyle modification:
    a. Establishment of sustainable exercise habits
    b. Weight management strategies
    c. Smoking management strategies

Therapeutic Interventions

1.Risk Factor Education: According to the SCORE-Turkey algorithm, the patient was classified as being at moderate cardiovascular risk. She was educated on healthy nutrition, smoking cessation, increasing physical activity, and weight management as part of lifestyle modification.

- The patient was referred to a smoking cessation center and advised to adhere to prescribed antihypertensive treatment and attend regular follow-up appointments.
- The healthcare team referred the patient to a registered dietitian for nutritional counseling and individualized dietary planning due to her overweight status and irregular dietary patterns.

The authors scheduled an individualized exercise training program and provided counseling on physical activity.

The patient's motivation level for engaging in physical activity was assessed. Based on the transtheoretical model of behavior change, she was determined to be in the **preparation stage**. To facilitate physical activity counseling, personal barriers to exercise were identified, and tailored strategies were developed to address them. A pedometer application was installed on the patient's mobile phone and advised to aim for a minimum of 7.500 steps per day.

Patients received training on energy conservation techniques designed to promote independence and comfort in performing daily activities. The patient was advised to carry out activities using proper posture, to prioritize and schedule physically demanding tasks during periods of peak energy, and to incorporate regular rest breaks between activities to prevent fatigue.

2. Breathing control training

Diaphragmatic and pursed lip breathing exercises were shown to the patient.

3. **Dyspnea-Relieving Positions**: The patient was instructed in body positions aimed at reducing dyspnea, including high Fowler's position, supported sitting, and standing positions that facilitate respiratory effort.
4. **Respiratory Muscle Training**

Type: Expiratory muscle strength training using a respiratory exercise device (Expiratory Muscle Strength Trainer 150 – EMST 150).

Protocol: Training was conducted at 30% of the patient's maximal expiratory pressure (MEP) for a duration of 8 weeks, with sessions scheduled 3 days per week. Each session lasted approximately 30 minutes and included 10 breaths per session.

5. Aerobic Exercise Training

Type: Continuous aerobic exercise training performed on a treadmill.

Training Structure: Each session included a 5-minute warm-up, 30 minutes of aerobic loading, and a 5-minute cool-down phase.

Intensity: Moderate-intensity aerobic exercise was conducted at 50% of the heart rate reserve (target: 143.6 beats/min), or according to subjective ratings of dyspnea (3–4 points) and fatigue

(5–6 points) on the Modified Borg Scale.

Duration: 30–40 minutes per session.

Frequency: Once daily, 3–5 days per week, for a total of 8 weeks (Figure 1).

6. Resistance Exercise Training

Type: Resistance training using an elastic resistance band targeting both upper and lower extremities.

Protocol: Flexion-abduction-external rotation movements following proprioceptive neuromuscular facilitation (PNF) full patterns using a red resistance band.

Intensity: Exercises were performed at approximately 40% of one-repetition maximum (1RM) or at a perceived dyspnea level of 3–4 and fatigue level of 5–6 on the Modified Borg Scale. Each session included 10 repetitions per set, for 2 sets.

Frequency: Once daily, 3–5 days per week.

Figure 1. Exercise Based Treatment Programs of the Bipolar disorder's patients

1st Week Program	
1. session	The patient underwent a detailed multidisciplinary evaluation, culminating in the development of a tailored cardiopulmonary rehabilitation program. The treatment plan specifically addresses: • Psychiatric comorbidities impacting cardiopulmonary function • Cardiac and respiratory manifestations associated with mood disorders • Physiotherapy interventions optimized for psychiatric patients Patient Education Components The patient received structured education regarding: 1. Cardiorespiratory complications in psychiatric populations 2. Physiological interactions between mental health and physical health 3. Evidence-based physiotherapy approaches for comorbid conditions
2nd session	Cardiopulmonary rehabilitation program was applied as planned
3th session	Cardiopulmonary rehabilitation program was performed and repeated
2-8. week	Respiratory muscle training: Mouth pressure was measured every week. New workloads for strength training were determined according to the new MEP obtained. Aerobic exercise training: New workloads equivalent to 50-60% of heart rate reserve were set each week. **Resistance Exercise Training:** Each week, the training load was adjusted to maintain a perceived exertion level of 5–6 points on the Modified Borg Scale, corresponding to a moderate level of fatigue.
Follow-Up	The patient was advised to attend monthly follow-up visits with healthcare professionals to monitor progress and ensure continuity of care within the cardiopulmonary rehabilitation program.

IMPORTANT CONSIDERATIONS DURING EXERCISE TRAINING

Vital signs were monitored before, during, and after all exercise sessions. Prior to initiating resistance exercise training, heart rate, blood pressure, and electrocardiographic (ECG) evaluations were conducted to ensure patient safety. To prevent the Valsalva maneuver—which can elevate intra-abdominal blood pressure—the patient was instructed to avoid breath-holding and excessive gripping of the resistance band. Resistance exercises were integrated with breathing techniques to promote safe performance.

During aerobic exercise training, the patient was routinely assessed for chest pain and dyspnea. Exercise sessions were terminated under the following conditions: an increase in heart rate exceeding 20 beats per minute, a decrease in heart rate greater than 10 beats per minute, a drop in systolic blood pressure greater than 10 mmHg, or if systolic/diastolic blood pressure exceeded 250 mmHg and 115 mmHg, respectively.

In patients with bipolar disorder, ECG monitoring was continued for up to 15 minutes post-exercise to ensure cardiovascular stability.

DISCUSSION AND CONCLUSION

In this section, authors examined the cardiopulmonary effects of bipolar disorder, a mental health condition that affects millions of individuals each year. Our findings indicate that bipolar disorder was associated with increased dyspnea, mild airway dysfunction, reduced expiratory muscle strength, decreased physical activity levels, and impaired exercise capacity. An 8-week exercise-based rehabilitation program can improve a patient's cardiac and pulmonary symptoms and contribute to well-being.

Huzmeli et al. 2024 demonstrated a decrease in exercise capacity and pulmonary function and respiratory muscle strength, and increased dyspnea. Although no impairment in inspiratory muscle strength was observed in our case study, a decrease in expiratory muscle strength was present and associated with dyspnea. While a previous study primarily reported reductions in peak expiratory flow (PEF) values, our findings indicated lower forced expiratory flow (FEF) values, which reflect small airway function. As previously mentioned this results may be related to the patient's obesity.

Previous studies have shown that obesity and physical inactivity are well-established risk factors for diabetes, metabolic syndrome, and cardiovascular disease—all of which disproportionately affect individuals with bipolar disorder. (Kilbourne et al., 2009; Thomson et al., 2015). In the present case involving an obese patient, clinical findings were consistent with previously documented risk factors in the literature. Based on these observations, a personalized cardiopulmonary rehabilitation program was designed. Consistent with the findings of Thomson et al. (2015), it is anticipated that the exercise intervention may facilitate neurogenesis and exert pleiotropic effects, including the enhancement of neuroplasticity, neurotransmission, and the regulation of neuronal growth processes. Similarly, it has been hypothesized that physical exercise, as a form of 'positive stress,' may enhance neurogenesis by increasing the expression of brain-derived neurotrophic factor (BDNF). Additionally, exercise training has been shown to stimulate the release of endogenous opioids, such as endorphins, which contribute to mood improvement. However, while improved mood and alleviation of affective symptoms are beneficial outcomes, these effects may present a double-edged sword in patients experiencing mania, warranting careful clinical consideration. Moreover, it is well established that as exercise capacity improves in individuals with bipolar disorder, fatigue tends to decrease, physical activity levels increase, and these changes collectively contribute to enhanced quality of life—particularly by positively impacting overall well-being (Ercan and Gündoğmuş 2022).

In this case, a structured, exercise-based program was implemented by considering the patient's cardiac and pulmonary symptoms. Consistent with literature, the intervention led to an improvement in exercise capacity. It is anticipated that this increase in physical capacity may contribute to enhanced well-being and a reduction in depressive symptoms.

Ruiz-Rull's (2024) study identified the presence of airway obstruction in individuals with bipolar disorder. Consistent with the findings of our case study, abnormal pulmonary function was observed, reinforcing prior evidence that approximately one-third of individuals with severe mental illness exhibit abnormal spirometry patterns. When these patterns reflect an obstructive component, they are often associated with factors such as smoking and abdominal obesity. Cardiovascular fitness may influence both mental and physical aspects of health-related quality of life (HRQoL) in individuals with bipolar disorder (Vancampfort et al., 2017). In this patient with bipolar disorder, a similar reduction in exercise capacity was observed (predicted %6MWT=0.67.88). IMT training can improve the cardiorespiratory fitness in mental disease and can improve the mental and physical HRQOl (Roldán et al., 2021). RMT effects may include (1) reduced respiratory muscle fatigue, (2) delayed respiratory muscle metaboreflex activation, (3) better maintenance of SaO_2 and blood flow to locomotor muscles. (Álvarez-Herms et al., 2019). Based on the findings of previous studies, an eight-week program of IMT combined with resistance training was implemented in our this case study. As a result of this intervention, we anticipate improvements in the patient's reduced exercise capacity, reductions in fatigue and dyspnea due to enhanced locomotor function, and an overall increase in physical activity levels—ultimately contributing to improved well-being .

Expiratory muscle strength plays a critical role in respiratory function and general health and contributes to ventilatory efficiency and exercise tolerance. During physical activity, strong expiratory muscles help manage intrathoracic pressure and reduce the breathing work, leading to improved aerobic performance and delayed onset of respiratory fatigue (Shei et al., 2016; McConnell & Romer, 2019). In individuals with chronic respiratory and neurological conditions, targeted expiratory muscle training (EMT) has been shown to improve dyspnea, fatigue, functional independence, and health-related quality of life (HRQoL) (Romer et al., 2022; Gosselink et al., 2018). In a study evaluating respiratory muscle strenght in individuals with mental illness, the measured values of MEP were found to be lower than predicted values, with a mean difference of -44.33 ± 27.06 cmH_2O for MEP (Birinci et al., 2019). Similarly, in our case, the patient demonstrated reduced expiratory muscle strength (MEP measured: 69 cmH_2O, the cut-off MEP: 81 cmH_2O). Consequently, an eight-week EMT program was planned. This case study is expected to enhance expiratory muscle strength, reduce fatigue, and improve functional capacity in individuals with bipolar disorder.

Psychiatric disorders, including depression, bipolar disorder, and schizophrenia, are frequently associated with decreased physical activity levels and an increased perception of dyspnea, even in the absence of primary respiratory disease. Dyspnea in individuals with mental illness may result from physiological deconditioning, altered respiratory control, somatic symptom amplification, or comorbid conditions such as obesity and smoking-related lung disease (Vancampfort et al., 2017; Falk et al., 2022). Patients with psychiatric disorders have reduced cardiorespiratory fitness and may have an increase in dyspnea perception during minimal exertion (Firth et al., 2021).

Recent studies suggest that program with structured physical activity can alleviate both dyspnea and psychiatric symptoms by improving respiratory muscle strength, reducing systemic inflammation, and enhancing neuroplasticity and mood regulation pathways (Stubbs et al., 2018; Schuch et al., 2020). Exercise-based rehabilitation programs tailored to individuals with mental illness have shown promising effects in improving exercise tolerance, decreasing fatigue and dyspnea, and ultimately enhancing quality of life and functional independence (Rosenbaum et al., 2022). Given the bidirectional correlation between physical inactivity and psychiatric symptom burden, incorporating respiratory assessments and graded physical activity interventions may be essential components of comprehensive care for individuals with severe mental illness.

Personalized exercise-based intervention programs are increasingly important in the treatment of mood disorders, including depression and bipolar disorder. Tailoring physical activity regimens to individual preferences, abilities, and clinical profiles improves adherence and therapeutic outcomes. A previous study has shown that personalized training combined with motivational interviewing and supervised activity significantly increased moderate-to-vigorous physical activity levels and improved depressive symptoms (Helbig et al., 2023). Another study found that personalized exercise plans integrated with psychological support can improve overall functioning and well-being in individuals with mild-to-moderate depression (Pascoe et al., 2021). These findings suggest that personalized exercise interventions are valuable as effective, sustainable, and patient-centered strategies for the management of bipolar disorder. While this case study adopts a similarly individualized approach to those employed in previous research, it distinguishes itself through its unique intervention design and implementation. Notably, as one of the few case studies exploring the combined application of expiratory muscle training (EMT) and resistance training in individuals with bipolar disorder, it offers a novel contribution to the existing literature and may broaden the current understanding of non-pharmacological treatment modalities in this population.

In conclusion, an eight-week personalized, exercise-based rehabilitation program may improve the perception of dyspnea and respiratory functions in individuals with bipolar disorder, enhance expiratory muscle strength, and increase both physical activity participation and exercise capacity. Future studies are recommended to investigate the effects of low, moderate, and high-intensity expiratory muscle training in larger populations within this patient group.

REFERENCES

Álvarez-Herms, J., Julià-Sánchez, S., Corbi, F., Odriozola-Martínez, A., & Burtscher, M. (2019). Putative Role of Respiratory Muscle Training to Improve Endurance Performance in Hypoxia: A Review. *Frontiers in Physiology*, *9*, 1970. DOI: 10.3389/fphys.2018.01970 PMID: 30697170

ATS Committee on Proficiency Standards for Clinical Pulmonary Function Laboratories. (2002). ATS statement: Guidelines for the six-minute walk test. *American Journal of Respiratory and Critical Care Medicine*, *166*(1), 111–117. DOI: 10.1164/ajrccm.166.1.at1102 PMID: 12091180

Bay, Ü. S., & Yılmaz, E. (2020). Ruhsal Bozukluklarda Fiziksel Aktivite ve Egzersizin Etkileri ile İlgili Yapılmış Çalışmaların İncelenmesi. *Mediterranean Journal of Sport Science*, *3*(2), 437–447. DOI: 10.38021/asbid.849274

Bentley, T. G. K., D'Andrea-Penna, G., Rakic, M., Arce, N., LaFaille, M., Berman, R., Cooley, K., & Sprimont, P. (2023). Breathing Practices for Stress and Anxiety Reduction: Conceptual Framework of Implementation Guidelines Based on a Systematic Review of the Published Literature. *Brain Sciences*, *13*(12), 1612. DOI: 10.3390/brainsci13121612 PMID: 38137060

Birinci, T., Mutlu, E. K., & Mustafaoğlu, R. (2019). Does Psychiatric Disorders Cause Reduction in Pulmonary Function and Respiratory Muscle Strength?: Case Series. *Thoracic Research and Practice*, *20*(1), 400–400.

Bissett, B., Gosselink, R., & van Haren, F. M. P. (2020). Respiratory Muscle Rehabilitation in Patients with Prolonged Mechanical Ventilation: A Targeted Approach. *Critical Care : the Official Journal of the Critical Care Forum*, *24*(1), 103. DOI: 10.1186/s13054-020-2783-0 PMID: 32204719

Brown, R. P., Gerbarg, P. L., & Muench, F. (2013). Breathing practices for treatment of psychiatric and stress-related medical conditions. *The Psychiatric Clinics of North America*, *36*(1), 121–140. DOI: 10.1016/j.psc.2013.01.001 PMID: 23538082

Craig, C. L., Marshall, A. L., Sjöström, M., Bauman, A. E., Booth, M. L., Ainsworth, B. E., Pratt, M., Ekelund, U., Yngve, A., Sallis, J. F., & Oja, P. (2003). International physical activity questionnaire: 12-country reliability and validity. *Medicine and Science in Sports and Exercise*, *35*(8), 1381–1395. DOI: 10.1249/01.MSS.0000078924.61453.FB PMID: 12900694

Darling-White, M., & Huber, J. E. (2017). The Impact of Expiratory Muscle Strength Training on Speech Breathing in Individuals With Parkinson's Disease: A Preliminary Study. *American Journal of Speech-Language Pathology, 26*(4), 1159–1166. DOI: 10.1044/2017_AJSLP-16-0132 PMID: 29114773

Elias, L. R., Miskowiak, K. W., Vale, A. M., Köhler, C. A., Kjærstad, H. L., Stubbs, B., Kessing, L. V., Vieta, E., Maes, M., Goldstein, B. I., & Carvalho, A. F. (2017). Cognitive Impairment in Euthymic Pediatric Bipolar Disorder: A Systematic Review and Meta-Analysis. *Journal of the American Academy of Child and Adolescent Psychiatry, 56*(4), 286–296. DOI: 10.1016/j.jaac.2017.01.008 PMID: 28335872

Ercan Doğu, S., & Gündoğmuş, A. G. (2022). The Relationship Between Physical Activity Level and Quality of Life in Individuals with Bipolar Disorder. *International Journal of Disabilities Sports & Health Sciences, 5*(2), 83–89. DOI: 10.33438/ijdshs.1137254

Erturk, N., Celik, A., Yaman, S. K., Yaman, H., Unal, F., & Kutukcu, E. C. (2024, December). Expiratory muscle strength training reduces oxidative stress and systemic inflammation in men with obstructive sleep apnea syndrome: A double-blinded, randomized parallel trial. *Sleep (Basel), 47*(12), zsae221. DOI: 10.1093/sleep/zsae221 PMID: 39297486

Falk, J., Saha, S., & McGrath, J. J. (2022). Respiratory disorders in people with severe mental illness: A review. *The Lancet. Psychiatry, 9*(3), 198–210. PMID: 35183279

First, M. B., Clarke, D. E., Yousif, L., Eng, A. M., Gogtay, N., & Appelbaum, P. S. (2023). DSM-5-TR: Rationale, Process, and Overview of Changes. *Psychiatric Services (Washington, D.C.), 74*(8), 869–875. DOI: 10.1176/appi.ps.20220334 PMID: 36510761

Firth, J., Firth, J. A., Stubbs, B., Vancampfort, D., Schuch, F. B., Hallgren, M., Veronese, N., Yung, A. R., & Sarris, J. (2018). Association Between Muscular Strength and Cognition in People With Major Depression or Bipolar Disorder and Healthy Controls. *JAMA Psychiatry, 75*(7), 740–746. DOI: 10.1001/jamapsychiatry.2018.0503 PMID: 29710135

Firth, J., Solmi, M., Wootton, R. E., Vancampfort, D., Schuch, F. B., Hoare, E., & Stubbs, B. (2021). A meta-review of "lifestyle psychiatry": The role of exercise, smoking, diet and sleep in the prevention and treatment of mental disorders. *World Psychiatry; Official Journal of the World Psychiatric Association (WPA), 20*(3), 388–403. DOI: 10.1002/wps.20873 PMID: 32931092

GBD 2019 Mental Disorders Collaborators (2022). Global, regional, and national burden of 12 mental disorders in 204 countries and territories, 1990-2019: a systematic analysis for the Global Burden of Disease Study 2019. *The lancet. Psychiatry, 9*(2), 137–150.

Gibbons, W. J., Fruchter, N., Sloan, S., & Levy, R. D. (2001). Reference values for a multiple repetition 6-minute walk test in healthy adults older than 20 years. *Journal of Cardiopulmonary Rehabilitation, 21*(2), 87–93. DOI: 10.1097/00008483-200103000-00005 PMID: 11314289

Göçen, H. B., & Özden, A. V. (2024). Autonomic Dysfunction in Psychiatric Disorders. Psikiyatride Güncel Yaklaşımlar -. *Psikiyatride Güncel Yaklasimlar, 16*(3), 401–409. DOI: 10.18863/pgy.1329118

Gosselink, R., De Vos, J., van den Heuvel, S. P., Segers, J., Decramer, M., & Kwakkel, G. (2011). Impact of inspiratory muscle training in patients with COPD: What is the evidence? *The European Respiratory Journal, 37*(2), 416–425. DOI: 10.1183/09031936.00031810 PMID: 21282809

Gosselink, R., De Vos, J., van den Heuvel, S. P., Segers, J., Decramer, M., & Kwakkel, G. (2018). Impact of inspiratory muscle training in patients with COPD: What is the evidence? *The European Respiratory Journal, 51*(2), 1701964. PMID: 21282809

Hayes, J. F., Miles, J., Walters, K., King, M., & Osborn, D. P. (2015). A systematic review and meta-analysis of premature mortality in bipolar affective disorder. *Acta Psychiatrica Scandinavica, 131*(6), 417–425. DOI: 10.1111/acps.12408 PMID: 25735195

Helbig, S., Zell, E., & Backes, A.. (2023). Effectiveness of a Personalized Exercise Program to Increase Physical Activity and Improve Mental Health in Patients with Depression: A Randomized Controlled Trial. *Frontiers in Psychiatry, 14*, 10338920.

HÜZMELİ. İ., & KATAYIFÇI, N., (2022). Solunum Kas Eğitimi. Solunumun Temel Değerlendirmesi (pp.283-301), Livre de Lyon.

Kang, G. E., Mickey, B. J., McInnis, M. G., Krembs, B. S., & Gross, M. M. (2018). Motor behavior characteristics in various phases of bipolar disorder revealed through biomechanical analysis: Quantitative measures of activity and energy variables during gait and sit-to-walk. *Psychiatry Research, 269*, 93–101. DOI: 10.1016/j.psychres.2018.08.062 PMID: 30145308

Kharabian Masouleh, S., Arélin, K., Horstmann, A., Lampe, L., Kipping, J. A., Luck, T., Riedel-Heller, S. G., Schroeter, M. L., Stumvoll, M., Villringer, A., & Witte, A. V. (2016). Higher body mass index in older adults is associated with lower gray matter volume: Implications for memory performance. *Neurobiology of Aging*, *40*, 1–10. DOI: 10.1016/j.neurobiolaging.2015.12.020 PMID: 26973099

Kilbourne, A. M., Morden, N. E., Austin, K., Ilgen, M., McCarthy, J. F., Dalack, G., & Blow, F. C. (2009). Excess heart-disease-related mortality in a national study of patients with mental disorders: Identifying modifiable risk factors. *General Hospital Psychiatry*, *31*(6), 555–563. DOI: 10.1016/j.genhosppsych.2009.07.008 PMID: 19892214

Kimhy, D., Vakhrusheva, J., Bartels, M. N., Armstrong, H. F., Ballon, J. S., Khan, S., Chang, R. W., Hansen, M. C., Ayanruoh, L., Lister, A., Castrén, E., Smith, E. E., & Sloan, R. P. (2015). The Impact of Aerobic Exercise on Brain-Derived Neurotrophic Factor and Neurocognition in Individuals With Schizophrenia: A Single-Blind, Randomized Clinical Trial. *Schizophrenia Bulletin*, *41*(4), 859–868. DOI: 10.1093/schbul/sbv022 PMID: 25805886

Laguna-Muñoz, D., Jiménez-Peinado, A., Jaén-Moreno, M. J., Camacho-Rodríguez, C., Del Pozo, G. I., Vieta, E., Caballero-Villarraso, J., Khan, M. I., Rico-Villademoros, F., & Sarramea, F. (2025). Respiratory disease in people with bipolar disorder: A systematic review and meta-analysis. *Molecular Psychiatry*, *30*(2), 777–785. DOI: 10.1038/s41380-024-02793-1 PMID: 39543369

Launders, N., Dotsikas, K., Marston, L., Price, G., Osborn, D. P. J., & Hayes, J. F. (2022). The impact of comorbid severe mental illness and common chronic physical health conditions on hospitalisation: A systematic review and meta-analysis. *PLoS One*, *17*(8), e0272498. DOI: 10.1371/journal.pone.0272498 PMID: 35980891

Laveneziana, P., Albuquerque, A., Aliverti, A., Babb, T., Barreiro, E., Dres, M., Dubé, B. P., Fauroux, B., Gea, J., Guenette, J. A., Hudson, A. L., Kabitz, H. J., Laghi, F., Langer, D., Luo, Y. M., Neder, J. A., O'Donnell, D., Polkey, M. I., Rabinovich, R. A., & Verges, S. (2019). ERS statement on respiratory muscle testing at rest and during exercise. *The European Respiratory Journal*, *53*(6), 1801214. DOI: 10.1183/13993003.01214-2018 PMID: 30956204

Lista-Paz, A., Langer, D., Barral-Fernández, M., Quintela-Del-Río, A., Gimeno-Santos, E., Arbillaga-Etxarri, A., Torres-Castro, R., Vilaró Casamitjana, J., Varas de la Fuente, A. B., Serrano Veguillas, C., Bravo Cortés, P., Martín Cortijo, C., García Delgado, E., Herrero-Cortina, B., Valera, J. L., Fregonezi, G. A. F., González Montañez, C., Martín-Valero, R., Francín-Gallego, M., & González-Doniz, L. (2023). Maximal Respiratory Pressure Reference Equations in Healthy Adults and Cut-off Points for Defining Respiratory Muscle Weakness. *Archivos de Bronconeumología, 59*(12), 813–820. DOI: 10.1016/j.arbres.2023.08.016 PMID: 37839949

Liu, Y., Yan, T., Chu, J. M., Chen, Y., Dunnett, S., Ho, Y. S., Wong, G. T., & Chang, R. C. (2019). The beneficial effects of physical exercise in the brain and related pathophysiological mechanisms in neurodegenerative diseases. *Laboratory Investigation, 99*(7), 943–957. DOI: 10.1038/s41374-019-0232-y PMID: 30808929

Mahler, D. A., & Wells, C. K. (1988). Evaluation of clinical methods for rating dyspnea. *Chest, 93*(3), 580–586. DOI: 10.1378/chest.93.3.580 PMID: 3342669

Manji, H. K., Quiroz, J. A., Payne, J. L., Singh, J., Lopes, B. P., Viegas, J. S., & Zarate, C. A. (2003). The underlying neurobiology of bipolar disorder. *World Psychiatry; Official Journal of the World Psychiatric Association (WPA), 2*(3), 136–146. PMID: 16946919

McConnell, A. Implementing respiratory muscle training. Chapter 6 in: Respiratory Muscle Training: Theory and Practice. Elsevier, 2013. DOI: 10.1016/B978-0-7020-5020-6.00006-6

McConnell, A. K., & Romer, L. M. (2019). Respiratory muscle training in healthy humans: Resolving the controversy. *International Journal of Sports Medicine, 40*(8), 497–504. PMID: 15162248

Mota, S., Güell, R., Barreiro, E., Solanes, I., Ramírez-Sarmiento, A., Orozco-Levi, M., Casan, P., Gea, J., & Sanchis, J. (2007). Clinical outcomes of expiratory muscle training in severe COPD patients. *Respiratory Medicine, 101*(3), 516–524. DOI: 10.1016/j.rmed.2006.06.024 PMID: 16942867

Neves, N. A. R. (2011). Técnicas de respiração para a redução do estresse em terapia cognitivo comportamental. *Arq Med Hosp Fac Cienc Med Santa Casa São Paulo, 56*(3), 158–168.

Oliva, V., Fico, G., De Prisco, M., Gonda, X., Rosa, A. R., & Vieta, E. (2025). Bipolar disorders: An update on critical aspects. *The Lancet Regional Health. Europe, 48*, 101135. DOI: 10.1016/j.lanepe.2024.101135 PMID: 39811787

Pascoe, M., Parker, A., & Van Vliet, H.. (2021). Individualized Exercise in the Treatment of Depression: The IDEA Randomized Controlled Trial Protocol. *Contemporary Clinical Trials*, *105*, 106389.

Pereira, C. S., Padoan, C. S., Garcia, L. F., Patusco, L., & Magalhães, P. V. S. (2019). Barriers and facilitators perceived by people with bipolar disorder for the practice of exercise: A qualitative study. *Trends in Psychiatry and Psychotherapy*, *41*(1), 1–8. DOI: 10.1590/2237-6089-2017-0069 PMID: 30994778

Roldán, A., Monteagudo, P., Cordellat, A., Sanchis-Soler, G., & Blasco-Lafarga, C. (2021). Inspiratory Muscle Strength and Cardiorespiratory Fitness Association With Health-Related Quality of Life in Healthy Older Adults. *Frontiers in Sports and Active Living*, *3*, 624947. DOI: 10.3389/fspor.2021.624947 PMID: 33817635

Romer, L. M., Polkey, M. I., & Verges, S. (2022). Respiratory muscle training and cardiovascular health: Current evidence and future directions. *Journal of Applied Physiology*, *132*(4), 1191–1202.

Rosenbaum, S., Tiedemann, A., Sherrington, C., Curtis, J., & Ward, P. B. (2022). Physical activity interventions for people with mental illness: A systematic review and meta-analysis. *Journal of Psychiatric Research*, *153*, 25–35.

Ruiz-Rull, C., Jaén-Moreno, M. J., Del Pozo, G. I., Gómez, C., Montiel, F. J., Alcántara, M., Carrión, L., Chauca, G. M., Feu, N., Guler, I., Rico-Villademoros, F., Camacho-Rodríguez, C., Gutierrez-Rojas, L., Mannino, D., & Sarramea, F. (2024). Low lung function in Bipolar Disorder and Schizophrenia: A hidden risk. *Frontiers in Physiology*, *15*, 1335798. DOI: 10.3389/fphys.2024.1335798 PMID: 38737830

Schuch, F. B., Vancampfort, D., Firth, J., Rosenbaum, S., Ward, P. B., Silva, E. S., & Stubbs, B. (2020). Physical activity and sedentary behavior in people with major depressive disorder: A systematic review and meta-analysis. Jaffray E. *Physical Therapy in Mental Health*, *15*(1), 62–74.

Serafim, S. D., da Ponte, F. D. R., Lima, F. M., Martins, D. S., Rosa, A. R., & Kunz, M. (2019). Effects of deep breathing in patients with bipolar disorder. *Perspectives in Psychiatric Care*, *55*(1), 119–125. DOI: 10.1111/ppc.12325 PMID: 30189115

Shei, R. J., Paris, H. L., Sogard, A. S., & Mickleborough, T. D. (2022). Time to Move Beyond a "One-Size Fits All" Approach to Inspiratory Muscle Training. *Frontiers in Physiology*, *12*, 766346. DOI: 10.3389/fphys.2021.766346 PMID: 35082689

Shei, R. J., Paris, H. L., Wilhite, D. P., Chapman, R. F., & Mickleborough, T. D. (2016). The role of inspiratory muscle training in athletic performance: A systematic review. *Sports Medicine (Auckland, N.Z.)*, *46*(5), 707–717.

Stubbs, B., Koyanagi, A., Schuch, F. B., Firth, J., Rosenbaum, S., Veronese, N., Solmi, M., Mugisha, J., & Vancampfort, D. (2016). Physical activity and depression: A large cross-sectional, population-based study across 36 low- and middle-income countries. *Acta Psychiatrica Scandinavica, 134*(6), 546–556. DOI: 10.1111/acps.12654 PMID: 27704532

Stubbs, B., Vancampfort, D., Firth, J., Hallgren, M., Schuch, F. B., Mugisha, J., & Rosenbaum, S. (2018). Physical activity and serious mental illness: A systematic review and meta-analysis of cardiorespiratory fitness. *Acta Psychiatrica Scandinavica, 138*(6), 464–478.

Stubbs, B., Vancampfort, D., Hallgren, M., Firth, J., Veronese, N., Solmi, M., Brand, S., Cordes, J., Malchow, B., Gerber, M., Schmitt, A., Correll, C. U., De Hert, M., Gaughran, F., Schneider, F., Kinnafick, F., Falkai, P., Möller, H. J., & Kahl, K. G. (2018). EPA guidance on physical activity as a treatment for severe mental illness: A meta-review of the evidence and Position Statement from the European Psychiatric Association (EPA), supported by the International Organization of Physical Therapists in Mental Health (IOPTMH). *European Psychiatry : the Journal of the Association of European Psychiatrists, 54*, 124–144. DOI: 10.1016/j.eurpsy.2018.07.004 PMID: 30257806

Svensson, M., Erhardt, S., Hållmarker, U., James, S., & Deierborg, T. (2022). A physically active lifestyle is associated with lower long-term incidence of bipolar disorder in a population-based, large-scale study. *International Journal of Bipolar Disorders, 10*(1), 26. DOI: 10.1186/s40345-022-00272-6 PMID: 36316595

Swartz, H. A., & Swanson, J. (2014). Psychotherapy for Bipolar Disorder in Adults: A Review of the Evidence. *Focus - American Psychiatric Publishing, 12*(3), 251–266. DOI: 10.1176/appi.focus.12.3.251 PMID: 26279641

Sylvia, L. G., Friedman, E. S., Kocsis, J. H., Bernstein, E. E., Brody, B. D., Kinrys, G., Kemp, D. E., Shelton, R. C., McElroy, S. L., Bobo, W. V., Kamali, M., McInnis, M. G., Tohen, M., Bowden, C. L., Ketter, T. A., Deckersbach, T., Calabrese, J. R., Thase, M. E., Reilly-Harrington, N. A., & Nierenberg, A. A. (2013). Association of exercise with quality of life and mood symptoms in a comparative effectiveness study of bipolar disorder. *Journal of Affective Disorders, 151*(2), 722–727. DOI: 10.1016/j.jad.2013.07.031 PMID: 23993440

Thomson, D., Turner, A., Lauder, S., Gigler, M. E., Berk, L., Singh, A. B., Pasco, J. A., Berk, M., & Sylvia, L. (2015). A brief review of exercise, bipolar disorder, and mechanistic pathways. *Frontiers in Psychology, 6*, 147. DOI: 10.3389/fpsyg.2015.00147 PMID: 25788889

Thomson, D., Turner, A., Lauder, S., Gigler, M. E., Berk, L., Singh, A. B., Pasco, J. A., Berk, M., & Sylvia, L. (2015). A brief review of exercise, bipolar disorder, and mechanistic pathways. *Frontiers in Psychology*, *6*, 147. DOI: 10.3389/fpsyg.2015.00147 PMID: 25788889

Vancampfort, D., Firth, J., Schuch, F. B., Rosenbaum, S., Mugisha, J., Hallgren, M., & Stubbs, B. (2017). Physical activity and sedentary behavior in people with major depressive disorder: A systematic review and meta-analysis. Jaffray E. *Physical Therapy in Mental Health*, *13*(3), 254–271.

Vancampfort, D., Hagemann, N., Wyckaert, S., Rosenbaum, S., Stubbs, B., Firth, J., Schuch, F. B., Probst, M., & Sienaert, P. (2017). Higher cardio-respiratory fitness is associated with increased mental and physical quality of life in people with bipolar disorder: A controlled pilot study. *Psychiatry Research*, *256*, 219–224. DOI: 10.1016/j.psychres.2017.06.066 PMID: 28646785

Vancampfort, D., Rosenbaum, S., Schuch, F., Ward, P. B., Richards, J., Mugisha, J., Probst, M., & Stubbs, B. (2017). Cardiorespiratory Fitness in Severe Mental Illness: A Systematic Review and Meta-analysis. *Sports Medicine (Auckland, N.Z.)*, *47*(2), 343–352. DOI: 10.1007/s40279-016-0574-1 PMID: 27299747

Van Dixhoorn, J. (2007). Whole-body breathing: A systems perspective on respiratory retraining. In Lehrer, P. M., Woolfolk, R. L., & Sime, W. E. (Eds.), *Principles and practice of stress management* (3rd ed., pp. 291–332). The Guilford Press.

Weiner, M., Warren, L., & Fiedorowicz, J. G. (2011). Cardiovascular morbidity and mortality in bipolar disorder. *Annals of Clinical Psychiatry*, *23*(1), 40–47. DOI: 10.1177/104012371102300107 PMID: 21318195

Chapter 6
Interfacing Chronic Illness and Psychological Resilience:
Case-Based Perspectives on Integrative Psychotherapeutic Interventions

Jennifer Marshall
http://orcid.org/0009-0007-7526-208X
Always Glow Psychology, USA

EXECUTIVE SUMMARY

Chronic physical illnesses frequently co-occur with mental health disorders, complicating patient care. This chapter examines the intersection of chronic illness and psychological resilience through a biopsychosocial lens. It reviews epidemiological data illustrating high rates of depression, anxiety, and trauma-related symptoms among individuals with conditions like diabetes, cancer, and rare diseases. Theoretical frameworks (biopsychosocial model, developmental, and family systems theories) inform the discussion. Three case studies (adolescent diabetes, adult cancer survivor, child with a rare disorder) demonstrate integrative psychotherapeutic interventions, cognitive-behavioral, trauma-focused, narrative, and family therapies tailored to whole-person care. Emphasis is placed on collaboration with medical teams via integrated care models to address both physical and mental needs. The chapter highlights how coordinated, holistic approaches bolster patient and family resilience, improving outcomes across the lifespan.

DOI: 10.4018/979-8-3373-3084-6.ch006

1. INTRODUCTION

Chronic physical illness and mental health disorders often go hand-in-hand. Epidemiological studies show that having a chronic medical condition significantly increases the likelihood of a comorbid psychiatric disorder (Adams et al., 2019; Jürisson et al., 2021). For example, one population study found that about 13% of individuals with at least one chronic disease also had an anxiety or mood disorder (Jürisson et al., 2021). In youth, a national U.S. cohort observed a two-year incidence of new mental health diagnoses of 11.5% in those with chronic physical conditions vs. 7.1% in peers without (a 51% relative increase). Such comorbidities are not just common, they worsen quality of life and complicate illness management. Depression or anxiety superimposed on a chronic illness is linked to poorer adherence to medical regimens, higher complication rates, and greater healthcare utilization (Gupta et al., 2024; Nair et al., 2021). In short, mental health is a central component of living with chronic illness, not a peripheral concern.

The biopsychosocial framework provides a guiding paradigm for understanding these phenomena (Engel, 1977). This model posits that health outcomes emerge from the interplay of biological factors (disease processes, genetics), psychological factors (emotions, coping behaviors), and social factors (family support, culture, socioeconomic status) (Engel, 1977). In contrast to a purely biomedical view, the biopsychosocial approach recognizes that a patient's experience of illness is shaped by mind–body interactions and environmental context. For instance, effectively managing diabetes or kidney disease depends not only on medications but also on the patient's stress levels, health beliefs, and support network (Nair et al., 2021). Adopting this holistic lens, the present chapter explores how psychological resilience can be fostered alongside medical treatment. Resilience refers to the ability to adapt and even grow in the face of adversity. Here, we aim to illustrate how collaborative, whole-person care can bolster resilience in patients and families coping with chronic illnesses.

The chapter proceeds as follows. First, we review key epidemiological trends and theoretical foundations relevant to chronic illness and mental health (Section 2). We then present three case studies (Section 3) – an adolescent with type 1 diabetes, an adult cancer survivor with trauma, and a child with a rare genetic disorder – to demonstrate integrative psychotherapeutic interventions in context. Each vignette highlights assessment, interventions (e.g., cognitive-behavioral therapy, narrative reframing, somatic techniques), outcomes, and cultural considerations. Next, we discuss strategies for integration with medical teams (Section 4), examining collaborative care models, interdisciplinary communication, ethical issues, and insurance factors in implementing integrative care. Finally, a brief conclusion (Section 5) summarizes take-home messages and future directions. Throughout, in-text citations and a reference list are provided per APA 7th edition guidelines, and a figure and table illustrate key concepts (see Figure 1 and Table 1). By combining up-to-date research with case-based perspectives, this chapter underscores the importance of attending to the psychological and social dimensions of chronic illness, and demonstrates practical approaches to do so.

2. EPIDEMIOLOGY AND THEORETICAL FOUNDATIONS

Prevalence and Impact: Chronic physical illnesses have a well-documented bidirectional relationship with mental health disorders across the lifespan (Gupta et al., 2024; National Cancer Institute [NCI], n.d.). In children and adolescents, having a chronic condition confers a markedly higher risk of developing a psychiatric condition. In the United States, Adams et al. (2019) reported that youth with chronic physical conditions had about a 50% greater risk of incident mental health diagnosis compared to those without such conditions. Specifically, over two years, 11.5% of youth with chronic illness developed a new mental disorder (commonly anxiety or depression), versus 7.1% of otherwise healthy youth. This elevated risk is partly mediated by illness-related activity limitations that disrupt normal development (e.g., school attendance, peer activities). By adulthood, the cumulative impact is substantial: for instance, individuals with diabetes have roughly double the odds of depression compared to non-diabetic individuals (Anderson et al., 2001). Meta-analyses indicate that up to 20–30% of patients with chronic illnesses like diabetes or heart disease experience clinical depression, a prevalence about twice that of the general population (Anderson et al., 2001; NCI, n.d.). Similar patterns are observed in diseases such as cancer and chronic lung disease. A National Cancer Institute review notes that depression affects approximately 25% of cancer patients, significantly higher than in cancer-free populations (NCI, n.d.). Anxiety and trauma-related symptoms are also common; one study found that about one-third of cancer survivors report at least moderate post-traumatic stress symptoms during or after treatment (Ochoa et al., 2017). Notably, when chronic illness and mental disorders co-occur, outcomes on both sides worsen. Patients with comorbid depression tend to have poorer adherence to treatment and disease control (e.g., worse glycemic control in diabetes) (Gupta et al., 2024), higher rates of complications and hospitalizations, and elevated mortality risk in some cases (Gupta et al., 2024; Nair et al., 2021). Among adolescents with type 1 diabetes, for example, depression has been associated with an 87% increased risk of diabetic ketoacidosis and doubled frequency of severe glycemic events compared to non-depressed peers (Gupta et al., 2024). In older adults, the accumulation of multiple chronic diseases further compounds depression risk: each additional illness increases the likelihood of depressive symptoms, reflecting an additive burden of stress and disability (DeLong et al., 2025). These epidemiological findings underscore that mental health is inseparable from physical health. Addressing this "whole health" reality is essential to improving quality of life and functional outcomes for individuals with chronic conditions.

Biopsychosocial and Developmental Frameworks: The biopsychosocial model introduced by Engel (1977) provides a conceptual foundation for integrative care. It asserts that to understand a patient's health, one must consider biological factors (e.g., disease pathology, medication effects), psychological factors (thoughts, emotions, behaviors), and social factors (family, culture, socioeconomic context) (Engel, 1977). In chronic illness, this means that effective management goes beyond treating the organ system alone. For instance, managing end-stage renal disease involves not only dialysis and medications but also psychological support for coping with life changes and social services to address transportation or financial barriers (Nair et al., 2021). Figure 1 illustrates the dynamic interplay of these domains in a chronic illness care pathway. Developmental psychology further refines this perspective by noting that the impact of chronic illness varies with the patient's life stage. A diagnosis in childhood or adolescence can disrupt normal developmental tasks (school engagement, identity formation, autonomy). Indeed, children with chronic conditions have approximately 2-3 times higher rates of emotional disorders like anxiety or depression compared to their healthy peers (Stein, 2022). Still, it is critical to recognize that most youth are resilient: as Stein (2022) observed, "the vast majority of children with chronic conditions do in fact thrive emotionally" *(*Stein, 2022*)*, given adequate support. This paradox, heightened risk yet potential for resilience, suggests the importance of early identification and intervention. Pediatric psychologists recommend routine mental health screening in specialty clinics (e.g., diabetes or cystic fibrosis clinics) so that issues can be caught early and addressed before worsening *(*Stein, 2022). In adulthood, chronic illness often intersects with vocational and family roles. The onset of illness in mid-life can threaten one's career, financial stability, and sense of identity as a provider, which can precipitate depression or demoralization. Older adults with chronic diseases may face social isolation or cognitive decline that further complicates illness management. At the same time, adults typically have more cognitive maturity and life experience to draw upon, which can aid in coping (e.g., utilizing problem-solving skills or past adversity mastery). Thus, a lifespan developmental view helps tailor interventions to the patient's age and stage.

Relational and Systemic Influences: Chronic illness is frequently described as a "family affair." Family systems theory emphasizes that an illness in one member reverberates through the entire family's functioning. In pediatric chronic illness, parental coping and the parent–child relationship are pivotal in the child's adjustment (Stein, 2022). Parents who maintain a positive outlook and effective problem-solving can model resilience for the child, whereas parental distress may heighten the child's anxiety. Sibling dynamics are also affected: siblings of children with serious illnesses or disabilities sometimes experience feelings of being "overshadowed" or neglected, or conversely take on caregiving roles beyond their years (Baker & Claridge, 2023). Qualitative research by Baker and Claridge (2023) found that families dealing with childhood chronic illness report unique challenges in family routines, sibling relationships, and marital stress, yet many also develop greater cohesion and resilience through the experience. In adult populations, a supportive spouse or family network can act as a buffer against depression. Studies of chronic cardiac patients, for example, show that those with strong family support have better medication adherence and fewer depressive symptoms than those socially isolated (Martire & Schulz, 2007). From a systems perspective, factors beyond the immediate family, such as healthcare systems, community resources, and culture, also play a role. Social determinants of health (like poverty, education, and insurance coverage) strongly influence mental health outcomes in chronic illness. A recent U.S. study noted that uninsured individuals with multiple chronic diseases had the highest rates of psychological distress (around 41%), far exceeding those who were insured (Adzrago et al., 2024). Barriers such as stigma or fragmented care systems can impede access to mental health care for chronic illness patients (Wenke et al., 2022). Conversely, community resources (support groups, religious communities, patient advocacy organizations) can provide crucial emotional support and practical assistance. In recognition of these multilevel influences, contemporary frameworks (e.g., "ecological" models of illness) call for interventions that span the individual, family, and system. For instance, the *Children's Oncology Group* endorses family-centered care in pediatric cancer, which involves psychosocial services for parents and siblings, not just the patient. In summary, a theoretical foundation that integrates biopsychosocial, developmental, and family systemic perspectives is essential for guiding interventions. It reminds clinicians to assess and address not only the disease itself, but also the emotional well-being of the patient, the functioning of the family, and the broader context in which care occurs. These principles will be evident in the case studies and approaches discussed in subsequent sections. *(Figure 1 provides a visual summary of the biopsychosocial integrative care model.)*

Figure 1. Biopsychosocial Integrative Care Flowchart.

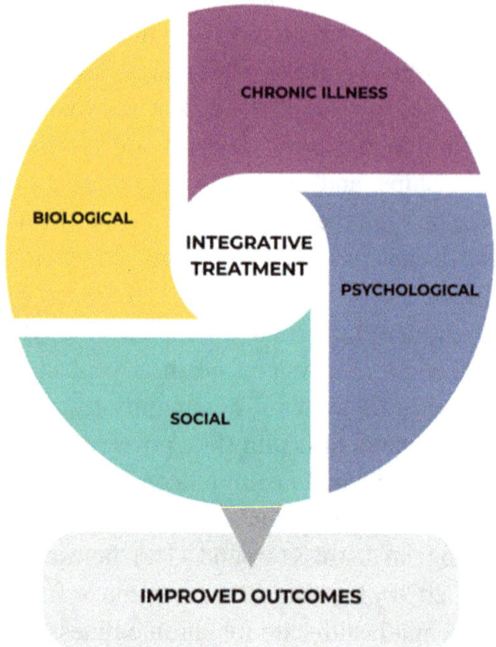

This figure illustrates how biological, psychological, and social factors intersect in chronic illness management.

3. CLINICAL CASE STUDIES

To ground these concepts, we present three case vignettes illustrating integrative psychotherapeutic interventions alongside medical care. Each case is drawn from a composite of clinical scenarios (with identifying details changed) and supported by relevant studies. We examine the patient's diagnoses, psychosocial issues, and treatment plan, noting how interventions are tailored to individual and cultural context. Table 1 summarizes the cases, interventions, outcomes, and key considerations.

Case 1: Adolescent With Type 1 Diabetes Mellitus (T1D)

Profile: *"A 15-year-old girl with T1D (diagnosed 5 years ago) is referred by her endocrinologist for depression and worsening glycemic control. She reports feeling 'burned out' by diabetes, increasingly isolating from friends because she feels different, and anxiety about long-term complications. Her hemoglobin A1c is 9.5% (above target), and she has missed multiple clinic appointments."* This scenario highlights common challenges in adolescents with chronic illness: the burden of daily disease management during a developmental stage focused on peer acceptance and autonomy.

Diagnostic considerations: The patient meets criteria for major depressive disorder (low mood, withdrawal, fatigue) in the context of diabetes. She also exhibits diabetes-specific distress, a well-recognized syndrome of frustration, fear, and burnout related to managing diabetes (Gupta et al., 2024). Depression and diabetes distress often overlap, and both are associated with poor adherence to glucose monitoring and insulin use (Gupta et al., 2024). Indeed, research shows depressed adolescents with T1D have significantly higher risks of acute complications – one study found an 87% higher incidence of diabetic ketoacidosis (DKA) among teens with T1D who had depression, compared to those without depression (Gupta et al., 2024). This patient's elevated A1c and disengagement from care are red flags for potential DKA or other complications. A thorough evaluation would include screening for any suicidal ideation or risky behaviors (e.g., insulin omission to lose weight, sometimes termed "diabulimia"). Culturally, her family background might influence her experience: for instance, attitudes toward mental health treatment or the role of family in diabetes care can vary across cultures. If she comes from a community where illness is a family-managed issue, involving her parents closely would be important; if she values independence, the approach might differ. Socioeconomic factors are also pertinent; insulin pumps and continuous glucose monitors are costly, and financial strain can exacerbate stress. These contextual factors will shape the intervention plan.

Interventions: A multifaceted cognitive-behavioral therapy (CBT) program is indicated to address both depression and diabetes self-management. CBT has shown efficacy in adolescents with T1D, being feasible and acceptable in this population (Rechenberg & Koerner, 2021). Rechenberg and Koerner's (2021) integrative review found that CBT interventions led to improvements in adolescents' depressive and anxiety symptoms, coping skills, and quality of life, with some studies noting better adherence and glycemic trends as well. In this patient's therapy, CBT would involve cognitive restructuring of negative beliefs ("I'll never be healthy" or "diabetes makes me a burden"), behavioral activation (re-engaging in enjoyable activities and diabetes routines), and problem-solving for treatment adherence. Importantly, diabetes education can be woven in so that she builds confidence in carb counting, insulin dosing, etc., rather than feeling overwhelmed. Sessions might include reviewing her glucose logs to identify patterns and collaboratively brainstorming solutions (turning this into a mastery experience). Because family dynamics are crucial, family-based therapy will be integrated. A behavioral family systems therapy approach can help address parent–teen conflict around diabetes tasks and improve communication (e.g., instead of nagging, parents learn to use supportive prompts; the teen practices expressing her need for autonomy). The family could set up a contract where the teen gets increased privileges as she meets self-care goals, aligning responsibility with growing independence. The inclusion of family is supported by evidence that involving caregivers can improve diabetes outcomes in youth (Stein, 2022). Another modality is narrative therapy: helping the patient "re-author" her personal illness narrative. For example, she might write a short story or letter to her diabetes, reframing it from an enemy into a challenge she is overcoming (transforming her identity from a victim of illness into a survivor or mentor). Such narrative reframing can empower adolescents, though formal research on diabetes is still emerging. Additionally, somatic and mindfulness techniques can be valuable for managing diabetes-related stress. Brief Acceptance and Commitment Therapy (ACT) exercises, focusing on acceptance of difficult feelings and commitment to values, have shown promise. A recent study of a 4-session ACT workshop for youth with T1D reported reduced stress levels and increased illness acceptance post-intervention. Teaching her mindfulness breathing to cope with needle anxiety or guiding her through a relaxation visualization during blood sugar checks may help lower her physiological arousal and frustration. The plan might also include referring her to a peer support group, either an in-person teen diabetes group or online forum, to combat her sense of isolation. Sometimes connecting with peers who "get it" dramatically reduces the feeling of being different. In summary, the therapeutic strategy is comprehensive: treat the depression, re-engage her in diabetes care behaviors, involve the family for support and conflict resolution, and build her resilience and coping toolkit.

Outcomes and evaluation: Progress will be monitored via both psychological measures and medical metrics. Depression severity can be tracked with a tool like the Patient Health Questionnaire-9 (PHQ-9) for adolescents, looking for reductions in scores over time. Diabetes-related distress can be measured with the Problem Areas In Diabetes – Teen version (PAID-T) (Gupta et al., 2024). Improved scores on these scales would indicate she's feeling less burdened. On the medical side, glycemic control (HbA1c) is a key outcome: the goal is to lower her A1c toward the target (e.g. from 9.5% down closer to the 7–8% range) as she improves adherence. It's worth noting that psychosocial interventions in diabetes have sometimes yielded modest improvements in A1c alongside mental health benefits (Rechenberg & Koerner, 2021). For instance, Gupta et al. (2024) piloted an internet-based CBT program for teens with T1D and found trends of improved PHQ-9 depression scores *and* slight HbA1c reductions after completion. Other tangible outcomes include frequency of blood glucose checks per day, which could be tracked via her glucometer or pump data. An increase in checking from one to four times daily would be an objective sign of better self-management. Additionally, family functioning can be assessed with a diabetes family conflict scale; ideally, scores would drop as conflict reduces.

Qualitatively, the hope would be to see the patient resume social activities (perhaps she starts attending her school's art club again or goes out with friends on weekends). Safety outcomes are critical too: no episodes of DKA or severe hypoglycemia over the intervention period would be a positive indicator. Regular pediatric endocrine visits (with a mental health provider integrated or on consult) can ensure these outcomes are reviewed and the care plan adjusted accordingly.

Cultural and socioeconomic considerations: tailoring the approach to her context is essential. If the patient is from a minority ethnic background, culturally sensitive materials (in her preferred language, reflecting foods her family eats, etc.) will enhance engagement. For example, incorporating her family's dietary traditions into the meal-planning aspect of diabetes management can help her feel understood and avoid alienating the family. If mental health carries stigma in her community, the therapist might frame sessions as "stress management coaching" to improve acceptability. Socioeconomically, the team should assist with any insurance or resource barriers. This might involve a social worker helping the family apply for diabetes supplies coverage, or connecting them with a nonprofit that provides free continuous glucose monitors to teens. Given her missed appointments, transportation could be an issue; if so, providing telehealth therapy sessions or clinic shuttle information would address that logistical need. Lastly, consider the school environment: ensuring she has a 504 plan at school for her diabetes (allowing flexibility to manage glucose in class, etc.) and that school staff are educated about her needs will reduce school-related stress. The therapist could even have a meeting with her school counselor to coordinate support. By being mindful of these cultural and socioeconomic factors, the intervention is more likely to succeed and truly meet the patient where she is.

Further reading (Case 1): Young-Hyman et al. (2016) – ADA position statement on psychosocial care in diabetes (Young-Hyman et al., 2016); *Rechenberg & Koerner (2021)* – review of CBT interventions in youth T1D (Rechenberg & Koerner, 2021); *Alassaf et al. (2023)* – study on depression prevalence in adolescents with T1D in Jordan (illustrating global context) (Alassaf et al., 2023).

Case 2: Adult Cancer Survivor With Post-Traumatic Stress

Profile: *"A 45-year-old woman, one year in remission from Stage III breast cancer, presents with severe anxiety about her health. She describes nightmares of being back in the chemotherapy chair, panic attacks triggered by routine follow-up scans, and avoidance of anything related to cancer (she skips oncology appointments and won't talk about her treatment experiences). She feels on edge and unable to fully move on, saying she's 'waiting for the other shoe to drop.' Her family notes she startles easily and has become distant."* This case typifies Cancer-Related Post-Traumatic Stress (PTS), which can meet criteria for PTSD in some survivors.

Cancer is a life-threatening ordeal involving repeated traumas (diagnosis, surgeries, chemotherapy, etc.), and a subset of survivors experience lasting psychological trauma from it (NCI, n.d.).

Diagnostic considerations: The patient's symptoms, intrusive memories (nightmares), hyperarousal (startle, constant fear), and avoidance align with Post-Traumatic Stress Disorder (PTSD). In the context of cancer, these are often referred to as cancer-related PTSD or post-traumatic stress symptoms (PTSS). It's important to differentiate normal adjustment distress from PTSD: many survivors have some anxiety, but this patient's persistent, severe reactions (e.g., avoiding care to not trigger panic) suggest a clinical PTSD syndrome. Prevalence estimates vary, but research indicates about 10–20% of cancer survivors have significant PTSD symptoms, though only a smaller fraction meet full diagnostic criteria (American Cancer Society, 2024; NCI, n.d.). *Conditioning* likely plays a role: during her treatment, neutral cues (the smell of antiseptic, the hospital waiting room) became associated with intense fear and helplessness. Now those formerly neutral cues elicit panic even though the worst is over (NCI, n.d.). This classical conditioning phenomenon is common in cancer PTSD; for example, survivors often report that certain sounds (like a chemo pump beeping) or smells instantly bring back waves of dread (NCI, n.d.).We should confirm she meets all PTSD criteria: beyond intrusion and avoidance, does she have negative alterations in mood/cognition (e.g., survivor's guilt, negative beliefs like "I'm permanently damaged")? And duration >1 month, significant impairment (yes, she's missing appointments and straining family relations). We should also assess for demoralization syndrome, an existential distress common in advanced cancer characterized by hopelessness and meaninglessness. It can overlap with PTSD or depression. This patient's vigilant "waiting for disaster" mindset might also indicate fear of cancer recurrence, a very prevalent concern among survivors that can approach phobic intensity. Culturally, different backgrounds respond to trauma in various ways. If she's from a culture that stigmatizes mental illness, she may somaticize her distress (perhaps she has a lot of physical complaints like body aches that could be masked depression/PTSD). Or she may feel pressure to be "grateful and positive" post-cancer, making her ashamed to admit to trauma symptoms. Understanding her cultural context will guide how we frame therapy (for instance, some cultures might respond better to a spiritual or community-support framing). Socioeconomic considerations include the fact that many cancer survivors face financial toxicity (job loss, medical debt), which can exacerbate anxiety. We should inquire if she's under financial or work-related stress since finishing treatment. Additionally, her family's dynamic changed during her illness; perhaps her spouse became a caregiver, and now their roles are in flux, contributing to marital tension. All these factors inform a tailored treatment plan.

Interventions: The cornerstone of treatment will be trauma-focused psychotherapy. An evidence-based option is Trauma-Focused Cognitive Behavioral Therapy (TF-CBT), sometimes also referred to as Cognitive Processing Therapy when addressing PTSD. Through CBT techniques, she can learn to gradually face cancer-related memories (rather than avoid them) and reframe catastrophic thoughts. For example, she might repeatedly imagine walking into the oncology clinic (in a safe therapy setting) to desensitize her triggers, a technique known as exposure. Cognitive techniques will target her belief that "the cancer will come back and kill me", gently challenging this and finding more balanced thoughts (e.g., "I'm cancer-free now, and if it ever returns, I have coped before and will get care immediately"). A case report in a bone marrow transplant survivor demonstrated how a short course of CBT (about 10 sessions) significantly reduced PTSD flashbacks and avoidance behaviors (Jarero et al., 2018). Another promising therapy is Eye Movement Desensitization and Reprocessing (EMDR). EMDR is a somatic-experiential therapy where the patient processes traumatic memories while engaging in bilateral eye movements or tapping. Some pilot studies with cancer survivors have shown positive outcomes. For instance, a *randomized trial in Italy* compared EMDR to standard talk therapy for cancer patients with PTSD, and found EMDR led to greater symptom reduction one month post-treatment (Jarero et al., 2018). A systematic review noted that across several small studies (total N=140 patients), even brief EMDR protocols (as few as 2 sessions) appeared to reduce cancer-related psychological distress, though more research is needed (Portigliatti Pomeri et al., 2021).

Given EMDR's efficiency, if a trained clinician is available, this could be offered; many survivors appreciate that EMDR doesn't require extensive verbal recounting of the trauma, which can be appealing if they feel "talked out" about cancer.

In addition to directly trauma-focused therapies, meaning-centered and narrative therapies are highly relevant. Ochoa et al. (2017) tested a Positive Psychotherapy group intervention aimed at facilitating post-traumatic growth (PTG) in distressed cancer survivors. Over 12 weeks, participants engaged in exercises to find positive meaning in their cancer experience (e.g. identifying personal strengths gained, writing letters of gratitude, sharing their story). The results were impressive: compared to a control group, those in therapy had significantly lower PTSD symptoms and distress, and higher PTG, with benefits maintained at 3- and 12-month follow-ups (Ochoa et al., 2017). This approach could help our patient shift from seeing herself as a helpless victim of cancer to perhaps a mentor or someone with a renewed life purpose (for example, some survivors find meaning by volunteering or raising awareness). We could do individual meaning-centered therapy by using guided journaling prompts like "How has surviving cancer changed what's important to you?" or "Write about a personal strength that emerged through your cancer journey." These can catalyze a narrative of resilience.

Acceptance and Commitment Therapy (ACT) is another integrative modality suited here. ACT focuses on accepting what one cannot control (e.g. uncertainty of recurrence) and committing to values-based action. Sarizadeh et al. (2021) conducted an RCT of an 8-week ACT group for Iranian breast cancer patients with demoralization and trauma symptoms, and found ACT significantly reduced demoralization and PTSD scores compared to controls. Techniques from ACT that we might use include mindfulness exercises (to ground her during waves of anxiety) and values clarification (identifying core values like family or faith, and encouraging engagement in those areas despite fear). For example, she might value being a loving mother. ACT would encourage her to act in the service of that value (like spending quality time with her children or planning a family trip) even while anxiety is present, rather than putting life on hold until she "feels safe" (which may never happen if avoidance continues).

Beyond individual therapy, involving her family or spouse is important. We could hold a few couples therapy sessions to address the strain in her marriage. Often, spouses don't know how to support a survivor with PTSD; they might unintentionally enable avoidance ("If the hospital scares you, you don't have to go") or feel shut out by her emotional numbing. In therapy, the couple can improve communication, the patient practicing sharing her fears with her husband instead of withdrawing, and the spouse learning to listen without immediately trying to "fix" or minimize her feelings. We may also enlist the spouse's help in exposure practice (e.g., he could accompany her to the clinic waiting room as a support during initial exposures). Education about PTSD for the family is key so they understand her behaviors (e.g., hypervigilance) are not personal or "crazy" but a trauma reaction. If children are involved, family sessions can also guide the patient on how to talk to her kids about her anxiety in a reassuring way. Kids will notice mom is different, and open communication at an age-appropriate level can prevent them from developing their anxieties.

Lastly, connecting her to a cancer support group or survivorship program can reduce isolation. Many survivors feel that only others who've "been there" truly understand. Hearing peers describe similar fears can normalize her experience and provide new coping ideas. Some support groups incorporate relaxation training or guest experts (like yoga instructors or oncologists doing Q&A), which could indirectly benefit her PTSD symptoms by building a support network and confidence in follow-up care. If she has spiritual or religious beliefs, involving a chaplain or spiritual counselor could help address existential questions (why did I survive? what's my life purpose now?). In summary, an integrative plan for this patient might include: trauma-focused CBT or EMDR to process memories, meaning-centered therapy to foster growth, ACT skills for handling uncertainty, couple/family sessions to enlist social support, and engagement with survivor community resources.

Outcomes and evaluation: We will measure improvement primarily by PTSD symptom scales. The PTSD Checklist (PCL-5), a self-report, is one convenient tool; clinically significant change might be, for example, a drop of 10+ points from baseline. If at baseline she scored, say, 60 (indicative of severe PTSD), we'd aim for scores below 40 (mild range) after treatment – or at least below 33, which is a common cutoff for probable PTSD. Another measure, the Impact of Event Scale (IES-R), could also gauge intrusion and avoidance reductions. In the Ochoa et al. trial, patients in therapy had marked decreases in PTSD symptom scores compared to controls (Ochoa et al., 2017); we hope to mirror such outcomes in individualized form. Post-traumatic growth (PTG) can be assessed with the Post-Traumatic Growth Inventory. We're not only aiming to reduce negatives but increase positives – e.g., an increase in PTG scores indicating she recognizes some positive changes (new priorities, deeper relationships) since surviving cancer. This would signify that instead of just feeling broken by the experience, she perceives some personal growth. We will also track anxiety and depression with something like the Hospital Anxiety and Depression Scale (HADS), since these often co-occur; a drop in HADS scores would complement PTSD improvements. From a medical perspective, a critical outcome is that she attends her follow-up appointments. Avoidance of care is dangerous, so success would be her showing up for scheduled oncology visits and screenings. We might monitor that via her self-report or coordinating with her oncologist (with consent). We'd also hope to see improvement in sleep (fewer nightmares, better duration) and in daily functioning (perhaps she returns to work, or takes on a meaningful project). If family strain was high, maybe a relationship satisfaction questionnaire for her and her spouse before and after could capture improved family functioning. Even qualitative feedback is valuable: if she says, "I still get scared sometimes, but it doesn't control me and I'm back to living my life," that is a victory. Given the nature of chronic PTSD, we'll likely schedule a follow-up booster or phone call a few months after therapy to ensure gains are maintained, especially around the time of the annual scan (a known trigger event). Overall, a multi-metric evaluation of symptoms, growth, healthcare engagement, and family well-being will give a full picture of her progress.

Cultural and socioeconomic considerations: Sensitivity to culture will guide our approach throughout. If she comes from a background where emotional expression is restrained, we might use less confrontational techniques initially (perhaps more written homework or metaphorical discussions if direct talk is uncomfortable). If mental health care is stigmatized, we ensure privacy and possibly involve a culturally matched counselor or interpreter if language is a barrier. Suppose she's Latina and more comfortable in Spanish. Connecting her with a Spanish-speaking survivors support group or resources from LIVESTRONG en Español could make a difference. We also consider gender roles: in some cultures, women feel they must stay strong and not burden the family with their mental struggles. We would validate her strength while gently conveying that seeking help is not a weakness, and in fact will help her fulfill her role (e.g., "to be the rock for your family, you need to heal yourself, and counseling can help with that"). On the socioeconomic front, it's crucial to address any financial or insurance obstacles. If she lost her job during treatment, does she have insurance now? If not, a social worker might help her apply for Medicaid or disability benefits. Are medication costs (for say, anxiety meds or sleep aids) an issue? If yes, we'd look for patient assistance programs. Also, given cancer follow-ups can be expensive (scans, travel to specialty centers), financial stress can fuel her anxiety ("what if I can't afford treatment if it comes back"). Part of therapy may involve financial planning referrals, or connecting her to a financial navigator (many cancer centers now have them). Ethically, we have to ensure that in involving family, we respect confidentiality and the patient's wishes about what to share – some cultures might want the whole family involved, others may have norms of not burdening children. We take her lead on how to incorporate family appropriately. We will also be aware of any health disparities she might have faced: if she is from a minority group that perhaps felt underserved or discriminated against in her cancer care, that trauma could compound her PTSD. We'd validate any such experiences and, if appropriate, discuss advocacy or patient-rights resources to empower her going forward. In sum, a culturally informed, resource-savvy approach will maximize the effectiveness of the interventions described.

Further reading (Case 2): National Cancer Institute PDQ (2022) – Patient guide on Cancer-Related Post-Traumatic Stress (NCI, n.d.); Ochoa et al. (2017) – Study on positive psychotherapy and posttraumatic growth in cancer survivors (Ochoa et al., 2017); Andersen et al. (2015) – Review of psychotherapy for PTSD in cancer survivors (including CBT, EMDR).

Case 3: Child With a Rare Genetic Disorder (and Family)

Profile: *"An 8-year-old boy was recently diagnosed with a rare metabolic disease (Pompe disease) that causes progressive muscle weakness and requires biweekly enzyme replacement infusions. He uses a wheelchair. His parents are struggling with the new diagnosis and report high stress levels. The child exhibits procedural anxiety (intense fear before each hospital infusion) and frequent sadness, saying things like 'Why am I the only kid who can't run?' His 5-year-old sister has begun acting out at home and school, possibly due to the shift of parental attention to the sick child."* This vignette captures common psychosocial facets of rare pediatric diseases: not only the child's psychological adjustment, but the entire family's adaptation is challenged.

Diagnostic considerations: The child does not have a mental disorder per se due to his medical condition, but he is showing signs of adjustment disorder with anxiety (worry and fear around medical procedures and hospital settings) and possibly some depressive features (sadness, feeling different). In rare diseases, formal psychiatric diagnoses in the child are less common than subclinical emotional and behavioral difficulties, but we remain vigilant: children with chronic illnesses have elevated rates of anxiety disorders and depression compared to healthy peers (Stein, 2022). Given his young age (8), his understanding of his condition and prognosis is limited; he might harbor misconceptions (young children sometimes think they caused their illness as punishment, etc.). Part of the assessment is checking his illness knowledge and fears. The parents could be assessed for their own mental health. Caregiver burden for rare diseases is enormous, and parental depression or PTSD is not uncommon after a diagnostic odyssey. They likely meet criteria for an adjustment disorder themselves, if not clinical depression, given the high stress ("I cry at least once a day," the mother says, hypothetically). The mention of parental stress also raises concern for caregiver fatigue or burnout. The sibling's behavioral issues are likely a reaction to changes at home – essentially, she might have an adjustment disorder as well, or simply be acting out to get attention. There is also a risk of sibling anxiety or jealousy; siblings of children with special needs sometimes feel guilt (thinking "I'm bad for being healthy" or "Did I somehow cause this?") or resentment ("All the attention goes to him"). We should assess the sister's perspective via the parents' or pediatrician's reports. Another element: the family's journey to diagnosis may have been long (many rare disease families go years without answers). They may have faced invalidation ("it's all in your head") or multiple misdiagnoses. That trauma of the diagnostic process can leave scars. Some parents of rare kids develop a form of medical trauma from repeated crises and encounters with an unresponsive health system. Culturally, consider if the family's cultural background has specific beliefs about illness or disability. In some cultures, a genetic condition might unfortunately carry stigma or even blame (relatives might whisper about parental wrongdoing or "curse"). Alternatively, some cultures have strong extended family support networks that rally in such times. Understanding where this family falls is key: do they have community/religious support, or are they isolated? Socioeconomically, rare diseases often bring financial strain: expensive treatments, one parent reducing work to become a full-time caregiver, and travel to specialized centers (Pompe might require going to a tertiary center far away). We must gauge if financial stress is high or if they have adequate insurance. If the father, say, had to quit his job to help, that's a big adjustment on top of the emotional burden. Also, education needs are crucial: the child likely qualifies for an Individualized Education Program (IEP) at school for accommodations (e.g., physical accessibility, adaptive PE). Are the parents navigating that process, and do they need advocacy help? Lastly, the rarity means the family may feel extremely isolated perhaps they've never met anyone with this disease; many people (even doctors) don't understand it. This isolation can breed hopelessness ("nobody knows what we're going through"). These considerations lay the groundwork for a targeted intervention plan.

Interventions: The care plan must be family-centered and multidisciplinary. For the child, employing play therapy and cognitive-behavioral techniques will address his anxiety and sadness in a developmentally appropriate way. A child life specialist at the infusion center can use medical play to help desensitize him: for example, playing pretend with a doll getting an "infusion," or a bravery chart where he places a sticker each time he completes a procedure. This helps make the hospital world more predictable and less scary. We can teach him simple coping self-talk (CBT for kids often uses phrases or imagery e.g., a "brave superhero" thought when he's afraid). Perhaps we create a ritual: before each infusion, he and a parent do a deep-breathing exercise and he listens to his favorite song or watches a cartoon during the IV start. These distraction and relaxation techniques can significantly reduce procedure-related distress (evidence supports using such non-pharmacological interventions to improve kids' medical procedure experiences). For his feelings of sadness about being different, narrative therapy can be powerful. One method is to help him create a "Hero Book" or storybook about himself: in it, he is the hero who fights a dragon (the illness) with special weapons (family, doctors, his own courage). By externalizing the illness as something separate from him (e.g., "Pompe is a dragon I'm learning to tame"), we reduce identity fusion with the disease. It also allows him to articulate fears and hopes in story form. Many kids respond well to such imaginative approaches and regain a sense of control and identity beyond "sick kid." Another tool is connecting him (virtually or in person) with other children with similar conditions, maybe via a rare disease family network or camp. Realizing he's not the "only one" is huge for children's psychosocial adjustment.

For the parents, providing psychological support is as critical as treating the child. Parent counseling or therapy can give them a space to process grief and anxiety. Often, when a child is diagnosed with a chronic disability, parents experience stages of grief (denial, anger, bargaining, etc.). The therapist can gently guide them through acceptance, acknowledging their feelings ("It's normal to feel overwhelmed and even angry that this happened") and helping them recognize their strengths ("Look at how you advocated to finally get a diagnosis that shows how resilient your family is"). Support groups for rare disease parents can be lifesaving; Pelentsov et al. (2016) documented that parents of children with rare diseases feel a profound need for peer support, which often isn't met. We'd connect these parents to a disease-specific foundation (e.g., a Pompe disease foundation or online forum) or a broader rare disease alliance where they can talk with others walking a similar path. Knowledge that "we are not alone" reduces isolation and provides practical coping tips from veteran parents. If the mother is exhibiting depressive symptoms or the father is experiencing chronic stress, we might incorporate some CBT or ACT strategies for caregivers. For example, brief CBT might involve scheduling pleasant activities for the parent (caregivers often completely sacrifice their own needs – encouraging the mom to go to her book club or the dad to resume a hobby once a week can replenish them). ACT techniques might help with uncontrollable worries about the child's future: we'd work on mindfulness (staying present-focused) and values (e.g., valuing being a good parent today rather than being paralyzed by what may happen in 10 years). Some rare disease centers are piloting telehealth therapy for parents due to the recognition of this need, so linking them with those services if available, is wise. Couple's counseling might also be considered if the parents' relationship is strained; many marriages suffer under the stress. Open communication and dividing caregiving tasks fairly can be facilitated in therapy.

Sibling support: It's crucial not to overlook the 5-year-old sister. We might bring her into a session for some therapeutic play that allows her to express her feelings. A simple technique is using drawings: ask her to draw her family or "how things are at home," it can reveal if she feels left out or angry. Then, the therapist (or parents with guidance) can validate her feelings ("I bet it's hard that so much attention goes to brother and you feel upset – that doesn't mean you're bad; your feelings make sense and mom and dad still love you just as much"). We'd coach parents to schedule special one-on-one time with the sibling regularly (even 15 minutes of exclusive "mom and me" play each day can improve a sibling's behavior). Also, positively involving the sibling in care can help – maybe she can be the "doctor's assistant" in a pretend game or help pick band-aid colors for her brother, so she feels included rather than shut out. If her behavioral issues at school continue, a child psychologist or school counselor might do some individual work with her (maybe a short course of play therapy focused on adjusting to the brother's illness).

School and systems: A case manager or social worker on the team should ensure the child has appropriate school interventions. For instance, an IEP might provide physical therapy at school, extra time to get between classes, or a personal aide if needed. Educating his classmates about his condition (with family consent) can promote inclusion; sometimes a brief presentation or a book about differences read in class can prevent bullying and encourage peers to be supportive. Many rare conditions are not visible or well-understood, leading to awkwardness or exclusion – proactive education fosters empathy.

Because rare diseases often involve complex care, care coordination is another vital service. If available, this family would benefit from a care coordinator or a "rare disease navigator" who can help them manage appointments across multiple specialists (e.g., neurologist, pulmonologist, geneticist), apply for insurance waivers or disability benefits, and access respite care services. In some healthcare systems, programs like the CARE-FAM-NET in Germany embed psychosocial care coordinators into rare disease teams (Wenke et al., 2022). These coordinators help bridge gaps between medical and mental health services, exactly what this family needs. If such a program isn't locally available, the medical social worker can partially fill that role by linking the family to external resources: for example, a nonprofit that provides respite care (trained volunteers or nurses who give parents a break), or charities that grant "wishes" or fun experiences to seriously ill children (to boost family morale).

Multidisciplinary collaboration is implied throughout: the mental health provider should be in close communication with the child's physicians, physical therapists, and school personnel (with consent). For instance, if the child's anxiety is causing him to refuse infusions, the psychologist could work with the medical team on a plan (maybe mild sedation combined with behavioral strategies, or scheduling therapy sessions on infusion days to coach him in vivo). Interdisciplinary team meetings even if by phone, ensure everyone is on the same page and reinforce a consistent approach (the last section of this chapter will expand on integrated care models).

In summary, the interventions span individual therapy for the child, therapy/support for parents and siblings, and systems-level coordination. The overarching goals are to reduce the child's distress, strengthen family coping and cohesion, and put supports in place so the family can sustain resilience through what is likely to be a long journey.

Outcomes and evaluation: Success in this case will be measured in multiple domains. For the child, we can use a standardized child anxiety scale (such as the Revised Children's Manifest Anxiety Scale or an appropriate medical procedure anxiety scale) before and after implementing coping strategies. A decrease in reported anxiety symptoms or observable distress during procedures (perhaps nurses rate his distress as much lower on a procedure checklist) would indicate improvement. We can also ask the child to rate his fear on a simple 1-10 scale each infusion; watching that number go down over time (say from 10 to 4) is a concrete outcome. His mood can be tracked with parent-report measures like the Child Behavior Checklist (CBCL), which has subscales for internalizing problems (anxiety/depression) – parents filling this out every few months could show a reduction in those scores. Additionally, the child's functioning is an important outcome: Are there fewer school absences? (If infusions or illness caused him to miss a lot, improvement means he's attending more consistently.) Is he engaging in social activities to the extent possible (maybe previously he stopped wanting playdates out of embarrassment; an outcome could be that he now has a friend over once a week and enjoys it). The child's own report

– e.g., “I don’t feel as scared about the hospital” or “I have fun at school now” – is valuable qualitative evidence of progress.

For the parents, outcomes include their stress and mental health levels. We might use a caregiver stress index or simply the Parenting Stress Index. If initially they scored in a high-stress range, a drop into the normal range post-intervention would be a positive sign. Parental depression or anxiety scales (like PHQ-9 or GAD-7) could be monitored if relevant; hopefully, scores decrease as they get support. Another crucial outcome is family quality of life. There are tools like the Family Quality of Life Scale or the PedsQL Family Impact Module that measure how the child’s health affects family functioning. Improvements there (e.g., parents report better family cohesion, more positive family activities) would indicate our family-centered approach is working. On a practical level, an outcome is whether they’ve successfully accessed resources: Did they obtain respite care? Did they secure an IEP and the necessary school supports? Often, these concrete wins (which can be checked off as yes/no outcomes) alleviate a lot of long-term stress. If insurance or equipment was an issue, an outcome is that they acquired the needed equipment (e.g., a home ventilator or wheelchair ramp – things that might have been pending).

We’d also look at the siblings’ adjustment. Teacher reports or behavioral logs can show if the sister’s behavior improved (for example, her frequency of tantrums or school disciplinary notes drops). Parent reports might indicate she seems happier or more secure (maybe she verbalizes less jealousy, or participates more in interactions with her brother rather than acting out).

Finally, because rare diseases evolve, we treat outcomes as ongoing. We might set a 6-month goal (child cooperating with infusions with minimal distress, parents feeling confident in care routines, sibling stabilized in behavior) and then revisit. Given the progressive nature of Pompe, new challenges will arise (perhaps later, the child will need ventilatory support or feeding tube, which will restart some anxiety or grief). So part of our outcome is also that the family feels equipped with coping skills for the future. An immeasurable but vital sign of success is if the parents say: “We know we can handle what comes next; we’ve gotten through before.” That kind of empowerment is the ultimate resilience indicator.

Cultural and socioeconomic considerations: Throughout the intervention, maintaining cultural humility is key. If the family is from a culture that involves extended family in child-rearing, we might include grandparents or an important elder in some sessions (with permission) to ensure alignment and get their support. If there are language needs, providing interpreters or bilingual therapists is non-negotiable for effective care. We’d also be aware of any cultural stigma: for example, if the parents are wary of labeling the child with any “mental” issues in documentation, we might frame therapy as “family support” or “coping skills training” rather than psychological therapy. On the socioeconomic side, ensuring the family is connected to all eligible services can vastly improve outcomes. We would check if they've applied for government programs like Supplemental Security Income (SSI) for the child (which can provide monthly financial support and automatically qualify him for Medicaid waivers for in-home services). If not, the social worker will guide them through it. Many rare diseases have foundations that provide grants or emergency funds – linking the family could alleviate financial crises (for instance, help with travel costs to an out-of-state specialist). If one parent had to leave work, perhaps the therapist could write a letter supporting a workplace accommodation for the other parent or connect them to legal resources if employment discrimination occurred. Education advocacy is another socioeconomic factor: parents with more resources often push for robust IEPs; if this family is less savvy or confident, the therapist might attend an IEP meeting or refer them to an education advocate.

Ethically, we handle issues of privacy with care: if we involve school or support agencies, we get clear consents and share information on a need-to-know basis to help the child. We also remain sensitive to the possibility of health disparities – perhaps the family struggled to get diagnosed due to systemic biases, or they have trouble trusting providers. Building a trusting therapeutic alliance is crucial; that might mean acknowledging past negative experiences with healthcare and validating their advocacy efforts. We should also consider the burden on the parents' relationship and personal time – sometimes an intervention is linking them to marital counseling or even helping arrange a date night (maybe a local charity offers free babysitting for special needs families periodically – that could be a godsend). Essentially, our approach tries to weave a safety net for the family, culturally and contextually attuned, so that they are not fighting this rare illness alone.

Further reading (Case 3): Wenke et al. (2022) – *Qualitative study on pathways to psychosocial care in rare pediatric diseases* (Wenke et al., 2022); Pelentsov et al. (2016) – *Study on support needs of parents caring for a child with a rare disease*; Besier et al. (2011) – *Impact of genetic chronic conditions on siblings and family (review).*

Table 1 below provides a high-level summary of the three cases, highlighting the chronic conditions, co-occurring psychosocial issues, interventions employed, key outcome measures, and special considerations.

Table 1. Summary of Case Studies

Case	Chronic Condition & Mental Health Issues	Key Interventions	Outcomes Tracked	Special Considerations
Adolescent with T1D	Type 1 Diabetes (5 yrs); *Depression*; Diabetes distress; High HbA1c	CBT for mood & adherence; Family therapy; Peer support; Mindfulness/ACT	PHQ-9A; PAID-T; HbA1c; glucose check frequency; DKA events	Low-income (insurance navigation); mental health stigma; 504 plan at school
Adult Cancer Survivor	Breast cancer remission; *PTSD* (nightmares, avoidance); Fear of recurrence; Family strain	Trauma-focused CBT; EMDR; Meaning centered therapy; Couples sessions	PCL-5; GAD-7; PTGI; appointment adherence; sleep quality	Financial toxicity; cultural taboos; child focused family sessions
Child with Rare Disease	Pompe disease; *Adjustment anxiety*; Parental stress; Sibling behavior issues	Play therapy & coping skills; Parent CBT/ support groups; Sibling "special time"; Care coordination/IEP	Child anxiety ratings; CBCL; Care Giver Stress Index; sibling teacher reports	Rural telehealth; language interpreter; rare disease grants/ resources

Note: Table 1 lists each vignette's core challenges, integrative interventions, outcome metrics, and contextual factors.

4. INTEGRATION WITH MEDICAL TEAMS

Managing the intersection of chronic illness and mental health requires close integration between behavioral health and medical care teams. Over the past two decades, integrated care models have gained traction as effective ways to treat co-morbid physical and mental conditions. One prominent example is the Collaborative Care Model (CoCM) in primary care. CoCM embeds a mental health care manager (often a psychologist or social worker) and a psychiatric consultant into the primary care setting to systematically identify and treat patients' behavioral health needs. There is robust evidence that collaborative, interdisciplinary care improves outcomes for patients with depression and coexisting chronic medical illnesses (Katon et al., 2010). In a landmark randomized trial, Katon and colleagues found that patients with diabetes and/or heart disease who received collaborative care for depression had significantly greater improvement in both depression symptoms and glycemic/ blood pressure control, compared to usual care. These findings have been replicated, demonstrating benefits such as higher depression remission rates, better medication adherence, and even reduced mortality in some studies of combined medical/behavioral interventions (Katon et al., 2010; Coventry et al., 2014). Economic analyses suggest integrated care is cost-effective as well – by preventing complications and reducing ER visits or hospitalizations, it offsets the costs of hiring behavioral staff

(Katon et al., 2010). Additionally, offering mental health services in the familiar medical home can reduce stigma and improve access, since patients are more likely to accept help in a primary care or specialty clinic they already visit than to go seek a separate mental health clinic (Katon et al., 2010).

Models of Collaborative Care: Integration can take different forms depending on the setting. In primary care, the CoCM typically functions with the primary care physician (PCP) as the team leader managing medical issues, a care manager tracking patients' mental health progress (often via phone check-ins, brief counseling, and registry management), and a psychiatrist providing regular case consultation on patients who aren't improving. This team meets weekly or biweekly to review cases – an approach that allows for systematic, measurement-based care (they adjust treatments if, say, PHQ-9 scores aren't improving after a few weeks) (Katon et al., 2010). The key is a treat-to-target philosophy: the team has defined goals (e.g., remission of depression, blood pressure under control) and if the patient isn't on track, they proactively change the plan (add therapy, switch meds, etc.) rather than waiting passively (Katon et al., 2010). Outside primary care, integrated care is spreading to specialty clinics. For example, many oncology centers now have psycho-oncology services embedded; cancer patients can see a mental health provider in the infusion center or exam clinic. In pediatrics, integrated behavioral health is becoming common in diabetes clinics, cystic fibrosis centers, etc., with psychologists on-site to address issues like regimen adherence or needle phobia in real time. Hospitals have long used consultation-liaison psychiatry for inpatients – that is, integration at the bedside for acute medical settings. Another variant is integrated pain management programs, where physicians, psychologists, physical therapists, and others co-create pain treatment plans. Regardless of setting, effective integrated teams share features: regular communication, shared care plans, and a culture of collaboration rather than siloed practice. As an example, consider our earlier Case 3 (child with Pompe disease): an ideal integrated approach might have a weekly team huddle including the geneticist, neurologist, physical therapist, social worker, and psychologist to coordinate the child's care plan and ensure consistency in messaging to the family.

Interdisciplinary Communication: Good communication is the linchpin of integration. Best practices include using a shared electronic health record (EHR) where all team members document their notes. That way, the psychologist's note about a patient's new coping strategy or stressor is visible to the physician, and the physician's note about a medical change (say a new medication) is known to the therapist. For instance, in Case 1, if the endocrinologist starts the teen on an insulin pump, the psychologist should know because it might impact the teen's self-image or require new learning that could frustrate her. Shared EHR notes facilitate this awareness (with the patient's consent – usually patients sign an integrated care consent acknowledging their providers will share info). Teams also often implement brief check-ins or "curbside" consults – e.g., the psychologist might pop into the doctor's office after a joint visit to quickly update, or vice versa. A structured version of this is a case conference: many clinics hold a meeting (monthly or so) where complex cases are discussed by the full team, generating holistic plans. Our cancer survivor patient, for example, could be discussed in a tumor board meeting that now also involves the psycho-oncologist, ensuring her PTSD is addressed alongside surveillance scans. Another communication tool is warm hand-offs: this is when, during a medical visit, the doctor personally introduces the patient to the behavioral health provider in the clinic (literally handing them off). This approach has been shown to greatly increase follow-through – it reduces the stigma and inertia of making a separate appointment. In primary care collaborative care, even though therapy might happen separately, the care manager often gives the PCP a quick summary to mention in appointments ("Dr. Smith, just so you know, Mr. Jones started counseling for his CHF-related depression, and he's set some walking goals"). When patients see that all providers are on the same page, it builds trust and adherence: they perceive the care team as united in helping them, so they are less likely to "split" or give conflicting info. However, teams must navigate confidentiality: sensitive matters (like a disclosure of domestic abuse to a therapist) may not be appropriate to put in the general chart unless safety requires action. Usually, teams develop guidelines about what types of information are always shared vs. kept more restricted. Following HIPAA, they share the minimum necessary info, and with patient awareness. An ethical guideline here is to regularly remind the patient that the team communicates. "Our team meets to talk about how to best support you, so I will update Dr. X that we met and some general things we're working on. I won't share anything you ask me not to, unless it's about safety." This transparency maintains trust.

Ethical and Legal Issues: Integrated care brings some unique ethical considerations. Confidentiality is one, as noted. Behavioral health providers typically keep psychotherapy notes private, but in an integrated setting, the expectation (and often formal consent) is that relevant information is shared with the team. Teams must still protect the patient's privacy by not oversharing beyond what helps medical care. For example, the psychologist might not detail marital conflicts in the chart, but would note that the patient is experiencing stress and a plan is in place to address it – enough for the physician to know context without breaching personal details. Clear role definition is also important ethically. Every team member should practice within their scope: e.g., a nurse might do basic depression screenings but will refer to a licensed therapist for actual psychotherapy; the primary doctor can prescribe antidepressants but shouldn't try to manage complex PTSD alone without consultation. Role clarity prevents things from falling through cracks ("I thought you were following up on that suicidal thought!" "No, I thought you were!" dangerous miscommunications to avoid). Teams often create protocols for scenarios, like if a patient expresses suicidal ideation to any team member, here's the step-by-step (assess immediacy, involve the psych consultant or crisis team, ensure safety, etc.). Another area is billing and legal documentation. Integrated care requires navigating billing codes – for example, in the US, Medicare introduced specific codes for collaborative care (CoCM) so that time spent by the behavioral manager and psychiatrist can be billed under the PCP. Ethically, one must ensure not to "double bill" or bill for services not provided. There are also state laws that vary on, say, what a psychologist vs. an MD can document or share. If the team spans multiple organizations (like a community mental health provider working with a private medical practice), they need proper Business Associate Agreements or releases to exchange info legally. Insurance parity laws (in the US, mental health parity) mandate equal coverage for mental health conditions – integrated care teams often advocate using these laws if insurers push back on covering behavioral services in a medical setting. For instance, if an insurance company states, "we won't pay for a psychologist in the endocrine clinic, the patient must go to a mental health clinic," the care team can appeal, citing parity (mental health care should be accessible and equivalent). This bleeds into insurance navigation issues: integrated programs sometimes need creative approaches to get paid. Many use the CoCM codes mentioned, or same-day billing (billing a medical and mental health visit on the same day, which some insurers disallow, but policies are changing). Some practices employ the behavioral clinician and treat their services as part of the overall cost of care, recouped by improved outcomes and payer quality bonuses rather than direct billing. An integrated care coordinator or practice manager usually works behind the scenes to manage these aspects so clinicians can focus on care.

On the patient side, integration helps with navigation immensely. Instead of the patient being on their own to find a therapist, the team arranges it. In some models, the behavioral specialist can accompany the patient to specialty referrals or at least ensure follow-up occurs. Case in point, our rare disease family (Case 3) likely felt overwhelmed coordinating neurologists, pulmonologists, therapists, and insurers – an integrated approach would lighten that load by having a navigator or team lead do a lot of that legwork. An ethically patient-centered approach here acknowledges that the healthcare system is complex; thus, part of our duty is to guide patients through it.

In summary, integrated care requires careful team communication, attention to confidentiality and scope, and often navigating administrative hurdles like billing and insurance. When these challenges are managed, however, the payoff is substantial: the patient receives care for mind and body in one coherent package. Our case examples would all benefit from integration: the teen with diabetes having her psychologist and endocrinologist coordinate on her goals; the cancer survivor's oncologist and therapist reinforcing each other's recommendations (the oncologist might prescribe an anxiolytic with input from the therapist, and encourage therapy as part of survivorship care); the rare disease family getting psychological support seamlessly alongside genetic counseling and medical treatment. Integrated care operationalizes the biopsychosocial model – it makes whole-person care a reality, not just an ideal (Jürisson et al., 2021). Health systems globally are increasingly moving in this direction, with collaborative care now implemented in many primary care clinics and specialty centers. While there are logistical and financial barriers to overcome, the trend is clear that the "interface" between medical and mental health professionals must be strong to optimally support patients and families dealing with chronic illness. As a result, training programs are emphasizing interprofessional education, and policy is slowly adapting to incentivize integrated practice. Future directions might include even more innovative integrations, such as digital platforms that allow shared care plans accessible to patients and all providers, or co-location of traditionally separate services (imagine a "one-stop" clinic for diabetes where you see an endocrinologist, dietitian, and psychologist in succession). Ultimately, the goal is a healthcare system where patients don't have to separate their mind and body, where every clinic is a place for whole-person healing.

5. CONCLUSION

Chronic illnesses and mental health conditions are deeply interconnected, affecting patients and families on multiple levels. This chapter highlighted how adopting a biopsychosocial, whole-person approach can transform care for individuals with co-occurring physical and psychological challenges. Key takeaways include the high prevalence of depression, anxiety, and trauma among those with chronic diseases and the subsequent impact on disease outcomes (Gupta et al., 2024; NCI, n.d.). However, through early identification and integrative interventions, patients can build resilience and even experience personal growth in the face of illness (Ochoa et al., 2017). The case studies demonstrated practical psychotherapeutic strategies – from CBT and family therapy to narrative and somatic techniques – tailored to different life stages and cultural contexts. These interventions yielded improvements not only in mental health symptoms but also in medical indicators like HbA1c and treatment adherence, reinforcing that treating the "whole person" benefits the whole outcome (Gupta et al., 2024; Rechenberg & Koerner, 2021). A recurring theme is the power of collaboration: resilient outcomes were facilitated when mental health professionals, medical teams, and family members worked in concert. Integrated care models exemplify this, breaking down silos so that patients receive unified, person-centered support. Looking ahead, healthcare systems should continue to remove barriers to integrated behavioral health services – through policy changes, training of interdisciplinary providers, and leveraging technology for coordination – so that every patient with a chronic illness has access to comprehensive care addressing both physical and psychological needs. In research, more longitudinal studies and trials of integrative interventions will help refine best practices and demonstrate long-term benefits (for example, does early psychosocial intervention in pediatric chronic illness lead to measurable health improvements decades later?). Finally, a cultural shift is needed in society to destigmatize mental health support in medical contexts; patients and families should feel as comfortable seeking therapy or counseling as they do asking about medications or surgeries. In conclusion, caring for chronic illness is not just about managing an organ system or lab value – it is about caring for a person and their loved ones. By embracing whole-person, collaborative care approaches, we bolster the innate resilience in patients and families, enabling them to not only manage illnesses but also lead fulfilling lives amidst adversity.

REFERENCES

Adams, J. S., Chien, A. T., & Wisk, L. E. (2019). Mental illness among youth with chronic physical conditions. *Pediatrics, 144*(1), e20181819. DOI: 10.1542/peds.2018-1819

Adzrago, D., Williams, D. R., & Williams, F. (2024). Multiple chronic diseases and psychological distress among adults in the United States: The intersectionality of chronic diseases, race/ethnicity, immigration, sex, and insurance coverage. *Social Psychiatry and Psychiatric Epidemiology, 60*, 181–199. DOI: 10.1007/s00127-024-02730-1

Alassaf, A., Gharaibeh, L., Zurikat, R. O., Farkouh, A., Ibrahim, S., Zayed, A. A., & Odeh, R. (2023). Prevalence of depression in patients with type 1 diabetes between 10 and 17 years of age in Jordan. *Journal of Diabetes Research, 2023*, 3542780. Advance online publication. DOI: 10.1155/2023/3542780

American Cancer Society. (2024, May 22). *Post-traumatic stress disorder (PTSD) after cancer.* https://www.cancer.org/cancer/survivorship/post-traumatic-stress-disorder-and-cancer.html

Anderson, R. J., Freedland, K. E., Clouse, R. E., & Lustman, P. J. (2001). The prevalence of comorbid depression in adults with diabetes: A meta-analysis. *Diabetes Care, 24*(6), 1069–1078. DOI: 10.2337/diacare.24.6.1069

Baker, K., & Claridge, A. M. (2023). "I have a Ph.D. in my daughter": Mother and child experiences of living with childhood chronic illness. *Journal of Child and Family Studies, 32*(9), 2625–2636. DOI: 10.1007/s10826-022-02506-8

DeLong, L. N., Fleetwood, K., Prigge, R., Galdi, P., Guthrie, B., & Fleuriot, J. (2025). Cluster and survival analysis of UK Biobank data reveals associations between physical multimorbidity clusters and subsequent depression. *Communications Medicine, 5*, 156. Advance online publication. DOI: 10.1038/s43856-025-00825-7

Engel, G. L. (1977). The need for a new medical model: A challenge for biomedicine. *Science, 196*(4286), 129–136. DOI: 10.1126/science.847460

Jarero, I., Givaudan, M., & Osorio, A. (2018). Randomized controlled trial on the provision of the EMDR integrative group treatment protocol adapted for ongoing traumatic stress to female patients with cancer-related posttraumatic stress disorder symptoms. *Journal of EMDR Practice and Research, 12*(3), 94–104. DOI: 10.1891/1933-3196.12.3.94

Jürisson, M., Pisarev, H., Uusküla, A., Lang, K., Oona, M., Elm, L., & Kalda, R. (2021). Physical–mental health comorbidity: A population-based cross-sectional study. *PLoS One*, *16*(12), e0260464. DOI: 10.1371/journal.pone.0260464

Katon, W. J., Lin, E. H., Von Korff, M., Ciechanowski, P., Ludman, E. J., Young, B., Peterson, D., Rutter, C. M., McGregor, M., & McCulloch, D. (2010). Collaborative care for patients with depression and chronic illnesses. *The New England Journal of Medicine*, *363*(27), 2611–2620. DOI: 10.1056/NEJMoa1003955

Martire, L. M., & Schulz, R. (2007). Involving family in psychosocial interventions for chronic illness. *Current Directions in Psychological Science*, *16*(2), 90–94. DOI: 10.1111/j.1467-8721.2007.00482.x

Nair, D., Cukor, D., Taylor, W. D., & Cavanaugh, K. L. (2021). Applying a biopsychosocial framework to achieve durable behavior change in kidney disease. *Seminars in Nephrology*, *41*(6), 487–504. DOI: 10.1016/j.semnephrol.2021.10.003

National Cancer Institute. (n.d.). *Depression (PDQ®)*. https://www.cancer.gov/about-cancer/coping/feelings/depression-hp-pdq

Ochoa, C., Casellas-Grau, A., Vives, J., Font, A., & Borràs, J. M. (2017). Positive psychotherapy for distressed cancer survivors: Posttraumatic growth facilitation reduces posttraumatic stress. *International Journal of Clinical and Health Psychology : IJCHP*, *17*(1), 28–37. DOI: 10.1016/j.ijchp.2016.09.002

Portigliatti Pomeri, A., La Salvia, A., Carletto, S., Oliva, F., & Ostacoli, L. (2021). EMDR in cancer patients: A systematic review. *Frontiers in Psychology*, *11*, 590204. DOI: 10.3389/fpsyg.2020.590204

Rechenberg, K., & Koerner, K. (2021). Cognitive behavioral therapy in adolescents with type 1 diabetes: An integrative review. *Journal of Pediatric Nursing*, *60*, 190–197. DOI: 10.1016/j.pedn.2021.03.021

Sarizadeh, M. S., Boogar, I. R., Talepasand, S., & Gharemanfard, F. (2021). Acceptance and commitment therapy for demoralization syndrome and cancer-related trauma: A randomized clinical trial. *International Journal of Cancer Management*, *14*(11), e114637. DOI: 10.5812/ijcm.114637

Stein, R. E. K. (2022). Mental health concerns and childhood chronic physical health conditions: A narrative review. *Pediatric Medicine*, *5*, 8. DOI: 10.21037/pm-20-107

Wenke, S., Jung, N., Forthmann, B., Maier, C., Hirschfeld, G., & Muehlan, H. (2022). Rare pediatric diseases and pathways to psychosocial care: A qualitative interview study with professional experts in Germany. *Orphanet Journal of Rare Diseases*, *17*(1), 361. DOI: 10.1186/s13023-021-02127-2

Young-Hyman, D., de Groot, M., Hill-Briggs, F., Gonzalez, J. S., Hood, K. K., & Peyrot, M. (2016). Psychosocial care for people with diabetes: A position statement of the American Diabetes Association. *Diabetes Care*, *39*(12), 2126–2140. DOI: 10.2337/dc16-2053

KEY TERMS AND DEFINITIONS

Biopsychosocial Model: A conceptual model proposing that biological, psychological, and social factors are all essential and interconnected determinants of health and disease. Under this model (first articulated by George Engel in 1977), illnesses are not viewed solely as biological malfunctions but as conditions influenced by a person's mental state, behaviors, family/support system, culture, and environment. In practice, using the biopsychosocial model means a clinician treating a patient with chronic pain would address not only the physical cause of pain but also the patient's coping strategies (psychological) and perhaps work or family dynamics (social) that affect the pain experience.

Collaborative Care Model: An evidence-based model of integrated care specifically designed to treat common mental health conditions (like depression and anxiety) in primary care and other general medical settings. Key features of the Collaborative Care Model (CoCM) include: a multi-disciplinary team (primary care provider, behavioral health care manager, and consulting psychiatrist), systematic screening and patient identification, measurement-based care plans (using scales to track progress), regular case reviews and psychiatric consultation for patients not improving, and stepped care adjustments until clinical goals are achieved. CoCM is typically population-based (managing a registry of patients). For example, in CoCM a family doctor's clinic might implement routine depression screening for all diabetes patients; a care manager follows up with those who screen positive to offer therapy and self-management support, while a psychiatrist meets with the care manager weekly to advise on any needed medication changes. This model has been shown to improve outcomes and is supported by specific billing codes in some healthcare systems.

Family-Centered Care: An approach to health care that views the *family* as an integral part of the patient's support system and actively involves family members in the care process. Originally prominent in pediatrics, it has become a guiding principle in managing pediatric chronic illnesses and other contexts. Family-centered care means respecting the family's knowledge of the patient, communicating openly with family members (with patient consent), and often including them in decision-making and care activities. It also means providing resources and education to the family unit, not just the patient. For instance, in family-centered care for a child with a disability, the healthcare team might coordinate therapy schedules to minimize disruption to family life, train parents in at-home exercises, address sibling questions, and adjust hospital policies (like flexible visiting hours) to accommodate family needs. The goal is to empower and support the family, recognizing that a well-supported family can greatly improve the patient's health outcomes and emotional well-being.

Integrative Care: A holistic approach to health care that *integrates* medical and psychological treatment, addressing the patient as a whole person. In practice, integrative care involves collaboration among different health professionals (physicians, psychologists, social workers, etc.) in developing and executing a unified care plan. The focus is on treating physical illness and co-occurring mental health or social issues simultaneously, rather than in separate silos. For example, an integrative care plan for diabetes might include insulin therapy, nutritional counseling, and cognitive-behavioral therapy for stress management, all coordinated by the care team.

Narrative Reframing: A therapeutic technique (common in narrative therapy) that involves changing the way a person tells the story of their life or illness to highlight strengths, meaning, or new perspectives. Essentially, it is "reframing" one's personal narrative. For example, a cancer survivor who initially narrates their experience as "I was completely destroyed by cancer" might, through therapy, reframe it to "I endured tremendous hardship and discovered my inner strength and what truly matters to me." This shift in the story can decrease feelings of victimhood and increase empowerment. Narrative reframing often involves writing exercises, metaphors, or conversations that help the individual view their situation through a more hopeful or constructive lens.

Psychological Resilience: The capacity to adapt to, withstand, or recover quickly from stress, adversity, or trauma. In the context of chronic illness, resilience refers to the patient's and family's ability to maintain psychological well-being and continue living a meaningful life despite the illness's challenges. Resilience is not a fixed trait but a set of coping processes and skills that can be developed – such as optimism, problem-solving, social support utilization, and finding purpose in the struggle. A resilient outcome might be a patient with a debilitating condition managing to find new ways to engage in valued activities and reporting a good quality of life, where others might have become overwhelmed.

Somatic Techniques: Therapeutic approaches that target the mind-body connection by using bodily or physical activities to help process emotions, reduce stress, or alleviate psychological symptoms. "Somatic" means relating to the body. These techniques include practices such as deep breathing exercises, progressive muscle relaxation, biofeedback, mindfulness meditation, yoga, or even EMDR (which uses guided eye movements). In trauma therapy, somatic techniques might involve grounding exercises to calm the body's fight-or-flight response. For someone with chronic illness, a somatic approach could include relaxation training to reduce chronic pain or anxiety (e.g. learning to deliberately relax muscle groups and slow breathing to signal safety to the brain). The underlying premise is that changing one's physiological state can positively influence mental state and vice versa.

Chapter 7
Case Studies in Clinical Psychiatry: Neurostimulation for Emotional and Affective Disorders

Kadir Uludag
http://orcid.org/0000-0003-3713-4670
Capital Medical University, China

EXECUTIVE SUMMARY

Neurostimulation has emerged as a significant therapeutic approach for various disabilities (e.g., emotional disability), revolutionizing the management and treatment of affected individuals. By delivering electrical impulses to the nervous system, it targets multiple types of disabilities, including those related to emotion. It has emerged as a significant therapeutic option for emotional disabilities, offering new hope for patients who do not respond adequately to traditional treatments. Emotional disabilities, such as major depressive disorder, anxiety disorders, and post - traumatic stress disorder, are characterized by dysregulated emotional states and disrupted neural circuits. Neurostimulation techniques, including deep brain stimulation (DBS), vagus nerve stimulation, transcranial magnetic stimulation (TMS), and transcranial direct - current stimulation (tDCS), target these underlying neural dysfunctions. DBS and vagus nerve stimulation, which are invasive and semi - invasive methods respectively, are often used for severe cases.

INTRODUCTION

Neurostimulation is commonly used in various fields such as Chronic pain management (e.g., spinal cord stimulation, peripheral nerve stimulation) (Magis &

DOI: 10.4018/979-8-3373-3084-6.ch007

Schoenen, 2012), Migraine treatment (Deer et al., 2014), Parkinson's disease (e.g., deep brain stimulation), Epilepsy (Yang et al., 2025), Depression and mood disorders (e.g., transcranial magnetic stimulation, vagus nerve stimulation), Obsessive-compulsive disorder (OCD) (e.g., deep brain stimulation), and Stroke rehabilitation (e.g., functional electrical stimulation). In addition, previous study concluded that TMS and tDCS offer therapeutic benefits for individuals with various mental health conditions, enhancing clinical outcomes—such as cognitive impairments in schizophrenia (Hyde et al., 2022). Furthermore, it maybe applied to help healthy individuals. Neurostimulation in healthy individuals refers to the application of various techniques that use electrical, magnetic, or chemical means to modulate the activity of the nervous system in people without neurological disorders. For example, previous study found that applying direct current stimulation to the prefrontal cortex has been found to be safe and can selectively enhance verbal fluency in healthy individuals (Iyer et al., 2005). Neurostimulation holds great promise for applications in healthy individuals, whether it's for cognitive or physical enhancement. The development of innovative tools, such as wearable devices, closed - loop systems, and imaging - guided techniques, is enhancing the precision and effectiveness of neurostimulation. However, as with any emerging technology, it is crucial to address the associated ethical considerations to ensure that these advancements are used in a responsible and beneficial manner.

Neurostimulation provides a unique approach to treating emotional disabilities such as depression, with its own set of advantages and limitations when compared to other treatment methods (e.g., antidepressants). It may help people with certain problems such as depression and pain. Brain Stimulation techniques like repetitive transcranial magnetic stimulation (rTMS) or transcranial direct - current stimulation (tDCS) can help restore this imbalance in brain activity (Nitsche et al., 2012). Neurostimulation methods could potentially influence vocal-related metrics. We have gathered a range of studies that examine the relationship between brain stimulation and alterations in voice (Table 1).

NEUROSTIMULATION FOR DEPRESSION

Several basic neurostimulation methods are used in the treatment of depression, including electroconvulsive therapy and rTMS. tDCS which utilizes a uniform direct current field with intensities, brings about enduring alterations in the brain (Paulus, 2011). Transcranial alternating current stimulation (tACS) is a non-invasive neuromodulation technique that delivers oscillating electrical currents to the scalp to entrain neural rhythms at specific frequencies. tACS is believed to alter ongoing brain oscillations in a manner that depends on the stimulation frequency (Lafleur et al., 2021). tACS may influence brain function and cognitive processes by aligning brain oscillations and promoting long-term synaptic plasticity (Elyamany, Leicht, Herrmann, & Mulert, 2021). In summary, non-invasive neurostimulation techniques such as tDCS and tACS offer promising avenues for modulating brain activity and treating depression. Their ability to induce lasting neural changes and influence cognitive processes highlights their potential for clinical application and further research.

Other findings showed that applying anodal tDCS to the left dorsolateral prefrontal cortex was related to an improvement in working memory function. This improvement was evidenced by an increase in recognition accuracy, and the subjects of this observation were stroke patients (Jo et al., 2009).

Also, we have listed specific studies related to brain stimulation and innovative methods related to voice analysis.

Table 1. Brain stimulation and innovative methods related to voice analysis

	Title of Study	Goal of Study	Results
Study 1	''Longitudinal Speech Change After Subthalamic Nucleus Deep Brain Stimulation in Parkinson's Disease Patients: A 2-Year Prospective Study''	A two - year prospective study was carried out by us on PD patients who had STN - DBS. We analyzed the alterations in speech function with the aim of identifying factors that could predict speech deterioration.	The effects of DBS on voice and speech quality show substantial differences across various studies. The anatomical region being stimulated likely plays a crucial part. This is because, in contrast to other regions, the stimulation of the pallidal area was predominantly linked to an enhancement in voice quality.
Study 2	''Effect of deep brain stimulation on glottal phonation in patients with Parkinson's disease and multiple sclerosis''	This current study looks into the impact of neurostimulatory procedures on the glottal phonation of three patients with Parkinson's disease and three patients with multiple sclerosis.	For the patients suffering from Parkinson's disease, it is demonstrated that the stimulation leads to a relative impairment of the glottal cycle. On the other hand, in the case of the patients with multiple sclerosis, a tendency towards hyperfunctional phonation is noted.
Study 3	''Transcranial direct-current stimulation in ultra-treatment-resistant schizophrenia''	The aim of this study was to assess both the effectiveness and safety of transcranial direct current stimulation (tDCS) in treating auditory hallucinations among hospitalized patients with ultra-treatment-resistant schizophrenia (TRS), and to evaluate how tDCS impacts cognitive functions.	Even though just a slight enhancement was observed in the scores related to auditory hallucinations for the group that received tDCS, this improvement held significance when contrasted with the situation where the control group received no standard treatment.

continued on following page

Table 1. Continued

	Title of Study	Goal of Study	Results
Study 4	Brain morphological changes in hypokinetic dysarthria of Parkinson's disease and use of machine learning to predict severity	As many as 90% of individuals with Parkinson's disease (PD) will ultimately develop the speech and voice disorder known as hypokinetic dysarthria (HD). Nevertheless, the brain morphological alterations linked to hypokinetic dysarthria have not been explored.	The morphological changes occurring in the brain are related to hypokinetic dysarthria (HD).
Study 5	Modulation of vocal pitch control through high-definition transcranial direct current stimulation of the left ventral motor cortex	We carried out an investigation to determine how high-definition transcranial direct current stimulation (HD-tDCS) applied to the left ventral motor cortex influences the neural mechanisms involved in the integration of sensory and motor functions during the control of voice motor actions.	neurostimulation of the left ventral motor cortex has an impact on the sensorimotor mechanisms that underlie the control of voice motor functions.

Table 2. Conceptual definitions of Emotional disorders

Perspective	Definition	Key Components	Relevance for Neurostimulation Research
Clinical (Diagnostic)	Emotional disorders are psychiatric conditions characterized by persistent disturbances in mood, affect, or anxiety that impair daily functioning.	Depression, anxiety, PTSD, mood instability, excessive fear	Identifies patient populations and treatment targets
Dimensional (Psychological)	Emotional disorders reflect maladaptive regulation of emotional responses across valence, arousal, and control domains.	Negative affect bias, poor emotional regulation, heightened stress reactivity	Supports symptom-based rather than diagnosis-based stimulation targets
Neurobiological	Emotional disorders arise from dysfunction in neural circuits governing emotion processing, reward, and cognitive control.	Limbic hyperactivity, prefrontal hypoactivity, network dysconnectivity	Guides stimulation sites (e.g., DLPFC, limbic circuits)
Cognitive–Behavioral	Emotional disorders involve distorted cognition, maladaptive behaviors, and reinforcement patterns that maintain emotional distress.	Rumination, avoidance, negative beliefs, impaired coping	Helps identify measurable behavioral outcomes of stimulation

continued on following page

Table 2. Continued

Perspective	Definition	Key Components	Relevance for Neurostimulation Research
Functional Model	Emotional disorders are conditions causing measurable impairment in social, occupational, and daily functioning due to emotional dysregulation.	Quality-of-life reduction, productivity loss, social impairment	Supports evaluation of real-world effectiveness of neuromodulation
Transdiagnostic	Emotional disorders are viewed as overlapping syndromes sharing common mechanisms such as negative valence sensitivity and impaired regulation networks.	Shared circuitry, common biomarkers, overlapping symptoms	Aligns with network-targeted and personalized stimulation approaches

Table 3. Markers of Depression

Category	Markers
Biological	Neurotransmitter imbalance
	Low serotonin levels
	Elevated cortisol
	Inflammation markers
Psychological	Persistent sadness
	Loss of interest
	Feelings of worthlessness
	Suicidal Thoughts
Behavioral	Social withdrawal
	Psychomotor changes
	Sleep disturbances
	Appetite changes
Cognitive	Impaired Concentration
	Memory difficulties
	Indeciveness
	Negative thinking

This table categorizes key markers associated with depression by domain.

- **Biological:** Includes genetic predispositions and chemical factors.

- **Psychological:** Covers emotional and cognitive symptoms.
- **Behavioral:** Lists observable changes in daily activities.
- **Cognitive:** Focuses on specific thought patterns and mental processes.

These categories help clinicians and researchers understand depression from multiple angles for accurate assessment (Table 3).

Neurostimulation, with its diverse techniques like DBS, vagus nerve stimulation, TMS, and tDCS, shows promise in managing emotional disabilities by targeting underlying neural dysfunctions, yet faces challenges such as variable patient response and side - effects, and voice analysis offers a novel way to assess its treatment efficacy as the field continues to grow but requires more research for optimization and long - term understanding.

VOICE AND BRAIN STIMULATION

Voice and brain stimulation techniques are increasingly explored for their potential to modulate vocal functions by influencing neural pathways that govern speech production and motor control.

Previous pioneering study conducted a systematic review to synthesize the effects of DBS on speech, voice, and language outcomes. Key findings revealed a heterogeneous and inconsistent pattern of results across different DBS studies, highlighting variability in how these functions are affected by the intervention. (Tabari et al., 2024). The effect of DBS on the quality of voice and speech shows differences across various studies. The anatomical area being stimulated likely plays a crucial part. This is because the stimulation of the pallidal area was predominantly linked to an enhancement in voice quality, as opposed to the stimulation of other regions (Baudouin et al., 2023). Other findings imply that both voice and fluency are impacted in distinct ways by DBS treatment, and that task conditions, when interacting with the functionality of the subcortical regions, have an effect on motor speech performance (Sidtis, Rogers, Godier, Tagliati, & Sidtis, 2010). Moreover, an acoustic analysis was carried out on the voices of 25 Parkinson's disease patients who underwent DBS to evaluate the effect of the treatment. Almost all the acoustic analysis parameters during the phonation of a prolonged /a/ showed improvement following DBS (Mate, Cobeta, Jiménez-Jiménez, & Figueiras, 2012). In another study, DBS was found to be effective in enhancing voice quality and improving voice-related quality of life in patients with vocal tremors (Lu et al., 2023).

Voice and brain stimulation techniques, particularly DBS, are being increasingly investigated for their impact on speech and vocal functions. While findings across studies are varied and sometimes inconsistent, evidence suggests that the effects of

DBS depend on the specific brain regions targeted, with stimulation of the pallidal area often linked to improvements in voice quality. Additionally, factors such as task conditions and subcortical functionality influence speech performance, and several studies report improvements in acoustic parameters and voice-related quality of life following DBS treatment.

COMPUTATIONAL ASPECTS OF BRAIN STIMULATION

The advancement of neurostimulation for emotional disorders is increasingly reliant on computational frameworks to enhance its precision, efficacy, and personalization. These approaches address core challenges such as inter-individual variability in neuroanatomy, unclear optimal stimulation targets, and the dynamic nature of brain states.

Key computational aspects include:

1. Personalized Electric Field Modeling: Using finite element method (FEM) models derived from individual structural MRI scans, researchers can simulate the distribution of electric (tDCS/tACS) or magnetic (TMS) fields in a patient's brain. This allows for the in-silico optimization of electrode placement or coil orientation to maximize dose at a target region (e.g., dorsolateral prefrontal cortex for depression) while minimizing off-target effects.
2. Network-Targeted Stimulation: Computational analysis of functional and effective connectivity from fMRI data is used to map dysfunctional emotional circuits. Instead of stimulating a single, generic cortical site, algorithms can identify personalized network nodes or pathways whose modulation is most likely to restore healthy network dynamics and alleviate specific symptoms.
3. Closed-Loop and Adaptive Protocols: Moving beyond fixed stimulation parameters, closed-loop systems use real-time computational analysis of physiological signals (e.g., EEG biomarkers of emotional state or voice acoustics) to dynamically adjust stimulation intensity, frequency, or timing. Reinforcement learning algorithms can "learn" the optimal stimulation strategy for an individual based on continuous feedback, adapting to their changing brain state.
4. Computational Voice Analysis as a Biomarker: As highlighted in the reviewed studies, voice is a sensitive output of neuromotor and emotional systems. Computational signal processing and machine learning can extract subtle vocal features (prosody, tremor, spectral components) that correlate with clinical state and stimulation effects. This provides an objective, quantifiable biomarker for real-time efficacy monitoring and long-term outcome prediction, enabling data-driven protocol optimization.

5. In-Silico Trials and Target Discovery: Large-scale computational brain models can simulate the effects of different stimulation protocols on neural population dynamics. This allows for the rapid, low-risk testing of novel stimulation paradigms and the identification of promising new targets before costly clinical trials.

In summary, computational neuroscience and engineering are transforming neurostimulation from a broadly applied tool into a targeted, precision medicine intervention. By integrating personalized biophysical models, network neuroscience, adaptive control algorithms, and digital biomarkers like voice, these approaches promise to reduce variability, improve outcomes, and unlock the full therapeutic potential of brain stimulation for emotional disorders.

CONCLUSION

Overall, neurostimulation holds great promise as a growing field in the treatment of emotional disabilities. However, to fully realize its potential, further research is essential. This research is needed to optimize its use, understand its long-term implications, and develop more effective and targeted treatment strategies for emotional disabilities. New tools such as voice analysis provide valuable insights into the treatment efficacy of brain stimulation, offering a fresh perspective on how brain stimulation impacts neural function and enabling the optimization of treatment protocols.

SUGGESTIONS

Future studies hold promise in exploring the intersection of AI technologies and neurostimulation, paving the way for innovative advancements. Emerging and future directions in this domain include the development of personalized stimulation protocols, where AI algorithms tailor interventions to individual neural profiles. AI-guided neurostimulation represents another frontier, leveraging machine learning to optimize stimulation parameters in real-time for enhanced efficacy. Noninvasive brain stimulation techniques for cognitive enhancement also warrant exploration, with AI potentially refining targeting and dosage to boost memory, attention, and other cognitive functions. Additionally, the integration of combined stimulation and pharmacological treatments could unlock synergistic effects, while applications in neurodevelopmental disorders such as ADHD and autism may offer new therapeutic avenues. Crucially, ethical and regulatory considerations in neuromodulation must be addressed alongside technological progress, ensuring responsible innovation that balances scientific potential with societal and ethical safeguards.

FIGURES

Figure 1. Graphical abstract

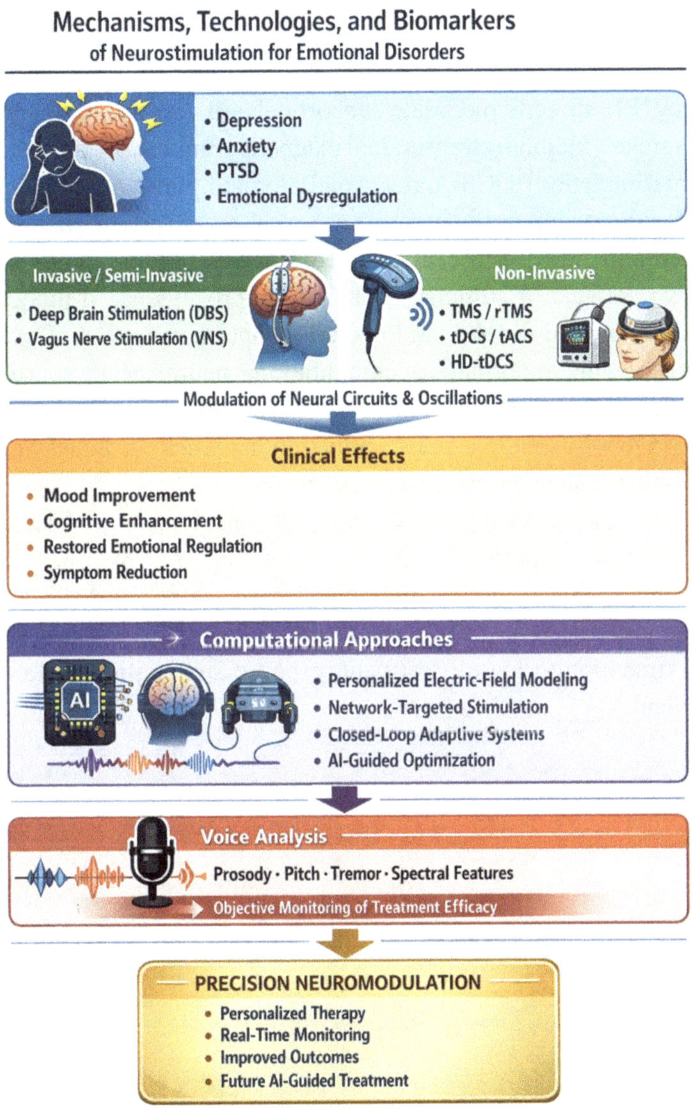

Figure 1 illustrates the conceptual framework linking neurostimulation techniques to the treatment of emotional disorders and highlights the role of computational approaches and voice analysis as emerging biomarkers of treatment efficacy.

The top section presents common emotional disorders, including depression, anxiety, post-traumatic stress disorder, and broader emotional dysregulation, which are associated with dysfunction in neural circuits such as limbic hyperactivity, prefrontal hypoactivity, and disrupted network connectivity.

The middle section summarizes major neurostimulation approaches. Invasive and semi-invasive methods, such as deep brain stimulation (DBS) and vagus nerve stimulation (VNS), directly modulate subcortical and network-level activity. Non-invasive techniques, including transcranial magnetic stimulation (TMS), transcranial direct-current stimulation (tDCS), transcranial alternating current stimulation (tACS), and high-definition tDCS, influence cortical excitability and oscillatory dynamics. These interventions aim to restore functional balance in emotional regulation circuits.

Downstream effects of stimulation include improvements in mood, cognitive performance, emotional control, and overall symptom reduction. The figure also highlights the growing importance of computational neuroscience approaches, such as individualized electric-field modeling, network-targeted stimulation, adaptive closed-loop protocols, and AI-guided optimization, which are transforming neuromodulation into a more personalized intervention.

A key feature of the framework is the inclusion of voice analysis as a digital biomarker. Acoustic properties of speech—including prosody, pitch, tremor, and spectral features—reflect both emotional state and neuromotor function and can therefore provide objective indicators of stimulation effects. These signals may support real-time monitoring of treatment response and facilitate data-driven protocol refinement.

Figure 2. Brain stimulation methods

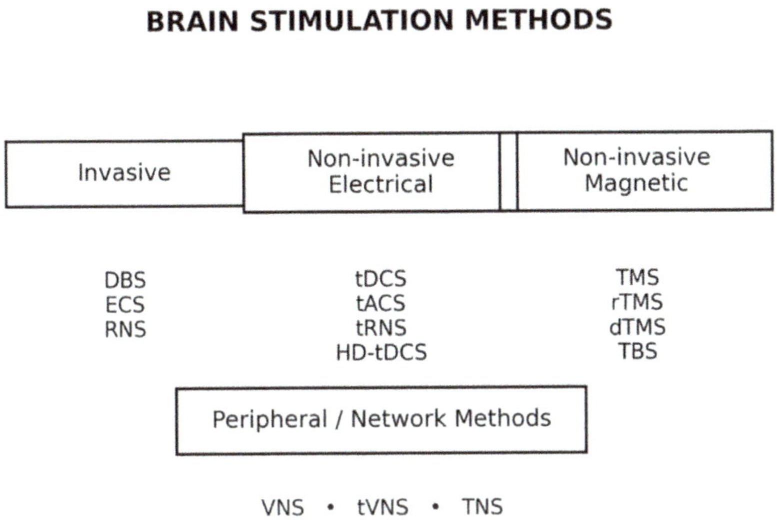

Brain stimulation approaches include invasive techniques, non-invasive electrical and magnetic methods, and peripheral neuromodulation strategies. These techniques differ in mechanism, level of invasiveness, and clinical application but share the goal of modulating neural circuits involved in cognition, emotion, and behavior (Figure 2).

Figure 3. Emotional disorders

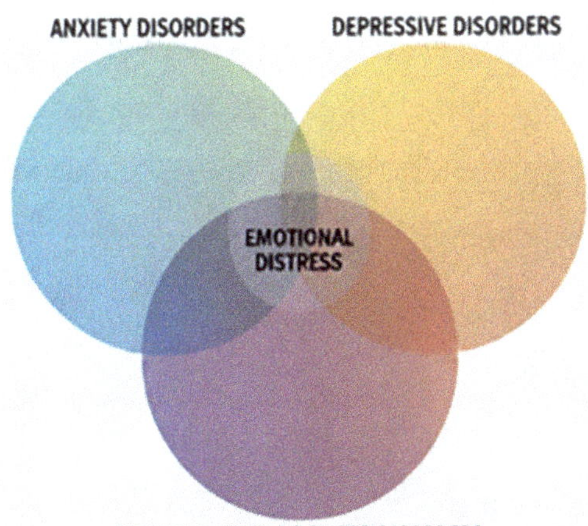

Figure 3 typically refers to the Mechanistic Overlap of emotional disorders.

Figure 4. Environmental factors related to mood disorders

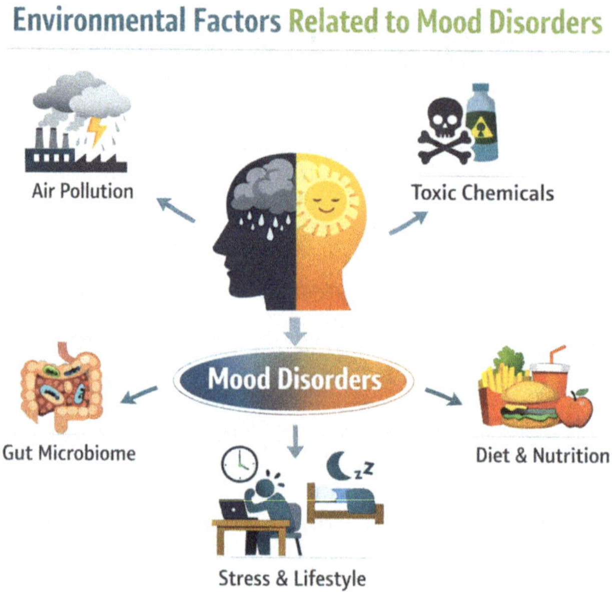

Environmental factors can affect mental health and increase the risk of mood disorders like depression and bipolar disorder. Things such as air pollution, toxic chemicals, and unhealthy diets can influence how the brain works. The gut microbiome also plays a role in mood through the gut–brain connection. In addition, stress, poor sleep, and lifestyle habits can impact emotional well-being. These factors work together and may contribute to changes in mood and mental health.

Figure 5. Ways to prevent mood disorders

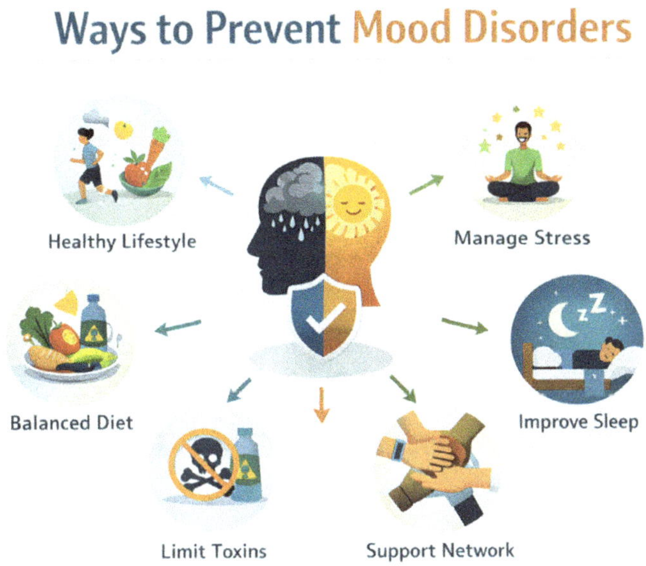

As shown in Figure 5, several lifestyle strategies can help reduce the risk of mood disorders. Maintaining a healthy lifestyle, including regular physical activity, supports overall brain health. Eating a balanced diet provides essential nutrients needed for proper brain function. Learning to manage stress through relaxation techniques or mindfulness can improve emotional stability. Getting adequate and consistent sleep is essential for mood regulation. Limiting exposure to toxins and harmful substances may also protect mental health. Finally, building a strong support network of family and friends provides emotional support and resilience.

Figure 6. Neurostimulation-related potential side effects

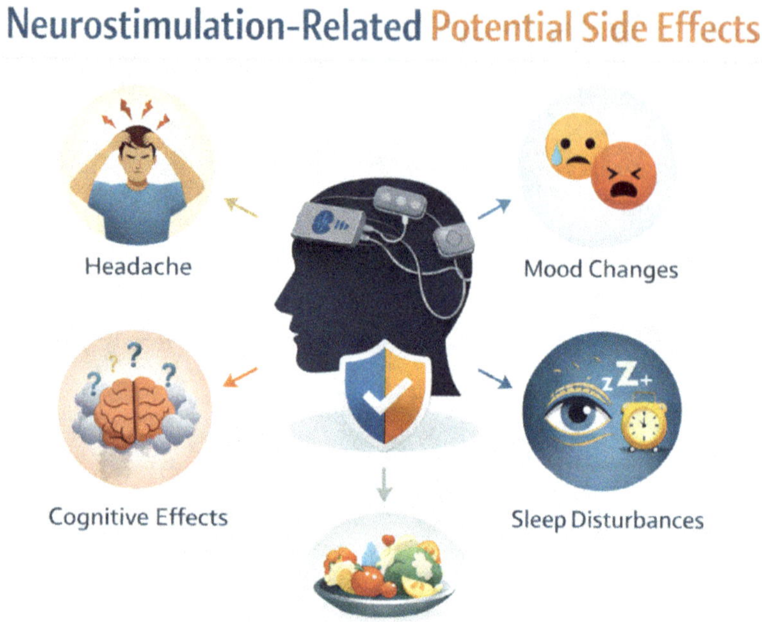

As illustrated in Figure 6, neurostimulation treatments are generally well tolerated, but some individuals may experience mild and temporary side effects. Common effects include headache and local discomfort during or after stimulation. Some patients may notice mood changes, such as irritability or emotional sensitivity. Cognitive effects, including mild concentration or memory difficulties, can occur in certain cases. Additionally, sleep disturbances may be reported during treatment. These side effects are typically manageable and should be monitored by a healthcare professional throughout the treatment process.

Figure 7. How neurostimulation works

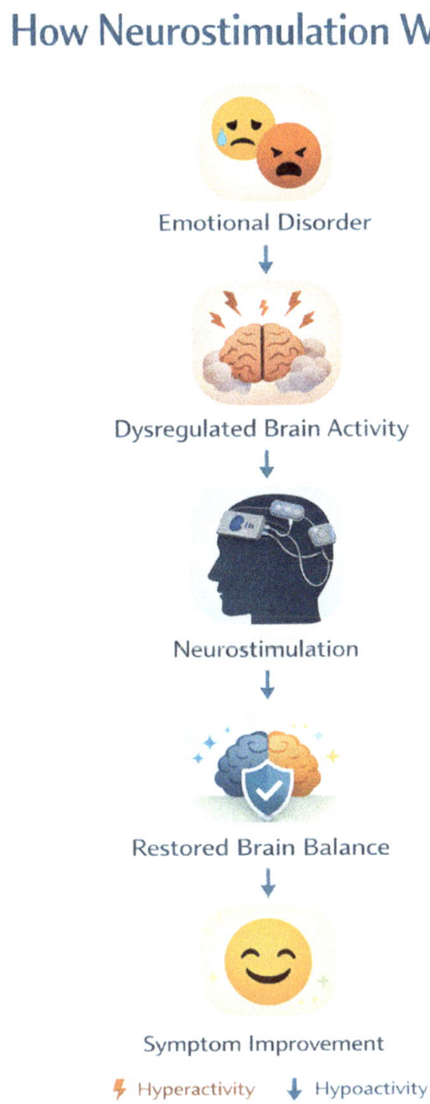

Figure 7 illustrates the mechanistic framework underlying neurostimulation in emotional disorders. Emotional disorders such as depression and anxiety are associated with dysregulated neural activity, typically characterized by limbic hyperactivity and prefrontal hypoactivity within emotion-regulation networks.

Neurostimulation techniques (e.g., DBS, TMS, tDCS, tACS, and VNS) modulate neural excitability and synaptic plasticity in targeted brain regions. By delivering controlled electrical or magnetic stimulation, these interventions aim to rebalance dysfunctional circuits, normalize network connectivity, and restore cortical–subcortical communication.

REFERENCES

Baudouin, R., Lechien, J. R., Carpentier, L., Gurruchaga, J.-M., Lisan, Q., & Hans, S. (2023). Deep brain stimulation impact on voice and speech quality in Parkinson's disease: A systematic review. *Otolaryngology - Head and Neck Surgery, 168*(3), 307–318. DOI: 10.1177/01945998221120189 PMID: 36040825

Deer, T. R., Mekhail, N., Petersen, E., Krames, E., Staats, P., Pope, J., Saweris, Y., Lad, S. P., Diwan, S., Falowski, S., Feler, C., Slavin, K., Narouze, S., Merabet, L., Buvanendran, A., Fregni, F., Wellington, J., & Levy, R. M. (2014). The appropriate use of neurostimulation: Stimulation of the intracranial and extracranial space and head for chronic pain. *Neuromodulation, 17*(6), 551–570. DOI: 10.1111/ner.12215 PMID: 25112890

Elyamany, O., Leicht, G., Herrmann, C. S., & Mulert, C. (2021). Transcranial alternating current stimulation (tACS): From basic mechanisms towards first applications in psychiatry. *European Archives of Psychiatry and Clinical Neuroscience, 271*(1), 135–156. DOI: 10.1007/s00406-020-01209-9 PMID: 33211157

Hyde, J., Carr, H., Kelley, N., Seneviratne, R., Reed, C., Parlatini, V., Garner, M., Solmi, M., Rosson, S., Cortese, S., & Brandt, V. (2022). Efficacy of neurostimulation across mental disorders: Systematic review and meta-analysis of 208 randomized controlled trials. *Molecular Psychiatry, 27*(6), 2709–2719. DOI: 10.1038/s41380-022-01524-8 PMID: 35365806

Iyer, M. B., Mattu, U., Grafman, J., Lomarev, M., Sato, S., & Wassermann, E. M. (2005). Safety and cognitive effect of frontal DC brain polarization in healthy individuals. *Neurology, 64*(5), 872–875. DOI: 10.1212/01.WNL.0000152986.07469.E9 PMID: 15753425

Jo, J. M., Kim, Y.-H., Ko, M.-H., Ohn, S. H., Joen, B., & Lee, K. H. (2009). Enhancing the working memory of stroke patients using tDCS. *American Journal of Physical Medicine & Rehabilitation, 88*(5), 404–409. DOI: 10.1097/PHM.0b013e3181a0e4cb PMID: 19620953

Lafleur, L.-P., Murray, A., Desforges, M., Pacheco-Barrios, K., Fregni, F., Tremblay, S., Saint-Amour, D., Lepage, J.-F., & Théoret, H. (2021). No aftereffects of high current density 10 Hz and 20 Hz tACS on sensorimotor alpha and beta oscillations. *Scientific Reports, 11*(1), 21416. DOI: 10.1038/s41598-021-00850-1 PMID: 34725379

Lu, F., Zhao, K., Wu, Y., Kong, Y., Gao, Y., & Zhang, L. (2023). Voice-related outcomes in deep brain stimulation in patients with vocal tremor: A systematic review and meta-analysis. *Journal of Voice*. Advance online publication. DOI: 10.1016/j.jvoice.2023.09.027 PMID: 37880051

Magis, D., & Schoenen, J. (2012). Advances and challenges in neurostimulation for headaches. *Lancet Neurology*, *11*(8), 708–719. DOI: 10.1016/S1474-4422(12)70139-4 PMID: 22814542

Mate, M. A., Cobeta, I., Jiménez-Jiménez, F. J., & Figueiras, R. (2012). Digital voice analysis in patients with advanced Parkinson's disease undergoing deep brain stimulation therapy. *Journal of Voice*, *26*(4), 496–501. DOI: 10.1016/j.jvoice.2011.03.006 PMID: 21704492

Nitsche, M. A., Koschack, J., Pohlers, H., Hullemann, S., Paulus, W., & Happe, S. (2012). Effects of frontal transcranial direct current stimulation on emotional state and processing in healthy humans. *Frontiers in Psychiatry*, *3*, 58. DOI: 10.3389/fpsyt.2012.00058 PMID: 22723786

Paulus, W. (2011). Transcranial electrical stimulation (tES–tDCS; tRNS, tACS) methods. *Neuropsychological Rehabilitation*, *21*(5), 602–617. DOI: 10.1080/09602011.2011.557292 PMID: 21819181

Sidtis, D. V. L., Rogers, T., Godier, V., Tagliati, M., & Sidtis, J. J. (2010). Voice and fluency changes as a function of speech task and deep brain stimulation. *Journal of Speech, Language, and Hearing Research: JSLHR*, *53*(5), 1167–1177. DOI: 10.1044/1092-4388(2010/09-0154) PMID: 20643796

Tabari, F., Berger, J. I., Flouty, O., Copeland, B., Greenlee, J. D., & Johari, K. (2024). Speech, voice, and language outcomes following deep brain stimulation: A systematic review. *PLoS One*, *19*(5), e0302739. DOI: 10.1371/journal.pone.0302739 PMID: 38728329

Yang, Y., Wei, P., Shi, J., Mao, Y., Zhang, J., Lei, D., & Li, W. (2025). Early assessment of responsive neurostimulation for drug-resistant epilepsy in China: A multicenter, self-controlled study. *Chinese Medical Journal*, *138*(4), 430–440. DOI: 10.1097/CM9.0000000000003292 PMID: 39593204

Chapter 8
Psychoneuroimmunology of Pelvic Pain

Issa Sulaiman Al-Amri
http://orcid.org/0000-0002-8238-8074
College of Arts and Sciences, Nizwa, Oman

Hoda Doustmohammadi
http://orcid.org/0009-0007-0280-8985
University of Nizw, Oman

Ashkan Delavari
http://orcid.org/0009-0007-0280-8985
University of Semnan, Iran

EXECUTIVE SUMMARY

Chronic Pelvic Pain (CPP) is pain lasting over three months, classified as a biopsychosocial disorder in ICD-11. Endometriosis and interstitial cystitis/bladder pain syndrome (IC/BPS) cause CPP, linking to depression and poor life quality. The Psychoneuroimmunological (PNI) model explains CPP's involvement with immune, nervous, and psychological systems. In endometriosis, ectopic implants trigger immune cell infiltration, increasing cytokines and NGF. IC/BPS shows inflammation with immune infiltration causing sensitization. Inflammatory signals activate microglia and astrocytes, triggering neuroinflammation. Stress affects the HPA axis, reducing anti-inflammatory responses and activating NLRP3 inflammasome. The gut-brain axis links dysbiosis to inflammation, while epigenetic mechanisms maintain neuronal hyperexcitability. Treatment must target the neuroimmune axis through pharmacologic and behavioral therapy for outcomes.

DOI: 10.4018/979-8-3373-3084-6.ch008

INTRODUCTION

A state of chronic pelvic pain may be viewed as a major and debilitating health issue, and it affects individuals of different backgrounds, impacting their lives in a substantial manner. Chronic pelvic pain may be defined as pain of pelvic origin, and it may be characterized by its presence or recurrence, persisting for a period of time exceeding three months. The ICD-11 classifies chronic pelvic pain as a separate entity of disease, and it is imperative to distinguish it from other circumstances where pelvic pain may be viewed as a symptom of another health issue.(Barke et al., 2022; Batulan et al., 2024; Siqueira-Campos et al.). This position is justified by the complex pathophysiology and the significant disease burden associated with chronic pain. Chronic pelvic pain is one of the most frequent causes of gynecologic visits and is strongly linked with prevalent mental health conditions such as posttraumatic stress disorder and major depressive disorder (Chen, 2023; Yamamoto et al., 2014). It is a multifactorial syndrome with multiple aetiologies, and endometriosis and interstitial cystitis/bladder pain syndrome (IC/BPS) are major contributors to chronic pelvic pain. Endometriosis, which is characterized by endometrial tissue located outside of the uterine cavity, is a major factor associated with chronic pelvic pain. Moreover, by acknowledging IC/BPS as a major contributor, there is a recognition of the relationship between urological and gynecological pain syndromes, as there is an interrelation between the two (Inzoli et al., 2024). The prevalence of these diseases is high; for instance, IC/BPS alone has been estimated to affect 3.3-7.9 million women in the United States (Yang et al., 2021). Endometriosis is a common disease that affects women throughout their lives (Siqueira-Campos et al.).

Figure 1. Chronic pelvic pain is a biopsychosocial condition involving pelvic pathology, psychological distress, and immune-nervous system interactions, which affect the quality of life.

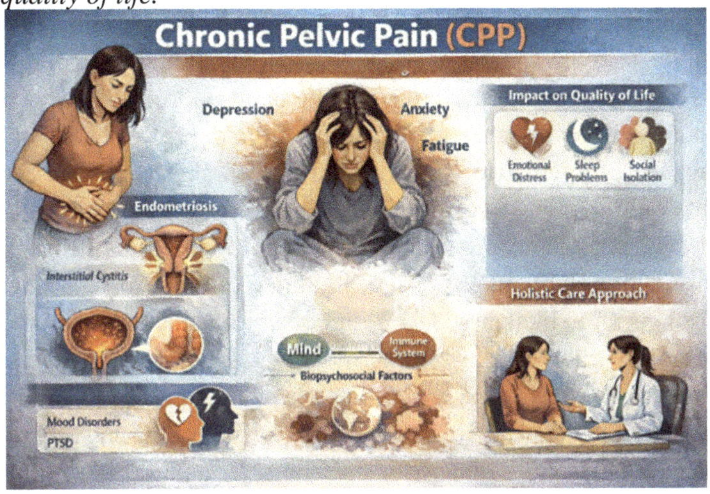

The importance of these diseases can also be understood not only based on the high prevalence rates but also considering the high level of distress that these diseases cause. The level of distress is indicated by the pain experienced, the presence of urinary symptoms, pain that occurs during sexual activities, and the changes that these diseases cause to the physical and mental aspects of HRQoL (Lin et al., 2021; Wang et al., 2021). One of the characteristics that defines chronic pelvic pain is the significantly high rates of comorbidity with mood and anxiety disorders. A considerable body of research has found that pelvic pain is significantly associated with psychological distress through several systematic reviews and meta-analyses. (Szypłowska et al., 2023; van Barneveld et al., 2022). In the setting of endometriosis, a systematic review reported that depressive symptoms had a varying prevalence of 9.8% to 98.5%, and anxiety from 11.5% to 87.5%(Szypłowska et al., 2023). Consolidated data indicate that 86% of women with endometriosis report depression, 29% experience moderately severe anxiety, and 68% encounter mood disorders in general(del Pino-Sedeño et al., 2024). These figures markedly exceed the global prevalence of depressive and anxiety disorders, which are approximately 4.4% and 7.3%, respectively. The association seems to be bidirectional and strong; a meta-analysis showed that women with endometriosis have significantly higher odds of experiencing both anxiety and depression than those without the condition(Delanerolle et al., 2021; Organization, 2017; van Barneveld et al., 2022).

Similar trends were observed for interstitial cystitis/bladder pain syndrome. Depression and anxiety are more prevalent among patients with IC/BPS than in the general population in all studies that reported on these comorbidities(Fischer-Grote et al., 2022). For instance, in a structural equation modeling study, it was found that 47.26% of patients with bladder pain syndrome/interstitial cystitis (BPS/IC) had depression, and 43.88% had anxiety, which clearly shows the emotional toll that these patients are under (Wu et al., 2025). In a separate study, people who have been diagnosed with interstitial cystitis/bladder pain syndrome have been shown to have a greater likelihood of currently suffering from depression and panic attacks. Furthermore, these psychiatric symptoms have been shown to have a significant link to quality of life. Interestingly, these psychiatric symptoms have been shown to coexist with IC/BPS, and insomnia and other somatic symptoms have been present. (Hsieh et al., 2021; Wu et al., 2025). The high rate of co-occurrence suggests that the relationship is more likely to be the result of a biological component rather than the reactive and psychological effects of living with chronic pain. The psychological effect of chronic pelvic pain is not simply a change in mood. The chronic and persistent nature of the pain, as well as the possibly frustrating and time-consuming process to attain an accurate diagnosis, contributes to considerable psychological stress. In addition, some level of social isolation is caused by the private and stigmatized nature of chronic pain. Moreover, lifestyle changes are caused by the need to manage pain and to regularly visit medical facilities (Mazza et al., 2024).

Loneliness is also heightened by the presence of fatigue, which in turn acts as a symptom. There exists an association between fatigue and increased TNFα levels in patients with chronic pelvic pain, which in turn establishes the connection between fatigue and systemic inflammation. (Karshikoff et al., 2021). In addition, cognitive distortions such as catastrophizing, the tendency to overestimate the threat value of pain, and feelings of helplessness due to pain are common in this group and have been established as important drivers that contribute to both the perception of pain and disability (Mazza et al., 2024; Sutherland et al., 2023). The toll that CPP takes on the individual to manage a chronic illness that involves pain, sleep disturbances, and distress places a heavy toll on the coping resources of the individual (Mazza et al., 2024). This impact is significant enough that the management of CPP now specifically includes attention to its psychological aspects, recognizing that untreated distress directly contributes to the worsening of physical symptoms and the efficacy of treatments [20]. This complex interaction between physical pain, emotional suffering, and functional impairment requires a biopsychosocial approach to treatment. The high prevalence rate argues for the necessity of researching a psychoneuroimmunological approach to understanding the interaction between the combined systems of the mind, nervous system, and immune system in creating and maintaining this disabling combination of symptoms.(Engeler et al., 2018).

INFLAMMATORY MECHANISMS AND CELLULAR PLAYERS IN PELVIC PATHOLOGIES

There is an increasing body of knowledge regarding the pathogenesis of chronic pelvic pain syndromes such as endometriosis and interstitial cystitis/chronic pelvic pain syndrome (IC/BPS). The emerging body of knowledge acknowledges the role of the dysfunctional neuroimmune interface as the key driver of pain perception. Pain is no longer seen as the passive endpoint of structural abnormalities but is propelled by an intricate inflammatory milieu. The inflammatory milieu is an intricate interplay of various inflammatory cells and mediators that interact with the nervous system. In the pathogenesis of endometriosis, the pro-inflammatory state is driven by the abnormal tissue of the endometrium present in the peritoneal cavity (Golinska et al., 2025). This is mediated by a variety of immune cells, including macrophages, neutrophils, and natural killer (NK) cells, that are unable to effectively remove the ectopic tissue (Chen & Li, 2023).

In this regard, the role of mast cells in the process under consideration cannot be overstated. Mast cells, as part of the human immune system, have granules and are located close to the neural fibers in the pelvic organs. There has been a considerable number of mast cells found in endometriotic lesions located close to the nerve fibers. The close location of the mast cells and the nerve fibers in the endometriotic lesions indicates a close interaction between the two (Golinska et al., 2025; Skaper et al., 2018). This close proximity of mast cells to nervous tissue makes them a key intermediary in the interface of the immune system and nervous system. When mast cells become activated, a state often induced by estrogen, a chemical commonly found in endometriomas of the ovaries, mast cells undergo a process of degranulation, where their cellular granules are released. This chemical environment directly sensitizes nociceptors, increasing pain perception (Chen & Li, 2023; Golinska et al., 2025). Mediators include histamine, serotonin, proteolytic enzymes such as tryptase, lipid metabolites such as prostaglandin D2, and NGF (Skaper et al., 2018); Golinska et al., 2025). Nerve Growth Factor (NGF), for instance, has been found to facilitate the process of axonal sprouting and to increase the excitability of the neuron. On the other hand, other pain mediators have been observed to activate the ion channels present in the sensory nerves, and for instance, they may react with the TRPV1 and TRPA1 channels, thus reducing the threshold of activation of these sensory nerves. Research findings have shown that the density of the nerve fibers present in the endometriotic lesions is significantly higher than in the control tissue. In addition, the distance between the gland structures and the nerve fibers is less in painful endometriosis (Chen & Li; Golinska et al., 2025). Inflammation in endometriosis is propagated by a network of soluble mediators, mainly proinflammatory cytokines. The main cytokines in this network are IL-6,

TNF-α, and IL-1β (Cuffaro et al., 2024; Graziottin et al., 2015). These factors are produced by endometriotic cells and infiltrating immune cells in the endometriotic lesions. These factors interact and play a role in the development and growth of endometriotic lesions, angiogenesis, and pain. Interleukin-6 has been shown to play a causal role in infertility in patients with endometriosis and to be a part of a signal transduction cascade involved in the growth and development of nerve fibers (Golinska et al., 2025). Another key mediator is PGE2, which has a major role in pain and inflammatory conditions. The inflammatory condition is not restricted to the peritoneal cavity only; in women suffering from endometriosis, the serum level of IL-6, TNF-α, and C-reactive protein has been found to be elevated. (Jiang et al., 2013; Yang et al., 2025). One study found that, among patients with endometriosis and co-morbid depression and anxiety, there are significantly elevated peripheral inflammatory markers, including interleukin-6 (IL-6), interleukin-1β (IL-1β), tumor necrosis factor-alpha (TNF-α), and C-reactive protein (CRP), compared with those with endometriosis alone. There is a direct relationship between inflammatory markers and psychological co-morbidity. There is also additional evidence of the relationship between pelvic inflammatory activity and psychological co-morbidity. (Yang et al., 2025). Sustained neuroinflammation is a pathophysiological mechanism of interstitial cystitis/bladder pain syndrome. This condition describes bladder pressure and pain exacerbated by filling, which impacts the quality of life (Lin et al., 2021; Moldwin et al.).

The bladder wall of patients with IC/BPS shows chronic inflammation through the infiltration and activation of immune cells (Graziottin et al., 2015). Immunophenotyping demonstrates B-cell- and T-cell responses, with IL-6 driving B-cell activation and diminishing T-regulatory cell suppression to maintain inflammation (Fallon et al., 2023). Mast cells are also involved in the formation of neuro-immune interactions near the bladder wall and the initiation of pain behaviors. The interaction between sensory cells and mast cells near the bladder wall maintains the cyclic process that results in bladder pain (Hayes et al., 2024; He et al., 2024). Pro-inflammatory cytokines play a critical role in the pathophysiology of diseases, including endometriosis and IC/BPS. Cytokines IL-1β, IL-6, and TNF-α have been implicated in the pathology of IC/BPS. There is active investigation of urinary measurements of these cytokines as non-invasive disease biomarkers (Graziottin et al., 2015; Jiang et al., 2021; Lin et al., 2021). The consistency between pelvic pain disorders suggests a mechanistic theme: a cycle in which local tissue inflammation, driven by resident immune cells such as mast cells and mediated by cytokines, induces nervous system sensitization that perpetuates the chronic, hypersensitive pain state of CPP. Dorsal root ganglia (which contain the cell bodies of primary sensory neurons) are critical. Resident immune cells in the DRG and interactions between macrophages and glial cells can directly modulate nociceptive signal pathways, contributing to the development of sensitization (Chen & Li, 2023; Meade & Garvey, 2022; Singto et al., 2025).

Figure 2. Neuroimmune interactions in chronic pelvic pain include local pelvic inflammation caused by immune cells and cytokines, which increase the sensitization of sensory nerves in endometriosis and interstitial cystitis/bladder painful syndrome (IC/BPS).

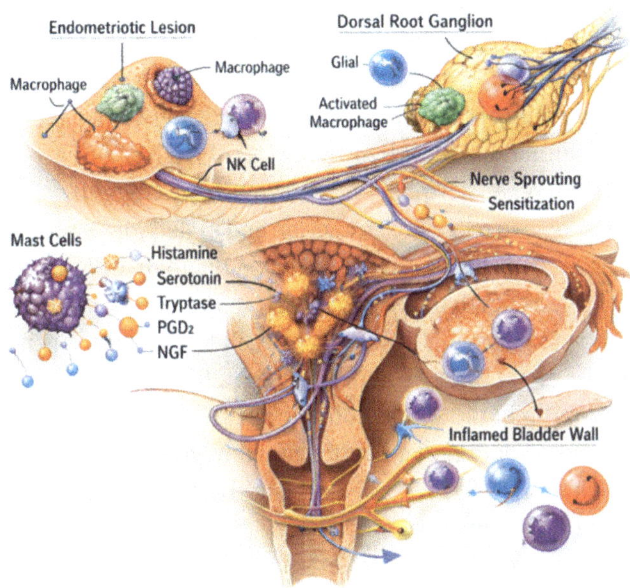

THE NEUROIMMUNE AXIS: BIDIRECTIONAL COMMUNICATION BETWEEN PELVIS AND BRAIN

CPP and mood disorders show a bidirectional neuro-immune association. the place where inflamed pelvic signals reach the central nervous system (CNS) to amplify pain and negative emotion. Psychological stress exacerbates peripheral inflammation and pain perception. This creates a self-sustaining pathological loop that is resistant to conventional treatment. Safety-related information is transmitted from the environment to the brain via mechanisms, including the passage of circulating cytokines, such as IL-1α, IL-1β, and TNF-α, across the blood-brain barrier (BBB) (Meade & Garvey, 2022; Walker et al., 2013). Upon entering the central nervous system (CNS), these cytokines can directly activate resident immune cells, namely microglia and astrocytes, and initiate a state of neuroinflammation. Upon entering the central nervous system (CNS), these cytokines can directly activate local immune cells, specifically microglia and astrocytes, thereby initiating neuroinflammation (Luo et al.; Skaper et al., 2018). The alternative pathway reliably produces secondary intermediates, including PGE2 and NO, which are synthesized in brain endothelial cells. Cytokines are generated at the brain endothelium and readily traverse the blood-brain barrier, exerting direct effects on neurons and glial cells (Walker et al., 2013). Cytokine signals from the peritoneal cavity activate sensory neurons in the hepatic vagus nerve, which project to the nucleus of the tractus solitarius (NTS) in the brainstem. Studies have confirmed that cutting this neural pathway (subdiaphragmatic vagotomy) prevents sickness behaviors, such as hyperalgesia and social withdrawal, after systemic inflammatory stimuli, proving its role in immune-to-brain signalling (Walker et al., 2013). When peripheral signals reach the CNS, they initiate a cascade of events that culminate in neuroinflammation and maladaptive plasticity. Microglia and macrophages of the brain and spinal cord are the main immune effector cells in this process. In response to cytokine signals from the periphery, microglia become "primed" and activated, moving from a surveillant to a reactive phenotype (Coluzzi et al., 2025; Skaper et al., 2018; Tizenberg et al., 2021).

Activated microglia in the spinal cord dorsal horn and pain-related areas of the brain, such as the anterior cingulate cortex and amygdala, release pro-inflammatory mediators, such as IL-1β, IL-6, TNF-α, and brain-derived neurotrophic factor (BDNF). This neuroinflammatory process modulates the neuronal function. BDNF secreted by microglia impairs the regulation of chloride ion homeostasis in spinal neurons, leading to disinhibition of pain transmission and the induction of central sensitization, a condition of increased neuronal excitability that is typical of many chronic pain conditions(Chen & Li, 2025; Dodds et al., 2016; Majima et al., 2018). This phenomenon extends beyond theoretical thought. Mouse models of endometriosis show extensive glial activation in the central nervous system, suggesting that chronic pelvic inflammation can lead to neuroinflammation in the brain and the spinal cord. Central sensitization reduces the threshold for pain, where normal stimuli are interpreted as pain (allodynia), and painful stimuli are perceived as more intense (hyperalgesia) (Chen & Li, 2025). Conversely, the brain-to-pelvis portion of the axis shows how psychological distress is an active participant in maintaining an inflammatory condition. Chronic stress and depression are known to disrupt the balance of two major physiological systems: the hypothalamic-pituitary-adrenal (HPA) axis and the autonomic nervous system (ANS)(GP, 2009; Li et al., 2025). Concurrently, psychological distress also initiates a change in the balance of the autonomic nervous system from parasympathetic dominance, also known as the "rest and digest" state, to sympathetic dominance, also known as the "fight or flight" response. The vagus nerve, the main parasympathetic nerve, plays an important anti-inflammatory role through the inflammatory reflex (Cerritelli et al., 2021; Gargus et al., 2025). When the level of vagal tone decreases, the inhibitory modulation of inflammation is removed, and the unregulated production of cytokines becomes possible. Psychological stress can prime the immune system for an exaggerated response. The inflammasome, an intracellular complex of multiple proteins that recognizes danger signals, plays a crucial role in mediating the relationship between psychological stress and the development of depression and inflammation(Iwata et al., 2013).

This primed state makes any following challenges prone to an exaggerated inflammatory response. A bidirectional feedback loop is shown in an endometriosis model where the ectopic lesions produce inflammatory mediators to activate mast cells and sensitize neurons. The activated mast cells, in turn, produce more inflammatory mediators, further sensitizing the neurons, thus creating a self-reinforcing cycle of inflammation. This model represents the psychoneuroimmunology (PNI) paradigm of the disease, where the pelvic pathology leads to a neuroimmune response that is then self-reinforced by psychological and physiological events, thus highlighting the need for a holistic therapeutic strategy (Golinska et al., 2025).

Figure 3. Bidirectional neuroimmune communication between pelvic inflammation and the brain. Peripheral immune signalling promotes central neuroinflammation and sensitization, whereas psychological stress and autonomic dysregulation feedback amplify pelvic inflammation.

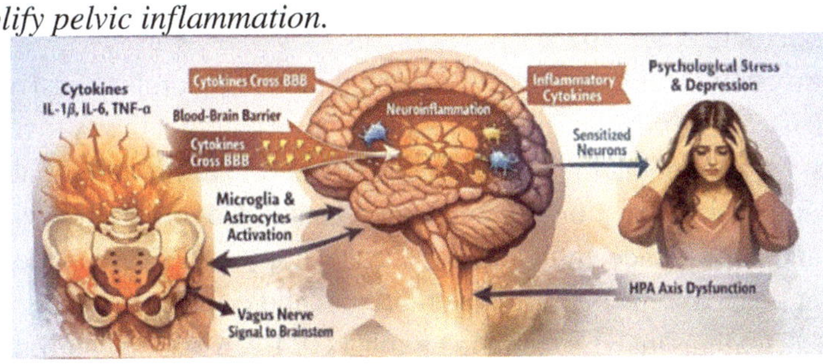

INTEGRATED THERAPEUTIC STRATEGIES TARGETING THE NEUROIMMUNE AXIS

Given the intricate interactions between pain, mood, and inflammation, effective management of chronic pelvic pain necessitates a comprehensive strategy that targets various points along the PNI axis. Conventional methods that focus on analgesia or surgical excision have proven to be of limited use, thus highlighting the importance of treatments that interact with the neuroimmune system. The development of pharmacological treatments is shifting from the use of broad-spectrum analgesics to drugs that act on specific inflammatory mediators. While both opioid and non-opioid pain medications are available, their use is limited due to side effects and nociplastic pain caused by central sensitization(Stanos et al., 2021). In relation to endometriosis, preclinical studies have identified promising repurposed drugs that target the JAK/STAT signaling pathway. This pathway is overexpressed in endometriotic lesions and is involved in linking immune activation to the development of nerve fibers(Golinska et al., 2025).

JAK inhibitors and mast cell stabilizers, such as Sodium Cromoglycate and Ketotifen, have shown promise in animal studies for treating symptoms by blocking this pathway and preventing mast cell degranulation, respectively(Golinska et al., 2025). Similarly, the noted effectiveness of anti-TNF agents in improving mood symptoms in patients with inflammatory bowel disease (IBD), a condition that has a high comorbidity with depression, offers a strong proof of concept for the use of peripheral cytokine modulation to treat both physical and psychological symptoms(Luo et al.). An area worth exploring further is herbal medicine, particularly Traditional Chinese Medicine (TCM). For example, the Yueju pill has been shown to have antidepressant-like effects in rat models, which could be related to the NF-kappaB signaling pathway, a key mediator of the inflammatory response TCM is a recognized treatment for neuropathic pain, and its use is recognized in official guidelines(Zhixiang et al., 2025).

Non-pharmacological therapies are a crucial part of a comprehensive strategy, many of which work through the psychosocial-neuroimmune pathway to re-establish homeostasis. Psychological therapies have a central role in the care of any chronic disease that imposes a heavy burden on mental health. Cognitive Behavioral Therapy (CBT) and Acceptance and Commitment Therapy (ACT) are evidence-based therapies that help patients manage the emotional and cognitive aspects of chronic pain (Luo et al.). Meta-analytic results show that CBT can lead to significant reductions in anxiety and depression scores in patients with inflammatory bowel disease (IBD), with some evidence suggesting that ACT may be similarly or more effective (Luo et al.). These therapies help patients develop adaptive coping strategies, reduce catastrophizing, and improve overall functioning in the face of pain (Sutherland et al., 2023). Physical therapies, specifically pelvic floor physical therapy, also play a critical role in that myofascial pain and dysfunction are common contributors to chronic pelvic pain (CPP) (Batulan et al., 2024; Lamvu, 2020). However, the most promising area of non-pharmacological therapy seems to lie in the realm of neuromodulation. Acupuncture, a traditional Chinese medicine modality, has been shown in randomized controlled trials to significantly reduce anxiety and depression in patients with chronic disease (Liu et al.).

The proposed mechanism is multisystemic and based on neuroimmunomodulation. There is evidence that acupuncture could help alleviate depression by normalizing feedback regulation in the hypothalamic-pituitary-adrenal (HPA) axis and by suppressing activation of CNS glial cells, thus reducing neuroinflammation (N. Li et al.; Zhang et al., 2025). Non-invasive neuromodulation therapies also hold great promise. Transcutaneous auricular vagus nerve stimulation (taVNS) is a therapy that targets the auricular branch of the vagus nerve through cutaneous stimulation of the ear; because of the central role of the vagus nerve in the inflammatory reflex, taVNS could reduce systemic inflammation by enhancing parasympathetic tone (Gargus et al.). A recent randomized comparative trial has shown that a combination of taVNS and electroacupuncture was effective in treating chronic pelvic pain (CPP), and this highlights the promise of complementary neuromodulatory approaches (S. Li et al.). Neuromodulation techniques that do not involve invasive procedures are also being investigated as potential novel methods for the therapy of CPP (Alam & Chen, 2023). This integrative framework unifies the fields of pharmacotherapy, neuromodulation, and psychological interventions. Thus, it signifies a paradigm shift from the management of symptoms to the facilitation of homeostatic restoration in the mind-body-immune axis.

EMERGING PARADIGMS AND FUTURE DIRECTIONS IN PELVIC PAIN RESEARCH

While the PNI model provides a rationale for the co-occurrence of pelvic pain and mood disorders, new paradigms offer additional understanding. The gut–brain axis, a communication network comprising the gastrointestinal system, microbiota, and central nervous system, is of major interest. (Hasan et al., 2025; Riehl et al., 2024). However, current evidence points out that alterations in gut microbiota, also called gut dysbiosis, can lead to a weakened gut barrier. The weakened gut barrier can cause a state of "leaky gut." Leaky gut is a state where bacterial components, e.g., lipopolysaccharide (LPS), enter the bloodstream. The entry of LPS into the bloodstream activates the innate immune system through a pathway involving Toll-like receptor 4 (TLR4). This results in the release of pro-inflammatory cytokines. (Cao et al., 2024). This inflammatory cascade signals the CNS, contributing to neuroinflammation and pain and depressive-like behaviours (Luo et al.; Ma et al., 2019). The vagus nerve has a crucial role in the gut-brain interaction, and it has been demonstrated that the efficacy of the action of probiotics in reducing stress is dependent on the presence of the vagal pathway. The modulation of the gut microbiome by diet, prebiotics, probiotics, or fecal transplantation may provide a key strategy in the development of new therapies for the treatment of chronic primary pain (CPP) and the associated psychiatric manifestations. (Luo et al.). Attention is focused on research regarding epigenetic changes as a potential mechanism for the long-term programming of pain and inflammation [42, 59]. Epigenetics refers to the study of heritable changes in gene expression that are not caused by alterations to the DNA sequence. These changes include DNA methylation, histone modifications, and non-coding RNAs, which can be influenced by environmental factors such as chronic stress and inflammation. In chronic pain conditions, there is DNA methylation change in the promoter region of genes involved in pain, such as OPRM1, where hypermethylation is associated with increased pain intensity. Histone deacetylases regulate pain signaling pathways by modulating synaptic transmission and neuronal excitability. Chronic pelvic pain and co-occurring mood disorders could persist through epigenetic modifications that keep neurons and glia in a hyperexcitable state. Drugs targeting these regulatory pathways may provide a therapeutic approach to reverse these epigenetic modifications (Cao et al., 2024). The discovery of intracellular pattern recognition receptors for innate immunity, particularly the inflammasome, has revealed the mechanisms of danger signal-induced inflammation. The NLRP3 inflammasome complex combines signals from pathogenic microorganisms, cell injury, and metabolic stress to trigger the expression of pro-inflammatory cytokines IL-1β and IL-18.(Cao et al., 2024). Activation of the NLRP3 inflammasome has been linked to hyperalgesia and neuropathic pain, which responds to stimuli such as ATP released from injured cells and ROS produced during the inflammatory response. Through the processing of various stimuli, including psychological stress, the inflammasome represents a promising target for therapy. Selective inhibitors of the NLRP3 inflammasome could interfere with the inflammation that underlies peripheral sensitization and neuroinflammation, potentially allowing the pain-depression cycle to be broken. The further study of pelvic pain requires the integration of these models into a peripheral neuroimmune (PNI) model, taking into consideration the gut microbiome, epigenetics, and innate immunity to provide a useful treatment for this condition (Cai et al., 2026).

CONCLUSION

Chronic pelvic pain, as a pathophysiological entity, can be best described as a biopsychosocial disorder with underlying chronic neuroimmune dysregulation. Such neuroimmune dysregulation is associated with the pathophysiological interaction of peripheral inflammatory mechanisms, central sensitization, and psychological symptomatology. For example, studies of endometriosis and interstitial cystitis/

bladder pain syndrome (IC/BPS) have identified the presence of a vicious cycle of pain, inflammatory, and mood states, all of which are interconnected through the peripheral neuroimmune system. The effective management of these patients, therefore, requires the implementation of an integrative therapeutic approach involving pharmacotherapy, neuromodulation, and psychological interventions. The establishment of the therapeutic paradigm, based on the latest understanding of the gut-brain axis, epigenetics, and innate immunity, offers great promise in the achievement of normal homeostasis in these patients.

REFERENCES

Alam, M. A.-O. X., & Chen, J. D. Z. (2023). Non-invasive neuromodulation: an emerging intervention for visceral pain in gastrointestinal disorders. (2332-8886 (Electronic)).

Barke, A., Korwisi, B., & Rief, W. (2022). Chronic Pain in the ICD-11: New Diagnoses That Clinical Psychologists Should Know About. *Clinical Psychology in Europe*, *4*(Special Issue), e9933. Advance online publication. DOI: 10.32872/cpe.9933 PMID: 36760323

Batulan, Z., Bhimla, A., Higginbotham, E. J., & National Academies of Sciences, E., and Medicine. (2024). Female-Specific and Gynecologic Conditions. In *Advancing Research on Chronic Conditions in Women*. National Academies Press (US).

Cai, X., Cai, X., Xie, Q., Xiao, X., Li, T., Zhou, T., & Sun, H. (2026). NLRP3 inflammasome and gut microbiota–brain axis: A new perspective on white matter injury after intracerebral hemorrhage. *Neural Regeneration Research*, *21*(1), 62–80. DOI: 10.4103/NRR.NRR-D-24-00917 PMID: 39885662

Cao, B., Xu, Q., Shi, Y., Zhao, R., Li, H., Zheng, J., Liu, F., Wan, Y., & Wei, B. (2024). Pathology of pain and its implications for therapeutic interventions. *Signal Transduction and Targeted Therapy*, *9*(1), 155. DOI: 10.1038/s41392-024-01845-w PMID: 38851750

Cerritelli, F., Frasch, M. G., Antonelli, M. C., Viglione, C., Vecchi, S., Chiera, M., & Manzotti, A. (2021). A review on the vagus nerve and autonomic nervous system during fetal development: Searching for critical windows. *Frontiers in Neuroscience*, *15*, 721605. DOI: 10.3389/fnins.2021.721605 PMID: 34616274

Chen, J. H. (2023). Management of Pelvic Pain, Dyspareunia, and Endometriosis. In *Handbook of Gynecology* (pp. 457–484). Springer. DOI: 10.1007/978-3-031-14881-1_78

Chen, Y., & Li, T. (2025). Unveiling the mechanisms of pain in endometriosis: Comprehensive analysis of inflammatory sensitization and therapeutic potential. *International Journal of Molecular Sciences*, *26*(4), 1770. DOI: 10.3390/ijms26041770 PMID: 40004233

Chen, Y., & Li, T. (2023). Unveiling the Mechanisms of Pain in Endometriosis: Comprehensive Analysis of Inflammatory Sensitization and Therapeutic Potential. LID - [doi] LID - 1770. (1422-0067 (Electronic)).DOI: 10.3390/ijms26041770

Coluzzi, F., Zeboudj, L., Scerpa, M. S., Giorgio, A., De Blasi, R. A., Malcangio, M., & Rocco, M. (2025). Microglial Activation in Nociplastic Pain: From Preclinical Models to PET Neuroimaging and Implications for Targeted Therapeutic Strategies. *International Journal of Molecular Sciences*, *26*(24), 11861. DOI: 10.3390/ijms262411861 PMID: 41465288

Cuffaro, F., Russo, E., & Amedei, A. (2024). Endometriosis, pain, and related psychological disorders: Unveiling the interplay among the microbiome, inflammation, and oxidative stress as a common thread. *International Journal of Molecular Sciences*, *25*(12), 6473. DOI: 10.3390/ijms25126473 PMID: 38928175

del Pino-Sedeño, T., Cabrera-Maroto, M., Abrante-Luis, A., González-Hernández, Y., & Ortiz Herrera, M. C. (2024). Effectiveness of psychological interventions in endometriosis: A systematic review with meta-analysis. *Frontiers in Psychology*, *15*, 1457842. DOI: 10.3389/fpsyg.2024.1457842 PMID: 39529727

Delanerolle, G., Ramakrishnan, R., Hapangama, D., Zeng, Y., Shetty, A., Elneil, S., & Phiri, P. (2021). A systematic review and meta-analysis of the Endometriosis and Mental-Health Sequelae; The ELEMI Project. *Women's Health (London, England)*, *17*, 17455065211019717. DOI: 10.1177/17455065211019717 PMID: 34053382

Dodds, K. N., Beckett, E. A., Evans, S. F., Grace, P. M., Watkins, L. R., & Hutchinson, M. R. (2016). Glial contributions to visceral pain: implications for disease etiology and the female predominance of persistent pain. (2158-3188 (Electronic)).

Engeler, D., Baranowski, A., Borovicka, J., Cottrell, A. M., Dinis, P., Elneil, S., . . . Goonewardene, S. (2018). EAU Guidelines, Full Text, Chronic Pelvic Pain 2018. European Association of Urology. Daniel Engeler, AP Baranowski, J. Borovicka, AQ Cottrell, P Dinis- Oliveira, S. Elneil, J Hughes, Bert Messelink, AC De Williams. Guidelines Associates: B Parsons, S Goonewardene. In.

Fallon, J., Stern, I. T., Laurent, M., Birder, L., Moldwin, R. M., & Stern, J. N. H. (2023). The immune system in Interstitial Cystitis/Bladder Pain Syndrome and therapeutic agents. *Continence*, *8*, 101057. https://doi.org/https://doi.org/10.1016/j.cont.2023.101057. DOI: 10.1016/j.cont.2023.101057

Fischer-Grote, L., Fössing, V., Aigner, M., Boeckle, M., & Fehrmann, E. (2022). Comorbidities of bladder pain syndrome in the context of the HITOP distress category: A systematic review and meta-analysis. *International Urogynecology Journal*, *33*(9), 2335–2356. DOI: 10.1007/s00192-022-05129-1 PMID: 35262767

Gargus, M., Ben-Azu, B., Landwehr, A., Dunn, J., Errico, J. P., & Tremblay, M. (2025). Mechanisms of vagus nerve stimulation for the treatment of neurodevelopmental disorders: a focus on microglia and neuroinflammation. (1662-4548 (Print)).

Golinska, M., Wolyniak, M., Kulesza, P., & Fendler, W. (2025). Neuroinflammation is responsible for pain in endometriosis-targeting the JAK-STAT pathway and mast cell activation. *Frontiers in Immunology, 16*, 1621178. DOI: 10.3389/fimmu.2025.1621178 PMID: 40948761

Golinska, M., Wołyniak, M., Kulesza, P., & Fendler, W. (2025). Neuroinflammation is responsible for pain in endometriosis - targeting the JAK-STAT pathway and mast cell activation. (1664-3224 (Electronic)).

GP, C. (2009). Stress and disorders of the stress system. *Nat Rev Endocrinol, 5*, 374-381.

Graziottin, A., Gambini, D., & Bertolasi, L. (2015). Genital and sexual pain in women. In Vodušek, D. B., & Boller, F. (Eds.), *Handbook of Clinical Neurology* (Vol. 130, pp. 395–412). Elsevier., https://doi.org/https://doi.org/10.1016/B978-0-444-63247-0.00023-7

Hasan, A., Scuderi, S. A., Capra, A. P., Giosa, D., Bonomo, A., Ardizzone, A., & Esposito, E. (2025). An Updated and Comprehensive Review Exploring the Gut–Brain Axis in Neurodegenerative Disorders and Neurotraumas: Implications for Therapeutic Strategies. *Brain Sciences, 15*(6), 654. DOI: 10.3390/brainsci15060654 PMID: 40563824

Hayes, B., Choi, H., Rathore, A., Bao, C., Shi, J., Huh, Y., Kim, M. W., Mencarelli, A., Bist, P., Ng, L. G., Shi, C., Nho, J. H., Kim, A., Yoon, H., Lim, D., Hannan, J. L., Purves, J. T., Hughes, F. M.Jr, Ji, R.-R., & Abraham, S. (2024). Recurrent infections drive persistent bladder dysfunction and pain via sensory nerve sprouting and mast cell activity. *Science Immunology, 9*(93), eadi5578. Advance online publication. DOI: 10.1126/sciimmunol.adi5578 PMID: 38427717

He, H. A.-O., Luo, H. A.-O., Qian, B. A.-O., Xu, H. A.-O., Zhang, G. A.-O., Zou, X. A.-O., & Zou, J. A.-O. (2024). Autonomic Nervous System Dysfunction Is Related to Chronic Prostatitis/Chronic Pelvic Pain Syndrome. (2287-4208 (Print)).

Hsieh, K.-L., Chin, H.-Y., Lo, T.-S., Long, C.-Y., Ho, C.-H., Huang, S. K.-H., Chuang, Y.-C., & Wu, M.-P. (2021). Interstitial cystitis/bladder pain syndrome patient is associated with subsequent increased risks of outpatient visits and hospitalizations: A population-based study. *PLoS One, 16*(9), e0256800. DOI: 10.1371/journal.pone.0256800 PMID: 34492065

Inzoli, A., Barba, M., Costa, C., Carazita, V., Cola, A., Fantauzzi, M.,...Frigerio, M. (2024). The Evil Twins of Chronic Pelvic Pain Syndrome: A Systematic Review and Meta-Analysis on Interstitial Cystitis/Painful Bladder Syndrome and Endometriosis. Healthcare, Iwata, M., Ota Kt Fau - Duman, R. S., & Duman, R. S. (2013). The inflammasome: pathways linking psychological stress, depression, and systemic illnesses. (1090-2139 (Electronic)).

Jiang, Y. H., Peng Ch Fau - Liu, H.-T., Liu Ht Fau - Kuo, H.-C., & Kuo, H. C. (2013). Increased pro-inflammatory cytokines, C-reactive protein and nerve growth factor expressions in serum of patients with interstitial cystitis/bladder pain syndrome. (1932-6203 (Electronic)).

Jiang, Y.-H., Jhang, J.-F., Hsu, Y.-H., Ho, H.-C., Wu, Y.-H., & Kuo, H.-C. (2021). Urine biomarkers in ESSIC type 2 interstitial cystitis/bladder pain syndrome and overactive bladder with developing a novel diagnostic algorithm. *Scientific Reports*, *11*(1), 914. DOI: 10.1038/s41598-020-80131-5 PMID: 33441752

Karshikoff, B., Martucci, K. T., & Mackey, S. (2021). Relationship Between Blood Cytokine Levels, Psychological Comorbidity, and Widespreadness of Pain in Chronic Pelvic Pain. *Frontiers in Psychiatry*, *12*, 651083. DOI: 10.3389/fpsyt.2021.651083 PMID: 34248700

Lamvu, G. (2020). Abstracts from the International Pelvic Pain Society (IPPS) Annual Scientific Meeting on Pelvic Pain 2019. *Pain Reports (Baltimore, Md.)*, *5*(2), e815. DOI: 10.1097/PR9.0000000000000815 PMID: 32440608

Li, M., She, K., Zhu, P., Li, Z., Liu, J., Luo, F., & Ye, Y. (2025). Chronic pain and comorbid emotional disorders: Neural circuitry and neuroimmunity pathways. *International Journal of Molecular Sciences*, *26*(2), 436. DOI: 10.3390/ijms26020436 PMID: 39859152

Li, N., Guo, Y., Gong, Y., Zhang, Y. A.-O., Fan, W., Yao, K.,...Lyu, Z. A.-O. The Anti-Inflammatory Actions and Mechanisms of Acupuncture from Acupoint to Target Organs via Neuro-Immune Regulation. (1178-7031 (Print)).

Li, S., Zhang, Z., Jiao, Y., Jin, G., Wu, Y., Xu, F.,...Rong, P. (n.d.). An assessor-blinded, randomized comparative trial of transcutaneous auricular vagus nerve stimulation (taVNS) combined with cranial electroacupuncture vs. citalopram for depression with chronic pain. (1664-0640 (Print)).

Lin, H.-Y., Lu, J.-H., Chuang, S.-M., Chueh, K.-S., Juan, T.-J., Liu, Y.-C., & Juan, Y.-S. (2021). Urinary biomarkers in interstitial cystitis/bladder pain syndrome and its impact on therapeutic outcome. *Diagnostics (Basel)*, *12*(1), 75. DOI: 10.3390/diagnostics12010075 PMID: 35054241

Liu, C., Zhao, Y., Qin, S., Wang, X., Jiang, Y., & Wu, W. Randomized controlled trial of acupuncture for anxiety and depression in patients with chronic insomnia. (2305-5839 (Print)).

Luo, K., Zhang, M., Tu, Q., Li, J., Wang, Y., Wan, S.,…Xia, L. From gut inflammation to psychiatric comorbidity: mechanisms and therapies for anxiety and depression in inflammatory bowel disease. (1742-2094 (Electronic)).

Ma, Q., Xing, C., Long, W., Wang, H. Y., Liu, Q., & Wang, R.-F. (2019). Impact of microbiota on central nervous system and neurological diseases: The gut-brain axis. *Journal of Neuroinflammation*, *16*(1), 53. DOI: 10.1186/s12974-019-1434-3 PMID: 30823925

Majima, T., Funahashi, Y., Kawamorita, N., Takai, S., Matsukawa, Y., Yamamoto, T., Yoshimura, N., & Gotoh, M. (2018). Role of microglia in the spinal cord in colon-to-bladder neural crosstalk in a rat model of colitis. *Neurourology and Urodynamics*, *37*(4), 1320–1328. DOI: 10.1002/nau.23484 PMID: 29350427

Mazza, M., Margoni, S., Mandracchia, G., Donofrio, G., Fischetti, A., Kotzalidis, G. D., & Moccia, L. (2024). This pain drives me crazy: Psychiatric symptoms in women with interstitial cystitis/bladder pain syndrome. *World Journal of Psychiatry*, *14*(6), 954–984. DOI: 10.5498/wjp.v14.i6.954 PMID: 38984334

Meade, E., & Garvey, M. (2022). The Role of Neuro-Immune Interaction in Chronic Pain Conditions; Functional Somatic Syndrome, Neurogenic Inflammation, and Peripheral Neuropathy. *International Journal of Molecular Sciences*, *23*(15), 8574. DOI: 10.3390/ijms23158574 PMID: 35955708

Moldwin, R. M., Nursey, V., Yaskiv, O., Dalvi, S., Macdonald, E. J., Funaro, M.,… Stern, J. A.-O. Immune cell profiles of patients with interstitial cystitis/bladder pain syndrome. (1479-5876 (Electronic)).

Organization, W. H. (2017). *Depression and other common mental disorders: global health estimates*.

Riehl, L., Fürst, J., Kress, M., & Rykalo, N. (2024). The importance of the gut microbiome and its signals for a healthy nervous system and the multifaceted mechanisms of neuropsychiatric disorders. *Frontiers in Neuroscience*, *17*, 1302957. DOI: 10.3389/fnins.2023.1302957 PMID: 38249593

Singto, T., Sergeeva, A., Filor, V., Vidak, J., Kleuser, B., Belik, V.,…Bäumer, W. (2025). Immune cells in dorsal root ganglia are associated with pruritus in a mouse model of allergic contact dermatitis and co-culture study. (1872-8421 (Electronic)).

Siqueira-Campos, V. A.-O., de Deus, M. A.-O., Poli-Neto, O. A.-O., Rosa, E. S. J. C. A.-O., de Deus, J. A.-O., & Conde, D. A.-O. X. Current Challenges in the Management of Chronic Pelvic Pain in Women: From Bench to Bedside. (1179-1411 (Print)).

Skaper, S. D., Facci, L., Zusso, M., & Giusti, P. (2018). An inflammation-centric view of neurological disease: Beyond the neuron. *Frontiers in Cellular Neuroscience*, *12*, 72. DOI: 10.3389/fncel.2018.00072 PMID: 29618972

Stanos, S. P., Tyburski, M. D., & Harden, R. N. (2021). 37 - Chronic Pain. In Cifu, D. X. (Ed.), *Braddom's Physical Medicine and Rehabilitation* (6th ed., pp. 748–773. e745). Elsevier., https://doi.org/https://doi.org/10.1016/B978-0-323-62539-5.00037 -0 DOI: 10.1016/B978-0-323-62539-5.00037-0

Sutherland, S., Grace Kelly, A., Ryden, A., Dmochowski, R. R., Reynolds, W. S., & McKernan, L. C. (2023). Compensatory coping and depression in women with interstitial cystitis/bladder pain syndrome. *Neurourology and Urodynamics*, *42*(1), 322–329. DOI: 10.1002/nau.25089 PMID: 36378850

Szypłowska, M., Tarkowski, R., & Kułak, K. (2023). The impact of endometriosis on depressive and anxiety symptoms and quality of life: A systematic review. *Frontiers in Public Health*, *11*, 1230303. DOI: 10.3389/fpubh.2023.1230303 PMID: 37744486

Tizenberg, B. N., Brenner, L. A., Lowry, C. A., Okusaga, O. O., Benavides, D. R., Hoisington, A. J.,... Postolache, T. A.-O. (2021). Biological and Psychological Factors Determining Neuropsychiatric Outcomes in COVID-19. (1535-1645 (Electronic)).

van Barneveld, E., Manders, J., van Osch, F. H., van Poll, M., Visser, L., van Hanegem, N., Lim, A. C., Bongers, M. Y., & Leue, C. (2022). Depression, anxiety, and correlating factors in endometriosis: A systematic review and meta-analysis. *Journal of Women's Health*, *31*(2), 219–230. DOI: 10.1089/jwh.2021.0021 PMID: 34077695

Walker, A. K., Kavelaars A Fau - Heijnen, C. J., Heijnen Cj Fau - Dantzer, R., & Dantzer, R. (2013). Neuroinflammation and comorbidity of pain and depression. (1521-0081 (Electronic)).

Wang, Y., Li, B., Zhou, Y., Wang, Y., Han, X., Zhang, S., He, Z., & Ouyang, L. (2021). Does endometriosis disturb mental health and quality of life? A systematic review and meta-analysis. *Gynecologic and Obstetric Investigation*, *86*(4), 315–335. DOI: 10.1159/000516517 PMID: 34352799

Wu, C., Wang, L., Zhou, X., Zhou, Y., Han, S., Dong, X., & Liu, H. (2025). Using structural equation modelling to explore the relationship between insomnia, anxiety and depression to the severity of BPS/IC: A cross-sectional study in Chongqing, China. *BMJ Open*, *15*(12), e099604. DOI: 10.1136/bmjopen-2025-099604 PMID: 41407415

Yamamoto, M. P., Carillo, J. F., & Howard, F. M. (2014). Chronic Abdominal Pain of Gynecologic Causes: Diagnosis and Treatment. In *Chronic Abdominal Pain: An Evidence-Based, Comprehensive Guide to Clinical Management* (pp. 103-113). Springer.

Yang, F. C., Zhou, Y., Zhang, S. Y., & Ma, R. (2025). Depression and anxiety in patients with endometriosis-associated chronic pain: Neuroimmune mechanisms mediated by inflammatory factors. (2220-3206 (Print)).

Yang, M.-H., Huang, J.-Y., Chen, S.-L., & Wei, J. C.-C. (2021). Association of interstitial cystitis/bladder pain syndrome with stress-related diseases: A nationwide population-based study. *Journal of Clinical Medicine*, *10*(23), 5669. DOI: 10.3390/jcm10235669 PMID: 34884371

Zhang, L., Luo, Y., Wei, T., Wang, D., He, Z. A.-O., Lan, L., & Zeng, F. A.-O. (2025). Acupuncture's Multisystem Neuroimmunomodulation: Central-Peripheral Interactions in Gastroenteric, Psychiatric, and Chronic Pain Disorders. (1755-5949 (Electronic)).

Zhixiang, C., Yan, L., Liu, X., Lingjie, X., Dong, H., Tao, S., & Yanqing, L. (2025). A Chinese Guideline for the Diagnosis and Treatment of Neuropathic Pain. *International Journal of Plant Research*, *1*(4), 56–86. DOI: 10.11648/j.ijpr.20250104.12

Compilation of References

Abubakari, M. S. (2021). The Internet of Things (IoT) as an Emerging Technological Solution for the Covid-19 Pandemic Mitigation: An Overview. In M. Khairudin, R. Asnawi, I. W. Djatmiko, P. Sudira, S. Hadi, & F. Arifin (Eds.), *Journal of Physics: Conference Series* (Vol. 1737, Issue 1). IOP Publishing Ltd. DOI: 10.1088/1742-6596/1737/1/012003

Adams, J. S., Chien, A. T., & Wisk, L. E. (2019). Mental illness among youth with chronic physical conditions. *Pediatrics*, *144*(1), e20181819. DOI: 10.1542/peds.2018-1819

Adzrago, D., Williams, D. R., & Williams, F. (2024). Multiple chronic diseases and psychological distress among adults in the United States: The intersectionality of chronic diseases, race/ethnicity, immigration, sex, and insurance coverage. *Social Psychiatry and Psychiatric Epidemiology*, *60*, 181–199. DOI: 10.1007/s00127-024-02730-1

Airainer, M., & Seifert, R. (2024). Lithium, the gold standard drug for bipolar disorder: Analysis of current clinical studies. *Naunyn-Schmiedeberg's Archives of Pharmacology*, *397*(12), 9723–9743. DOI: 10.1007/s00210-024-03210-8 PMID: 38916833

Akaishi, T., Tarasawa, K., Fushimi, K., Hamada, H., Saito, M., Kobayashi, N., Kikuchi, S., Tomita, H., Ishii, T., Fujimori, K., & Yaegashi, N. (2023). Risk Factors Associated with Peripartum Suicide Attempts in Japan. *JAMA Network Open*, *6*(1), e2250661. Advance online publication. DOI: 10.1001/jamanetworkopen.2022.50661 PMID: 36633845

Alam, M. A.-O. X., & Chen, J. D. Z. (2023). Non-invasive neuromodulation: an emerging intervention for visceral pain in gastrointestinal disorders. (2332-8886 (Electronic)).

Alassaf, A., Gharaibeh, L., Zurikat, R. O., Farkouh, A., Ibrahim, S., Zayed, A. A., & Odeh, R. (2023). Prevalence of depression in patients with type 1 diabetes between 10 and 17 years of age in Jordan. *Journal of Diabetes Research, 2023*, 3542780. Advance online publication. DOI: 10.1155/2023/3542780

Álvarez-Herms, J., Julià-Sánchez, S., Corbi, F., Odriozola-Martínez, A., & Burtscher, M. (2019). Putative Role of Respiratory Muscle Training to Improve Endurance Performance in Hypoxia: A Review. *Frontiers in Physiology*, *9*, 1970. DOI: 10.3389/fphys.2018.01970 PMID: 30697170

Alvir, J. M. J., Lieberman, J. A., Safferman, A. Z., Schwimmer, J. L., & Schaaf, J. A. (1993). Clozapine-induced agranulocytosis—Incidence and risk factors in the United States. *The New England Journal of Medicine*, *329*(3), 162–167. DOI: 10.1056/NEJM199307153290303 PMID: 8515788

Alzheimer's Association. (2023). 2023 Alzheimer's Disease Facts and Figures. Alzheimer's & Dementia, 19(4), 1-50. doi:.DOI: 10.1002/alz.13177

American Cancer Society. (2024, May 22). *Post-traumatic stress disorder (PTSD) after cancer.* https://www.cancer.org/cancer/survivorship/post-traumatic-stress-disorder-and-cancer.html

American Psychiatric Association. (2013). Diagnostic and Statistical Manual of Mental Disorders (DSM-5). 5th Edition. Arlington, VA: American Psychiatric Publishing.

American Psychiatric Association. (2022). Personality disorders. In *Diagnostic and statistical manual of mental disorders* (5th ed., text rev.; pp. 629–684). https://doi.org/DOI: 10.1176/appi.books.9780890425787

Anderson, R. J., Freedland, K. E., Clouse, R. E., & Lustman, P. J. (2001). The prevalence of comorbid depression in adults with diabetes: A meta-analysis. *Diabetes Care*, *24*(6), 1069–1078. DOI: 10.2337/diacare.24.6.1069

Andrès, E., Zimmer, J., Mecili, M., Weitten, T., Alt, M., & Maloisel, F. (2011). Clinical presentation and management of drug-induced agranulocytosis. *Expert Review of Hematology*, *4*(2), 143–151. DOI: 10.1586/ehm.11.12 PMID: 21495924

Ashdown-Franks, G., Firth, J., Carney, R., Carvalho, A. F., Hallgren, M., Koyanagi, A., Rosenbaum, S., Schuch, F. B., Smith, L., Solmi, M., Vancampfort, D., & Stubbs, B. (2020). Exercise as Medicine for Mental and Substance Use Disorders: A Meta-review of the Benefits for Neuropsychiatric and Cognitive Outcomes. In *Sports Medicine* (Vol. 50, Issue 1). DOI: 10.1007/s40279-019-01187-6

Atri, A., Dickerson, B. C., Clevenger, C., Karlawish, J., Knopman, D., Lin, P., Norman, M., Onyike, C., Sano, M., Scanland, S., & Carrillo, M. (2024). Alzheimer's Association clinical practice guideline for the Diagnostic Evaluation, Testing, Counseling, and Disclosure of Suspected Alzheimer's Disease and Related Disorders (DETeCD-ADRD): Executive summary of recommendations for primary care. Alzheimer's & Dementia, alz.14333. DOI: 10.1002/alz.14333

ATS Committee on Proficiency Standards for Clinical Pulmonary Function Laboratories. (2002). ATS statement: Guidelines for the six-minute walk test. *American Journal of Respiratory and Critical Care Medicine*, *166*(1), 111–117. DOI: 10.1164/ajrccm.166.1.at1102 PMID: 12091180

Baker, K., & Claridge, A. M. (2023). "I have a Ph.D. in my daughter": Mother and child experiences of living with childhood chronic illness. *Journal of Child and Family Studies*, *32*(9), 2625–2636. DOI: 10.1007/s10826-022-02506-8

Barke, A., Korwisi, B., & Rief, W. (2022). Chronic Pain in the ICD-11: New Diagnoses That Clinical Psychologists Should Know About. *Clinical Psychology in Europe*, *4*(Special Issue), e9933. Advance online publication. DOI: 10.32872/cpe.9933 PMID: 36760323

Batulan, Z., Bhimla, A., Higginbotham, E. J., & National Academies of Sciences, E., and Medicine. (2024). Female-Specific and Gynecologic Conditions. In *Advancing Research on Chronic Conditions in Women*. National Academies Press (US).

Baudouin, R., Lechien, J. R., Carpentier, L., Gurruchaga, J.-M., Lisan, Q., & Hans, S. (2023). Deep brain stimulation impact on voice and speech quality in Parkinson's disease: A systematic review. *Otolaryngology - Head and Neck Surgery*, *168*(3), 307–318. DOI: 10.1177/01945998221120189 PMID: 36040825

Bay, Ü. S., & Yılmaz, E. (2020). Ruhsal Bozukluklarda Fiziksel Aktivite ve Egzersizin Etkileri ile İlgili Yapılmış Çalışmaların İncelenmesi. *Mediterranean Journal of Sport Science*, *3*(2), 437–447. DOI: 10.38021/asbid.849274

Bentley, T. G. K., D'Andrea-Penna, G., Rakic, M., Arce, N., LaFaille, M., Berman, R., Cooley, K., & Sprimont, P. (2023). Breathing Practices for Stress and Anxiety Reduction: Conceptual Framework of Implementation Guidelines Based on a Systematic Review of the Published Literature. *Brain Sciences*, *13*(12), 1612. DOI: 10.3390/brainsci13121612 PMID: 38137060

Birinci, T., Mutlu, E. K., & Mustafaoğlu, R. (2019). Does Psychiatric Disorders Cause Reduction in Pulmonary Function and Respiratory Muscle Strength?: Case Series. *Thoracic Research and Practice*, *20*(1), 400–400.

Biso, L., Aringhieri, S., Carli, M., Scarselli, M., & Longoni, B. (2024). Therapeutic drug monitoring in psychiatry: Enhancing treatment precision and patient outcomes. *Pharmaceuticals (Basel, Switzerland)*, *17*(5), 642. DOI: 10.3390/ph17050642 PMID: 38794212

Bissett, B., Gosselink, R., & van Haren, F. M. P. (2020). Respiratory Muscle Rehabilitation in Patients with Prolonged Mechanical Ventilation: A Targeted Approach. *Critical Care : the Official Journal of the Critical Care Forum*, *24*(1), 103. DOI: 10.1186/s13054-020-2783-0 PMID: 32204719

Blackman, G., Lisshammar, J. E. L., Zafar, R., Pollak, T. A., Pritchard, M., Cullen, A. E., Rogers, J., Carter, B., Griffiths, K., Nour, M., David, A. S., McGuire, P., Stewart, R., & MacCabe, J. (2021). Clozapine Response in Schizophrenia and Hematological Changes. *Journal of Clinical Psychopharmacology*, *41*(1), 19–24. DOI: 10.1097/JCP.0000000000001329 PMID: 33347018

Bleich, L., Grohmann, R., Greil, W., Dabbert, D., Erfurth, A., Toto, S., & Seifert, J. (2024). Clozapine-associated adverse drug reactions in 38,349 psychiatric inpatients: Drug surveillance data from the AMSP project between 1993 and 2016. *Journal of Neural Transmission (Vienna, Austria)*, *131*(9), 1117–1134. DOI: 10.1007/s00702-024-02818-7 PMID: 39136776

Bostock, E. C. S., Kirkby, K. C., & Taylor, B. V. M. (2017). The current status of the ketogenic diet in psychiatry. In *Frontiers in Psychiatry* (Vol. 8). Issue MAR., DOI: 10.3389/fpsyt.2017.00043

Bozzatello, P., Blua, C., Rocca, P., & Bellino, S. (2021). Mental health in childhood and adolescence: The role of polyunsaturated fatty acids. *Biomedicines*, *9*(8), 850. Advance online publication. DOI: 10.3390/biomedicines9080850 PMID: 34440053

Brown, R. P., Gerbarg, P. L., & Muench, F. (2013). Breathing practices for treatment of psychiatric and stress-related medical conditions. *The Psychiatric Clinics of North America*, *36*(1), 121–140. DOI: 10.1016/j.psc.2013.01.001 PMID: 23538082

Bruijnzeel, D., Suryadevara, U., & Tandon, R. (2014). Antipsychotic treatment of schizophrenia: An update. *Asian Journal of Psychiatry*, *11*, 3–7. DOI: 10.1016/j.ajp.2014.08.002 PMID: 25216917

Burns, A. V., & Marder, S. (2023). Schizophrenia spectrum and other psychotic disorders. In IsHak, W. W. (Ed.), *Atlas of psychiatry* (pp. 469–492). Springer., DOI: 10.1007/978-3-031-15401-0_15

Cai, X., Cai, X., Xie, Q., Xiao, X., Li, T., Zhou, T., & Sun, H. (2026). NLRP3 inflammasome and gut microbiota–brain axis: A new perspective on white matter injury after intracerebral hemorrhage. *Neural Regeneration Research, 21*(1), 62–80. DOI: 10.4103/NRR.NRR-D-24-00917 PMID: 39885662

Cao, B., Xu, Q., Shi, Y., Zhao, R., Li, H., Zheng, J., Liu, F., Wan, Y., & Wei, B. (2024). Pathology of pain and its implications for therapeutic interventions. *Signal Transduction and Targeted Therapy, 9*(1), 155. DOI: 10.1038/s41392-024-01845-w PMID: 38851750

Černe Kolarič, J., Plemenitaš Ilješ, A., Kraner, D., Gönc, V., Lorber, M., Mlinar Reljić, N., Fekonja, Z., & Kmetec, S. (2024). Long-term impact of community psychiatric care on quality of life amongst people living with schizophrenia: A systematic review. *Health Care, 12*(17), 1750. DOI: 10.3390/healthcare12171750 PMID: 39273773

Cerritelli, F., Frasch, M. G., Antonelli, M. C., Viglione, C., Vecchi, S., Chiera, M., & Manzotti, A. (2021). A review on the vagus nerve and autonomic nervous system during fetal development: Searching for critical windows. *Frontiers in Neuroscience, 15*, 721605. DOI: 10.3389/fnins.2021.721605 PMID: 34616274

Chen, J. H. (2023). Management of Pelvic Pain, Dysparcunia, and Endometriosis. In *Handbook of Gynecology* (pp. 457–484). Springer. DOI: 10.1007/978-3-031-14881-1_78

Chen, Y., & Li, T. (2025). Unveiling the mechanisms of pain in endometriosis: Comprehensive analysis of inflammatory sensitization and therapeutic potential. *International Journal of Molecular Sciences, 26*(4), 1770. DOI: 10.3390/ijms26041770 PMID: 40004233

Chung, J., & Teo, J. (2022). Mental Health Prediction Using Machine Learning: Taxonomy, Applications, and Challenges. In *Applied Computational Intelligence and Soft Computing* (Vol. 2022). DOI: 10.1155/2022/9970363

Cohen, D., Bogers, J. P., van Dijk, D., Bakker, B., & Schulte, P. F. (2012). Beyond white blood cell monitoring: Screening in the initial phase of clozapine therapy. *The Journal of Clinical Psychiatry, 73*(10), 1887. DOI: 10.4088/JCP.11r06977 PMID: 23140648

Collares, S. F., de Ávila Júnior, A. M., Martins, T. C., Rezende, V. H. M., Romano-Silva, M. A., Santos, R. M. S., & de Miranda, D. M. (2025). Systematic review and meta-analysis of weight gain and metabolic changes in children and adolescents using second-generation antipsychotics. *Pharmacology, Biochemistry, and Behavior, 251*, 174012. DOI: 10.1016/j.pbb.2025.174012 PMID: 40180054

Coluzzi, F., Zeboudj, L., Scerpa, M. S., Giorgio, A., De Blasi, R. A., Malcangio, M., & Rocco, M. (2025). Microglial Activation in Nociplastic Pain: From Preclinical Models to PET Neuroimaging and Implications for Targeted Therapeutic Strategies. *International Journal of Molecular Sciences*, *26*(24), 11861. DOI: 10.3390/ijms262411861 PMID: 41465288

Correll, C. U., & Schooler, N. R. (2020). Negative symptoms in schizophrenia: A review and clinical guide for recognition, assessment, and treatment. *Neuropsychiatric Disease and Treatment*, *16*, 519–534. DOI: 10.2147/NDT.S225643 PMID: 32110026

Craig, C. L., Marshall, A. L., Sjöström, M., Bauman, A. E., Booth, M. L., Ainsworth, B. E., Pratt, M., Ekelund, U., Yngve, A., Sallis, J. F., & Oja, P. (2003). International physical activity questionnaire: 12-country reliability and validity. *Medicine and Science in Sports and Exercise*, *35*(8), 1381–1395. DOI: 10.1249/01.MSS.0000078924.61453.FB PMID: 12900694

Cuffaro, F., Russo, E., & Amedei, A. (2024). Endometriosis, pain, and related psychological disorders: Unveiling the interplay among the microbiome, inflammation, and oxidative stress as a common thread. *International Journal of Molecular Sciences*, *25*(12), 6473. DOI: 10.3390/ijms25126473 PMID: 38928175

Darling-White, M., & Huber, J. E. (2017). The Impact of Expiratory Muscle Strength Training on Speech Breathing in Individuals With Parkinson's Disease: A Preliminary Study. *American Journal of Speech-Language Pathology*, *26*(4), 1159–1166. DOI: 10.1044/2017_AJSLP-16-0132 PMID: 29114773

Davis, N., Harris, L., & Cunningham, U. (2019). Professional ecologies shaping technology adoption in early childhood education with multilingual children. *British Journal of Educational Technology*, *50*(3), 1320–1339. Advance online publication. DOI: 10.1111/bjet.12774

De Berardis, D., Rapini, G., Olivieri, L., Di Nicola, D., Tomasetti, C., Valchera, A., & Di Nicola, M. (2018). Safety of antipsychotics for the treatment of schizophrenia: A focus on the adverse effects of clozapine. *Therapeutic Advances in Drug Safety*, *9*(5), 237–256. DOI: 10.1177/2042098618756261 PMID: 29796248

de Freitas, D. F., Patel, I., Kadra-Scalzo, G., Pritchard, M., Shetty, H., Broadbent, M., Patel, R., Downs, J., Segev, A., Khondoker, M., MacCabe, J. H., Bhui, K., & Hayes, R. D. (2022). Ethnic inequalities in clozapine use among people with treatment-resistant schizophrenia: A retrospective cohort study using data from electronic clinical records. *Social Psychiatry and Psychiatric Epidemiology*, *57*(7), 1341–1355. DOI: 10.1007/s00127-022-02257-3 PMID: 35246709

De Nayer, A., De Hert, M., Scheen, A., Van Gaal, L., Peuskens, J., De Nayer, A., De Hert, M., Scheen, A., Van Gaal, L., & Peuskens, J.on behalf of the Consensus Groupon behalf of the Consensus Group. (2005). Belgian consensus on metabolic problems associated with atypical antipsychotics. *International Journal of Psychiatry in Clinical Practice*, *9*(2), 130–137. DOI: 10.1080/13651500510018310 PMID: 24930795

Deer, T. R., Mekhail, N., Petersen, E., Krames, E., Staats, P., Pope, J., Saweris, Y., Lad, S. P., Diwan, S., Falowski, S., Feler, C., Slavin, K., Narouze, S., Merabet, L., Buvanendran, A., Fregni, F., Wellington, J., & Levy, R. M. (2014). The appropriate use of neurostimulation: Stimulation of the intracranial and extracranial space and head for chronic pain. *Neuromodulation*, *17*(6), 551–570. DOI: 10.1111/ner.12215 PMID: 25112890

del Pino-Sedeño, T., Cabrera-Maroto, M., Abrante-Luis, A., González-Hernández, Y., & Ortiz Herrera, M. C. (2024). Effectiveness of psychological interventions in endometriosis: A systematic review with meta-analysis. *Frontiers in Psychology*, *15*, 1457842. DOI: 10.3389/fpsyg.2024.1457842 PMID: 39529727

Delanerolle, G., Ramakrishnan, R., Hapangama, D., Zeng, Y., Shetty, A., Elneil, S., & Phiri, P. (2021). A systematic review and meta-analysis of the Endometriosis and Mental-Health Sequelae; The ELEMI Project. *Women's Health (London, England)*, *17*, 17455065211019717. DOI: 10.1177/17455065211019717 PMID: 34053382

DeLong, L. N., Fleetwood, K., Prigge, R., Galdi, P., Guthrie, B., & Fleuriot, J. (2025). Cluster and survival analysis of UK Biobank data reveals associations between physical multimorbidity clusters and subsequent depression. *Communications Medicine*, *5*, 156. Advance online publication. DOI: 10.1038/s43856-025-00825-7

Deng, Y., & He, J. (2023). A Comparison between before and during the Pandemic in Nonsuicidal Self-Injury Behaviors of Bipolar Disorder. *The Journal of Nervous and Mental Disease*, *211*(12), 896–901. Advance online publication. DOI: 10.1097/NMD.0000000000001572 PMID: 36044661

Dodds, K. N., Beckett, E. A., Evans, S. F., Grace, P. M., Watkins, L. R., & Hutchinson, M. R. (2016). Glial contributions to visceral pain: implications for disease etiology and the female predominance of persistent pain. (2158-3188 (Electronic)).

Drzyzga, Ł., Obuchowicz, E., Marcinowska, A., & Herman, Z. S. (2006). Cytokines in schizophrenia and the effects of antipsychotic drugs. *Brain, Behavior, and Immunity*, *20*(6), 532–545. DOI: 10.1016/j.bbi.2006.02.002 PMID: 16580814

Dubey, P., Thakur, B., Rodriguez, S., Cox, J., Sanchez, S., Fonseca, A., Reddy, S., Clegg, D., & Dwivedi, A. K. (2021). A systematic review and meta-analysis of the association between maternal polycystic ovary syndrome and neuropsychiatric disorders in children. In *Translational Psychiatry* (Vol. 11, Issue 1). DOI: 10.1038/s41398-021-01699-8

Duffy, A., Goodday, S., Keown-Stoneman, C., & Grof, P. (2019). The emergent course of bipolar disorder: Observations over two decades from the Canadian high-risk offspring cohort. *The American Journal of Psychiatry*, *176*(9), 720–729. Advance online publication. DOI: 10.1176/appi.ajp.2018.18040461 PMID: 30525908

Elias, L. R., Miskowiak, K. W., Vale, A. M., Köhler, C. A., Kjærstad, H. L., Stubbs, B., Kessing, L. V., Vieta, E., Maes, M., Goldstein, B. I., & Carvalho, A. F. (2017). Cognitive Impairment in Euthymic Pediatric Bipolar Disorder: A Systematic Review and Meta-Analysis. *Journal of the American Academy of Child and Adolescent Psychiatry*, *56*(4), 286–296. DOI: 10.1016/j.jaac.2017.01.008 PMID: 28335872

Ellis, G., & Sevda Lis, N. (2019). Understanding and improving multidisciplinary team working in geriatric medicine. Age and Ageing, 48(4), 498–505. DOI: 10.1093/ageing/afz021

Elyamany, O., Leicht, G., Herrmann, C. S., & Mulert, C. (2021). Transcranial alternating current stimulation (tACS): From basic mechanisms towards first applications in psychiatry. *European Archives of Psychiatry and Clinical Neuroscience*, *271*(1), 135–156. DOI: 10.1007/s00406-020-01209-9 PMID: 33211157

Engeler, D., Baranowski, A., Borovicka, J., Cottrell, A. M., Dinis, P., Elneil, S., . . . Goonewardene, S. (2018). EAU Guidelines, Full Text, Chronic Pelvic Pain 2018. European Association of Urology. Daniel Engeler, AP Baranowski, J. Borovicka, AQ Cottrell, P Dinis- Oliveira, S. Elneil, J Hughes, Bert Messelink, AC De Williams. Guidelines Associates: B Parsons, S Goonewardene. In.

Engel, G. L. (1977). The need for a new medical model: A challenge for biomedicine. *Science*, *196*(4286), 129–136. DOI: 10.1126/science.847460

Ercan Doğu, S., & Gündoğmuş, A. G. (2022). The Relationship Between Physical Activity Level and Quality of Life in Individuals with Bipolar Disorder. *International Journal of Disabilities Sports & Health Sciences*, *5*(2), 83–89. DOI: 10.33438/ijdshs.1137254

Erturk, N., Celik, A., Yaman, S. K., Yaman, H., Unal, F., & Kutukcu, E. C. (2024, December). Expiratory muscle strength training reduces oxidative stress and systemic inflammation in men with obstructive sleep apnea syndrome: A double-blinded, randomized parallel trial. *Sleep (Basel)*, *47*(12), zsae221. DOI: 10.1093/sleep/zsae221 PMID: 39297486

Faber, S. C., Roy, A. K., Michaels, T. I., & Williams, M. T. (2023). The weaponization of medicine: Early psychosis in the Black community and the need for racially informed mental healthcare. *Frontiers in Psychiatry*, *14*, 1098292. DOI: 10.3389/fpsyt.2023.1098292 PMID: 36846217

Falk, J., Saha, S., & McGrath, J. J. (2022). Respiratory disorders in people with severe mental illness: A review. *The Lancet. Psychiatry*, *9*(3), 198–210. PMID: 35183279

Fallon, J., Stern, I. T., Laurent, M., Birder, L., Moldwin, R. M., & Stern, J. N. H. (2023). The immune system in Interstitial Cystitis/Bladder Pain Syndrome and therapeutic agents. *Continence*, *8*, 101057. https://doi.org/https://doi.org/10.1016/j.cont.2023.101057. DOI: 10.1016/j.cont.2023.101057

Feldman, H. H., & Gauthier, S. (2008). Management of Alzheimer's Disease: Practical Insights and Emerging Therapies. Journal of Clinical Psychiatry, 69(11), 1704-1711. DOI: 10.4088/JCP.v69n1104

Ferensztajn-Rochowiak, E., & Rybakowski, J. K. (2023). Long-term lithium therapy: Side effects and interactions. *Pharmaceuticals (Basel, Switzerland)*, *16*(1), 74. DOI: 10.3390/ph16010074 PMID: 36678571

First, M. B., Clarke, D. E., Yousif, L., Eng, A. M., Gogtay, N., & Appelbaum, P. S. (2023). DSM-5-TR: Rationale, Process, and Overview of Changes. *Psychiatric Services (Washington, D.C.)*, *74*(8), 869–875. DOI: 10.1176/appi.ps.20220334 PMID: 36510761

Firth, J., Firth, J. A., Stubbs, B., Vancampfort, D., Schuch, F. B., Hallgren, M., Veronese, N., Yung, A. R., & Sarris, J. (2018). Association Between Muscular Strength and Cognition in People With Major Depression or Bipolar Disorder and Healthy Controls. *JAMA Psychiatry*, *75*(7), 740–746. DOI: 10.1001/jamapsychiatry.2018.0503 PMID: 29710135

Firth, J., Solmi, M., Wootton, R. E., Vancampfort, D., Schuch, F. B., Hoare, E., & Stubbs, B. (2021). A meta-review of "lifestyle psychiatry": The role of exercise, smoking, diet and sleep in the prevention and treatment of mental disorders. *World Psychiatry; Official Journal of the World Psychiatric Association (WPA)*, *20*(3), 388–403. DOI: 10.1002/wps.20873 PMID: 32931092

Fischer-Grote, L., Fössing, V., Aigner, M., Boeckle, M., & Fehrmann, E. (2022). Comorbidities of bladder pain syndrome in the context of the HITOP distress category: A systematic review and meta-analysis. *International Urogynecology Journal, 33*(9), 2335–2356. DOI: 10.1007/s00192-022-05129-1 PMID: 35262767

Gahona-Villegas, J. R., Reyes-Jurado, P., & Ríos-Méndez, R. E. (2023). Renovascular arterial hypertension in children. Three case report. *Acta Pediátrica de México, 44*(3). Advance online publication. DOI: 10.18233/apm.v44i3.2264

Gargus, M., Ben-Azu, B., Landwehr, A., Dunn, J., Errico, J. P., & Tremblay, M. (2025). Mechanisms of vagus nerve stimulation for the treatment of neurodevelopmental disorders: a focus on microglia and neuroinflammation. (1662-4548 (Print)).

GBD 2019 Mental Disorders Collaborators (2022). Global, regional, and national burden of 12 mental disorders in 204 countries and territories, 1990-2019: a systematic analysis for the Global Burden of Disease Study 2019. *The lancet. Psychiatry, 9*(2), 137–150.

Gibbons, W. J., Fruchter, N., Sloan, S., & Levy, R. D. (2001). Reference values for a multiple repetition 6-minute walk test in healthy adults older than 20 years. *Journal of Cardiopulmonary Rehabilitation, 21*(2), 87–93. DOI: 10.1097/00008483-200103000-00005 PMID: 11314289

Göçen, H. B., & Özden, A. V. (2024). Autonomic Dysfunction in Psychiatric Disorders. Psikiyatride Güncel Yaklaşımlar -. *Psikiyatride Güncel Yaklasimlar, 16*(3), 401–409. DOI: 10.18863/pgy.1329118

Golinska, M., Wołyniak, M., Kulesza, P., & Fendler, W. (2025). Neuroinflammation is responsible for pain in endometriosis - targeting the JAK-STAT pathway and mast cell activation. (1664-3224 (Electronic)).

Golinska, M., Wolyniak, M., Kulesza, P., & Fendler, W. (2025). Neuroinflammation is responsible for pain in endometriosis-targeting the JAK-STAT pathway and mast cell activation. *Frontiers in Immunology, 16*, 1621178. DOI: 10.3389/fimmu.2025.1621178 PMID: 40948761

González-Rodríguez, A., & Seeman, M. V. (2020). Addressing delusions in women and men with delusional disorder: Key points for clinical management. *International Journal of Environmental Research and Public Health, 17*(12), 4583. DOI: 10.3390/ijerph17124583 PMID: 32630566

Gordon, S., Mote, J., & Fulford, D. (2023). Qualitative analysis of paranoia reported in clinical interviews with Black and White adults with schizophrenia. *Psychiatric Services (Washington, D.C.)*, *74*(12), 1257–1264. DOI: 10.1176/appi.ps.20220089 PMID: 37254507

Gosselink, R., De Vos, J., van den Heuvel, S. P., Segers, J., Decramer, M., & Kwakkel, G. (2011). Impact of inspiratory muscle training in patients with COPD: What is the evidence? *The European Respiratory Journal*, *37*(2), 416–425. DOI: 10.1183/09031936.00031810 PMID: 21282809

Goto, A., Yoshimi, A., Nagai, T., Ukigai, M., Mouri, A., Ozaki, N., & Noda, Y. (2017). Human neutrophils show decreased survival upon long-term exposure to clozapine. *Human Psychopharmacology*, *32*(6), e2629. DOI: 10.1002/hup.2629 PMID: 28913970

GP, C. (2009). Stress and disorders of the stress system. *Nat Rev Endocrinol, 5*, 374-381.

Graziottin, A., Gambini, D., & Bertolasi, L. (2015). Genital and sexual pain in women. In Vodušek, D. B., & Boller, F. (Eds.), *Handbook of Clinical Neurology* (Vol. 130, pp. 395–412). Elsevier., https://doi.org/https://doi.org/10.1016/B978-0-444-63247-0.00023-7

Guinart, D., de Filippis, R., Rosson, S., Patil, B., Prizgint, L., Talasazan, N., Meltzer, H., Kane, J. M., & Gibbons, R. D. (2021). Development and validation of a computerized adaptive assessment tool for discrimination and measurement of psychotic symptoms. *Schizophrenia Bulletin*, *47*(3), 644–652. DOI: 10.1093/schbul/sbaa168 PMID: 33164091

Gurtner, M., Smith, M., Gage, R., Howey-Brown, A., Wang, X., Latavao, T., Deng, J. D., Zwanenburg, S. P., Stanley, J., & Signal, L. (2022). Objective Assessment of the Nature and Extent of Children's Internet-Based World: Protocol for the Kids Online Aotearoa Study. *JMIR Research Protocols*, *11*(10), e39017. Advance online publication. DOI: 10.2196/39017 PMID: 36129809

Hamina, A., Taipale, H., Lieslehto, J., Lähteenvuo, M., Tanskanen, A., Mittendorfer-Rutz, E., & Tiihonen, J. (2024). Comparative effectiveness of antipsychotics in patients with schizophrenia spectrum disorder. *JAMA Network Open*, *7*(10), e2438358–e2438358. DOI: 10.1001/jamanetworkopen.2024.38358 PMID: 39382894

Hannaway, D. (2024). Digital learning in childhood: Possibilities for pedagogical transformation in South Africa. *South African Journal of Childhood Education*, *14*(1). Advance online publication. DOI: 10.4102/sajce.v14i1.1422

Hasan, A., Scuderi, S. A., Capra, A. P., Giosa, D., Bonomo, A., Ardizzone, A., & Esposito, E. (2025). An Updated and Comprehensive Review Exploring the Gut–Brain Axis in Neurodegenerative Disorders and Neurotraumas: Implications for Therapeutic Strategies. *Brain Sciences*, *15*(6), 654. DOI: 10.3390/brainsci15060654 PMID: 40563824

Hayes, B., Choi, H., Rathore, A., Bao, C., Shi, J., Huh, Y., Kim, M. W., Mencarelli, A., Bist, P., Ng, L. G., Shi, C., Nho, J. H., Kim, A., Yoon, H., Lim, D., Hannan, J. L., Purves, J. T., Hughes, F. M.Jr, Ji, R.-R., & Abraham, S. (2024). Recurrent infections drive persistent bladder dysfunction and pain via sensory nerve sprouting and mast cell activity. *Science Immunology*, *9*(93), eadi5578. Advance online publication. DOI: 10.1126/sciimmunol.adi5578 PMID: 38427717

Hayes, J. F., Miles, J., Walters, K., King, M., & Osborn, D. P. (2015). A systematic review and meta-analysis of premature mortality in bipolar affective disorder. *Acta Psychiatrica Scandinavica*, *131*(6), 417–425. DOI: 10.1111/acps.12408 PMID: 25735195

He, H. A.-O., Luo, H. A.-O., Qian, B. A.-O., Xu, H. A.-O., Zhang, G. A.-O., Zou, X. A.-O., & Zou, J. A.-O. (2024). Autonomic Nervous System Dysfunction Is Related to Chronic Prostatitis/Chronic Pelvic Pain Syndrome. (2287-4208 (Print)).

Helbig, S., Zell, E., & Backes, A.. (2023). Effectiveness of a Personalized Exercise Program to Increase Physical Activity and Improve Mental Health in Patients with Depression: A Randomized Controlled Trial. *Frontiers in Psychiatry*, *14*, 10338920.

Hippius, H. (1999). A historical perspective of clozapine. *The Journal of Clinical Psychiatry*, *60*(12), 22–23. PMID: 10372606

Hofmann, S. G., Asnaani, A., Vonk, I. J. J., Sawyer, A. T., & Fang, A. (2012). The efficacy of cognitive behavioral therapy: A review of meta-analyses. In *Cognitive Therapy and Research* (Vol. 36, Issue 5). DOI: 10.1007/s10608-012-9476-1

Hsieh, K.-L., Chin, H.-Y., Lo, T.-S., Long, C.-Y., Ho, C.-H., Huang, S. K.-H., Chuang, Y.-C., & Wu, M.-P. (2021). Interstitial cystitis/bladder pain syndrome patient is associated with subsequent increased risks of outpatient visits and hospitalizations: A population-based study. *PLoS One*, *16*(9), e0256800. DOI: 10.1371/journal.pone.0256800 PMID: 34492065

HÜZMELİ. İ., & KATAYIFÇI, N., (2022). Solunum Kas Eğitimi. Solunumun Temel Değerlendirmesi (pp.283-301), Livre de Lyon.

Hyde, J., Carr, H., Kelley, N., Seneviratne, R., Reed, C., Parlatini, V., Garner, M., Solmi, M., Rosson, S., Cortese, S., & Brandt, V. (2022). Efficacy of neurostimulation across mental disorders: Systematic review and meta-analysis of 208 randomized controlled trials. *Molecular Psychiatry*, *27*(6), 2709–2719. DOI: 10.1038/s41380-022-01524-8 PMID: 35365806

Inouye, S. K., van Dyck, C. H., Alessi, C. A., Balkin, S., Siegal, A. P., & Horwitz, R. I. (1990). The delirium syndrome: The incidence, mortality, and long-term consequences of delirium in hospitalized elderly patients. Journal of the American Geriatrics Society, 38(12), 1425-1432. doi:. 1990.tb01758.xDOI: 10.1111/j.1532-5415

Inzoli, A., Barba, M., Costa, C., Carazita, V., Cola, A., Fantauzzi, M.,…Frigerio, M. (2024). The Evil Twins of Chronic Pelvic Pain Syndrome: A Systematic Review and Meta-Analysis on Interstitial Cystitis/Painful Bladder Syndrome and Endometriosis. Healthcare, Iwata, M., Ota Kt Fau - Duman, R. S., & Duman, R. S. (2013). The inflammasome: pathways linking psychological stress, depression, and systemic illnesses. (1090-2139 (Electronic)).

Islam, F., Hain, D., Lewis, D., Law, R., Brown, L. C., Tanner, J.-A., & Müller, D. J. (2022). Pharmacogenomics of Clozapine-induced agranulocytosis: A systematic review and meta-analysis. *The Pharmacogenomics Journal*, *22*(4), 230–240. DOI: 10.1038/s41397-022-00281-9 PMID: 35710824

Iyer, M. B., Mattu, U., Grafman, J., Lomarev, M., Sato, S., & Wassermann, E. M. (2005). Safety and cognitive effect of frontal DC brain polarization in healthy individuals. *Neurology*, *64*(5), 872–875. DOI: 10.1212/01.WNL.0000152986.07469.E9 PMID: 15753425

Jarero, I., Givaudan, M., & Osorio, A. (2018). Randomized controlled trial on the provision of the EMDR integrative group treatment protocol adapted for ongoing traumatic stress to female patients with cancer-related posttraumatic stress disorder symptoms. *Journal of EMDR Practice and Research*, *12*(3), 94–104. DOI: 10.1891/1933-3196.12.3.94

Jiang, Y. H., Peng Ch Fau - Liu, H.-T., Liu Ht Fau - Kuo, H.-C., & Kuo, H. C. (2013). Increased pro-inflammatory cytokines, C-reactive protein and nerve growth factor expressions in serum of patients with interstitial cystitis/bladder pain syndrome. (1932-6203 (Electronic)).

Jiang, Y.-H., Jhang, J.-F., Hsu, Y.-H., Ho, H.-C., Wu, Y.-H., & Kuo, H.-C. (2021). Urine biomarkers in ESSIC type 2 interstitial cystitis/bladder pain syndrome and overactive bladder with developing a novel diagnostic algorithm. *Scientific Reports*, *11*(1), 914. DOI: 10.1038/s41598-020-80131-5 PMID: 33441752

Jo, J. M., Kim, Y.-H., Ko, M.-H., Ohn, S. H., Joen, B., & Lee, K. H. (2009). Enhancing the working memory of stroke patients using tDCS. *American Journal of Physical Medicine & Rehabilitation*, *88*(5), 404–409. DOI: 10.1097/PHM.0b013e3181a0e4cb PMID: 19620953

Jung, M., Lim, C., Lee, C., Kim, S., & Kim, J. (2021). Human dietitians vs. Artificial intelligence: Which diet design do you prefer for your children? *The Journal of Allergy and Clinical Immunology*, *147*(2), AB117. Advance online publication. DOI: 10.1016/j.jaci.2020.12.430

Jürisson, M., Pisarev, H., Uusküla, A., Lang, K., Oona, M., Elm, L., & Kalda, R. (2021). Physical–mental health comorbidity: A population-based cross-sectional study. *PLoS One*, *16*(12), e0260464. DOI: 10.1371/journal.pone.0260464

Kang, G. E., Mickey, B. J., McInnis, M. G., Krembs, B. S., & Gross, M. M. (2018). Motor behavior characteristics in various phases of bipolar disorder revealed through biomechanical analysis: Quantitative measures of activity and energy variables during gait and sit-to-walk. *Psychiatry Research*, *269*, 93–101. DOI: 10.1016/j.psychres.2018.08.062 PMID: 30145308

Karshikoff, B., Martucci, K. T., & Mackey, S. (2021). Relationship Between Blood Cytokine Levels, Psychological Comorbidity, and Widespreadness of Pain in Chronic Pelvic Pain. *Frontiers in Psychiatry*, *12*, 651083. DOI: 10.3389/fpsyt.2021.651083 PMID: 34248700

Katon, W. J., Lin, E. H., Von Korff, M., Ciechanowski, P., Ludman, E. J., Young, B., Peterson, D., Rutter, C. M., McGregor, M., & McCulloch, D. (2010). Collaborative care for patients with depression and chronic illnesses. *The New England Journal of Medicine*, *363*(27), 2611–2620. DOI: 10.1056/NEJMoa1003955

Kay, S. R., Fiszbein, A., & Opler, L. A. (1987). The Positive and Negative Syndrome Scale (PANSS) for schizophrenia. *Schizophrenia Bulletin*, *13*(2), 261–276. DOI: 10.1093/schbul/13.2.261 PMID: 3616518

Kharabian Masouleh, S., Arélin, K., Horstmann, A., Lampe, L., Kipping, J. A., Luck, T., Riedel-Heller, S. G., Schroeter, M. L., Stumvoll, M., Villringer, A., & Witte, A. V. (2016). Higher body mass index in older adults is associated with lower gray matter volume: Implications for memory performance. *Neurobiology of Aging*, *40*, 1–10. DOI: 10.1016/j.neurobiolaging.2015.12.020 PMID: 26973099

Kilbourne, A. M., Morden, N. E., Austin, K., Ilgen, M., McCarthy, J. F., Dalack, G., & Blow, F. C. (2009). Excess heart-disease-related mortality in a national study of patients with mental disorders: Identifying modifiable risk factors. *General Hospital Psychiatry*, *31*(6), 555–563. DOI: 10.1016/j.genhosppsych.2009.07.008 PMID: 19892214

Kimhy, D., Vakhrusheva, J., Bartels, M. N., Armstrong, H. F., Ballon, J. S., Khan, S., Chang, R. W., Hansen, M. C., Ayanruoh, L., Lister, A., Castrén, E., Smith, E. E., & Sloan, R. P. (2015). The Impact of Aerobic Exercise on Brain-Derived Neurotrophic Factor and Neurocognition in Individuals With Schizophrenia: A Single-Blind, Randomized Clinical Trial. *Schizophrenia Bulletin*, *41*(4), 859–868. DOI: 10.1093/schbul/sbv022 PMID: 25805886

Kirchner, S. K., Roeh, A., Nolden, J., & Hasan, A. (2018). Diagnosis and treatment of schizotypal personality disorder: Evidence from a systematic review. *npj. Schizophrenia*, *4*(1), 20. DOI: 10.1038/s41537-018-0062-8 PMID: 30282970

Lafleur, L.-P., Murray, A., Desforges, M., Pacheco-Barrios, K., Fregni, F., Tremblay, S., Saint-Amour, D., Lepage, J.-F., & Théoret, H. (2021). No aftereffects of high current density 10 Hz and 20 Hz tACS on sensorimotor alpha and beta oscillations. *Scientific Reports*, *11*(1), 21416. DOI: 10.1038/s41598-021-00850-1 PMID: 34725379

Laguna-Muñoz, D., Jiménez-Peinado, A., Jaén-Moreno, M. J., Camacho-Rodríguez, C., Del Pozo, G. I., Vieta, E., Caballero-Villarraso, J., Khan, M. I., Rico-Villademoros, F., & Sarramea, F. (2025). Respiratory disease in people with bipolar disorder: A systematic review and meta-analysis. *Molecular Psychiatry*, *30*(2), 777–785. DOI: 10.1038/s41380-024-02793-1 PMID: 39543369

Lamvu, G. (2020). Abstracts from the International Pelvic Pain Society (IPPS) Annual Scientific Meeting on Pelvic Pain 2019. *Pain Reports (Baltimore, Md.)*, *5*(2), e815. DOI: 10.1097/PR9.0000000000000815 PMID: 32440608

Langa, K. M., & Levine, D. A. (2014). The Diagnosis and Management of Mild Cognitive Impairment: A Review. JAMA, 312(23), 2551-2561. doi:DOI: 10.1001/jama.2014.15204

Launders, N., Dotsikas, K., Marston, L., Price, G., Osborn, D. P. J., & Hayes, J. F. (2022). The impact of comorbid severe mental illness and common chronic physical health conditions on hospitalisation: A systematic review and meta-analysis. *PLoS One*, *17*(8), e0272498. DOI: 10.1371/journal.pone.0272498 PMID: 35980891

Laveneziana, P., Albuquerque, A., Aliverti, A., Babb, T., Barreiro, E., Dres, M., Dubé, B. P., Fauroux, B., Gea, J., Guenette, J. A., Hudson, A. L., Kabitz, H. J., Laghi, F., Langer, D., Luo, Y. M., Neder, J. A., O'Donnell, D., Polkey, M. I., Rabinovich, R. A., & Verges, S. (2019). ERS statement on respiratory muscle testing at rest and during exercise. *The European Respiratory Journal, 53*(6), 1801214. DOI: 10.1183/13993003.01214-2018 PMID: 30956204

Le, T., & Ruffalo, M. L. (2025). Psychotherapy for delusional disorder: Theoretical models and therapeutic techniques. *American Journal of Psychotherapy, 78*(4), 251–255. DOI: 10.1176/appi.psychotherapy.20240061 PMID: 40495539

Leucht, S., Arbter, D., Engel, R. R., Kissling, W., & Davis, J. M. (2009). How effective are second-generation antipsychotic drugs? A meta-analysis of placebo-controlled trials. *Molecular Psychiatry, 14*(4), 429–447. DOI: 10.1038/sj.mp.4002136 PMID: 18180760

Li, N., Guo, Y., Gong, Y., Zhang, Y. A.-O., Fan, W., Yao, K.,…Lyu, Z. A.-O. The Anti-Inflammatory Actions and Mechanisms of Acupuncture from Acupoint to Target Organs via Neuro-Immune Regulation. (1178-7031 (Print)).

Li, S., Zhang, Z., Jiao, Y., Jin, G., Wu, Y., Xu, F.,…Rong, P. (n.d.). An assessor-blinded, randomized comparative trial of transcutaneous auricular vagus nerve stimulation (taVNS) combined with cranial electroacupuncture vs. citalopram for depression with chronic pain. (1664-0640 (Print)).

Licht, R. W. (2012). Lithium: Still a major option in the management of bipolar disorder. *CNS Neuroscience & Therapeutics, 18*(3), 219–226. DOI: 10.1111/j.1755-5949.2011.00260.x PMID: 22070642

Li, M., She, K., Zhu, P., Li, Z., Liu, J., Luo, F., & Ye, Y. (2025). Chronic pain and comorbid emotional disorders: Neural circuitry and neuroimmunity pathways. *International Journal of Molecular Sciences, 26*(2), 436. DOI: 10.3390/ijms26020436 PMID: 39859152

Lim, K., Peh, O.-H., Yang, Z., Rekhi, G., Rapisarda, A., See, Y.-M., Abdul Rashid, N. A., Ang, M.-S., Lee, S.-A., Sim, K., Huang, H., Lencz, T., Lee, J., & Lam, M. (2021). Large-scale evaluation of the Positive and Negative Syndrome Scale (PANSS) symptom architecture in schizophrenia. *Asian Journal of Psychiatry, 62*, 102732. DOI: 10.1016/j.ajp.2021.102732 PMID: 34118560

Lin, D., Joshi, K., Keenan, A., Shepherd, J., Bailey, H., Berry, M., Wright, J., Meakin, S., Benson, C., & Kim, E. (2021). Associations between relapses and psychosocial outcomes in patients with schizophrenia in real-world settings in the United States. *Frontiers in Psychiatry, 12*, 695672. DOI: 10.3389/fpsyt.2021.695672 PMID: 34764891

Lin, H.-Y., Lu, J.-H., Chuang, S.-M., Chueh, K.-S., Juan, T.-J., Liu, Y.-C., & Juan, Y.-S. (2021). Urinary biomarkers in interstitial cystitis/bladder pain syndrome and its impact on therapeutic outcome. *Diagnostics (Basel), 12*(1), 75. DOI: 10.3390/diagnostics12010075 PMID: 35054241

Lista-Paz, A., Langer, D., Barral-Fernández, M., Quintela-Del-Río, A., Gimeno-Santos, E., Arbillaga-Etxarri, A., Torres-Castro, R., Vilaró Casamitjana, J., Varas de la Fuente, A. B., Serrano Veguillas, C., Bravo Cortés, P., Martín Cortijo, C., García Delgado, E., Herrero-Cortina, B., Valera, J. L., Fregonezi, G. A. F., González Montañez, C., Martín-Valero, R., Francín-Gallego, M., & González-Doniz, L. (2023). Maximal Respiratory Pressure Reference Equations in Healthy Adults and Cut-off Points for Defining Respiratory Muscle Weakness. *Archivos de Bronconeumología, 59*(12), 813–820. DOI: 10.1016/j.arbres.2023.08.016 PMID: 37839949

Liu, C., Zhao, Y., Qin, S., Wang, X., Jiang, Y., & Wu, W. Randomized controlled trial of acupuncture for anxiety and depression in patients with chronic insomnia. (2305-5839 (Print)).

Liu, J., Zhao, W., & Wang, Y. (2025). Lights and shadows of clozapine on the immune system in schizophrenia: A narrative literature review. *Metabolic Brain Disease, 40*(2), 128. DOI: 10.1007/s11011-025-01558-1 PMID: 39954151

Liu, X. (2024). Ethical research on the artificial intelligence training system for preschoolers under the guidance of child-centered theory. *Applied and Computational Engineering, 32*(1), 171–176. Advance online publication. DOI: 10.54254/2755-2721/32/20230206

Liu, Y., Yan, T., Chu, J. M., Chen, Y., Dunnett, S., Ho, Y. S., Wong, G. T., & Chang, R. C. (2019). The beneficial effects of physical exercise in the brain and related pathophysiological mechanisms in neurodegenerative diseases. *Laboratory Investigation, 99*(7), 943–957. DOI: 10.1038/s41374-019-0232-y PMID: 30808929

Li, X.-H., Zhong, X.-M., Lu, L., Zheng, W., Wang, S., Rao, W., Wang, S., Ng, C. H., Ungvari, G. S., Wang, G., & Xiang, Y.-T. (2020). The prevalence of agranulocytosis and related death in clozapine-treated patients: A comprehensive meta-analysis of observational studies. *Psychological Medicine, 50*(4), 583–594. DOI: 10.1017/S0033291719000369 PMID: 30857568

Lu, F., Zhao, K., Wu, Y., Kong, Y., Gao, Y., & Zhang, L. (2023). Voice-related outcomes in deep brain stimulation in patients with vocal tremor: A systematic review and meta-analysis. *Journal of Voice*. Advance online publication. DOI: 10.1016/j.jvoice.2023.09.027 PMID: 37880051

Luo, K., Zhang, M., Tu, Q., Li, J., Wang, Y., Wan, S.,...Xia, L. From gut inflammation to psychiatric comorbidity: mechanisms and therapies for anxiety and depression in inflammatory bowel disease. (1742-2094 (Electronic)).

Madej, K. (2024). Representation of Disability in Children's Video Games. In *Representation of Disability in Children's Video Games*. DOI: 10.4324/9781003430445

Magis, D., & Schoenen, J. (2012). Advances and challenges in neurostimulation for headaches. *Lancet Neurology*, *11*(8), 708–719. DOI: 10.1016/S1474-4422(12)70139-4 PMID: 22814542

Mahler, D. A., & Wells, C. K. (1988). Evaluation of clinical methods for rating dyspnea. *Chest*, *93*(3), 580–586. DOI: 10.1378/chest.93.3.580 PMID: 3342669

Majima, T., Funahashi, Y., Kawamorita, N., Takai, S., Matsukawa, Y., Yamamoto, T., Yoshimura, N., & Gotoh, M. (2018). Role of microglia in the spinal cord in colon-to-bladder neural crosstalk in a rat model of colitis. *Neurourology and Urodynamics*, *37*(4), 1320–1328. DOI: 10.1002/nau.23484 PMID: 29350427

Malhi, G. S., Tanious, M., Das, P., Coulston, C. M., & Berk, M. (2013). Potential mechanisms of action of lithium in bipolar disorder: Current understanding. *CNS Drugs*, *27*(2), 135–153. DOI: 10.1007/s40263-013-0039-0 PMID: 23371914

Mamah, D. (2011). *The Washington Early Recognition Center Affectivity and Psychosis (WERCAP) Screen*. Washington University School of Medicine in St. Louis. Retrieved from https://werc.wustl.edu/Content/pdfs/WERCAP%20Screen%202022.pdf

Mamah, D., Owoso, A., Sheffield, J. M., & Bayer, C. (2014).

Manji, H. K., Quiroz, J. A., Payne, J. L., Singh, J., Lopes, B. P., Viegas, J. S., & Zarate, C. A. (2003). The underlying neurobiology of bipolar disorder. *World Psychiatry; Official Journal of the World Psychiatric Association (WPA)*, *2*(3), 136–146. PMID: 16946919

Ma, Q., Xing, C., Long, W., Wang, H. Y., Liu, Q., & Wang, R.-F. (2019). Impact of microbiota on central nervous system and neurological diseases: The gut-brain axis. *Journal of Neuroinflammation*, *16*(1), 53. DOI: 10.1186/s12974-019-1434-3 PMID: 30823925

Martire, L. M., & Schulz, R. (2007). Involving family in psychosocial interventions for chronic illness. *Current Directions in Psychological Science*, *16*(2), 90–94. DOI: 10.1111/j.1467-8721.2007.00482.x

Mate, M. A., Cobeta, I., Jiménez-Jiménez, F. J., & Figueiras, R. (2012). Digital voice analysis in patients with advanced Parkinson's disease undergoing deep brain stimulation therapy. *Journal of Voice*, *26*(4), 496–501. DOI: 10.1016/j.jvoice.2011.03.006 PMID: 21704492

Mazza, M., Margoni, S., Mandracchia, G., Donofrio, G., Fischetti, A., Kotzalidis, G. D., & Moccia, L. (2024). This pain drives me crazy: Psychiatric symptoms in women with interstitial cystitis/bladder pain syndrome. *World Journal of Psychiatry*, *14*(6), 954–984. DOI: 10.5498/wjp.v14.i6.954 PMID: 38984334

McConnell, A. Implementing respiratory muscle training. Chapter 6 in: Respiratory Muscle Training: Theory and Practice. Elsevier, 2013. DOI: 10.1016/B978-0-7020-5020-6.00006-6

McConnell, A. K., & Romer, L. M. (2019). Respiratory muscle training in healthy humans: Resolving the controversy. *International Journal of Sports Medicine*, *40*(8), 497–504. PMID: 15162248

McKnight, R. F., Adida, M., Budge, K., Stockton, S., Goodwin, G. M., & Geddes, J. R. (2012). Lithium toxicity profile: A systematic review and meta-analysis. *Lancet*, *379*(9817), 721–728. DOI: 10.1016/S0140-6736(11)61516-X PMID: 22265699

Meade, E., & Garvey, M. (2022). The Role of Neuro-Immune Interaction in Chronic Pain Conditions; Functional Somatic Syndrome, Neurogenic Inflammation, and Peripheral Neuropathy. *International Journal of Molecular Sciences*, *23*(15), 8574. DOI: 10.3390/ijms23158574 PMID: 35955708

Merrill, R. M. (2022). Mental Health Conditions According to Stress and Sleep Disorders. *International Journal of Environmental Research and Public Health*, *19*(13), 7957. Advance online publication. DOI: 10.3390/ijerph19137957 PMID: 35805615

Merritt, C. C., Halverson, T. F., Elliott, T., Jarskog, L. F., Pedersen, C. A., & Penn, D. L. (2023). Racial disparities and predictors of functioning in schizophrenia. *The American Journal of Orthopsychiatry*, *93*(3), 177–187. DOI: 10.1037/ort0000661 PMID: 36931838

Moldwin, R. M., Nursey, V., Yaskiv, O., Dalvi, S., Macdonald, E. J., Funaro, M.,… Stern, J. A.-O. Immune cell profiles of patients with interstitial cystitis/bladder pain syndrome. (1479-5876 (Electronic)).

Moody, G., & Miller, B. J. (2018). Total and differential white blood cell counts and hemodynamic parameters in first-episode psychosis. *Psychiatry Research, 260*, 307–312. DOI: 10.1016/j.psychres.2017.11.086 PMID: 29223800

Moreno-Küstner, B., Martín, C., & Pastor, L. (2018). Prevalence of psychotic disorders and its association with methodological issues: A systematic review and meta-analyses. *PLoS One*, *13*(4), e0195687. DOI: 10.1371/journal.pone.0195687 PMID: 29649252

Morris, N. (2014). Silenced in Childhood: A Survivor of Abuse Finds her Voice through Group Dramatherapy. *Dramatherapy : the Journal of the British Association of Dramatherapy*, *36*(1), 3–17. Advance online publication. DOI: 10.1080/02630672.2014.926958

Mota, S., Güell, R., Barreiro, E., Solanes, I., Ramírez-Sarmiento, A., Orozco-Levi, M., Casan, P., Gea, J., & Sanchis, J. (2007). Clinical outcomes of expiratory muscle training in severe COPD patients. *Respiratory Medicine*, *101*(3), 516–524. DOI: 10.1016/j.rmed.2006.06.024 PMID: 16942867

Muñoz-Negro, J. E., & Cervilla, J. A. (2016). A systematic review on the pharmacological treatment of delusional disorder. *Journal of Clinical Psychopharmacology*, *36*(6), 684–690. DOI: 10.1097/JCP.0000000000000595 PMID: 27811554

Nair, D., Cukor, D., Taylor, W. D., & Cavanaugh, K. L. (2021). Applying a biopsychosocial framework to achieve durable behavior change in kidney disease. *Seminars in Nephrology*, *41*(6), 487–504. DOI: 10.1016/j.semnephrol.2021.10.003

Nassar, A., & Azab, A. N. (2014). Effects of lithium on inflammation. *ACS Chemical Neuroscience*, *5*(6), 451–458. DOI: 10.1021/cn500038f PMID: 24803181

National Cancer Institute. (n.d.). *Depression (PDQ®)*. https://www.cancer.gov/about-cancer/coping/feelings/depression-hp-pdq

Neves, N. A. R. (2011). Técnicas de respiração para a redução do estresse em terapia cognitivo comportamental. *Arq Med Hosp Fac Cienc Med Santa Casa São Paulo*, *56*(3), 158–168.

Newman, W. J., & Newman, B. M. (2016). Rediscovering clozapine: After a turbulent history, current guidance on initiating and monitoring. *Current Psychiatry*, *15*(7), 42–46.

Ng, D. C. E., Liew, C. H., Tan, K. K., Awang, E. H., Nazri, F. N. A., Maran, A. K. T., Mohan, V. A. C., Ramachandran, D., Chok, M., Teh, C. H., Mohamad Nor, A., Baharuddin, S., & Khoo, E. J. (2024). Clinical comparison of HMPV and RSV infections in hospitalised Malaysian children: A propensity score matched study. *The Clinical Respiratory Journal, 18*(3), e13747. Advance online publication. DOI: 10.1111/crj.13747 PMID: 38529669

Nitsche, M. A., Koschack, J., Pohlers, H., Hullemann, S., Paulus, W., & Happe, S. (2012). Effects of frontal transcranial direct current stimulation on emotional state and processing in healthy humans. *Frontiers in Psychiatry, 3*, 58. DOI: 10.3389/fpsyt.2012.00058 PMID: 22723786

Novick, D., Montgomery, W., Treuer, T., Moneta, M. V., & Haro, J. M. (2017). Real-world Effectiveness of Antipsychotics for the Treatment of Negative Symptoms in Patients with Schizophrenia with Predominantly Negative Symptoms. *Pharmacopsychiatry, 50*(02), 56–63. DOI: 10.1055/s-0042-112818 PMID: 28208190

Ochoa, C., Casellas-Grau, A., Vives, J., Font, A., & Borràs, J. M. (2017). Positive psychotherapy for distressed cancer survivors: Posttraumatic growth facilitation reduces posttraumatic stress. *International Journal of Clinical and Health Psychology : IJCHP, 17*(1), 28–37. DOI: 10.1016/j.ijchp.2016.09.002

Oliva, V., Fico, G., De Prisco, M., Gonda, X., Rosa, A. R., & Vieta, E. (2025). Bipolar disorders: An update on critical aspects. *The Lancet Regional Health. Europe, 48*, 101135. DOI: 10.1016/j.lanepe.2024.101135 PMID: 39811787

Oloyede, E., Nettey, V., Dzahini, O., Silva, E., Majkic, N., Montford, P., Secchi, A., Whiskey, E., & Taylor, D. (2025). Low awareness of clozapine-induced agranulocytosis in a mixed-method survey of 354 patients and carers. *Schizophrenia, 11*(1), 129. DOI: 10.1038/s41537-025-00639-5 PMID: 41168211

Onitsuka, T., Hirano, Y., Nakazawa, T., Ichihashi, K., Miura, K., Inada, K., Mitoma, R., Yasui-Furukori, N., & Hashimoto, R. (2022). Toward recovery in schizophrenia: Current concepts, findings, and future research directions. *Psychiatry and Clinical Neurosciences, 76*(7), 282–291. DOI: 10.1111/pcn.13342 PMID: 35235256

Opgen-Rhein, C., & Dettling, M. (2008). Clozapine-Induced Agranulocytosis and its Genetic Determinants. *Pharmacogenomics, 9*(8), 1101–1111. DOI: 10.2217/14622416.9.8.1101 PMID: 18681784

Opie, J. E., Esler, T. B., Clancy, E. M., Wright, B., Painter, F., Vuong, A., Booth, A. T., Newman, L., Johns-Hayden, A., Hameed, M., Hooker, L., Olsson, C., & McIntosh, J. E. (2024). Universal Digital Programs for Promoting Mental and Relational Health for Parents of Young Children: A Systematic Review and Meta-Analysis. In *Clinical Child and Family Psychology Review* (Vol. 27, Issue 1). DOI: 10.1007/s10567-023-00457-0

Organization, W. H. (2017). *Depression and other common mental disorders: global health estimates.*

Paron, K. (2024). Exploring Child-Patient Autonomy: Findings from an Ethnographic Study of Clinic Visits by Children. *Child Indicators Research, 17*(1), 99–121. Advance online publication. DOI: 10.1007/s12187-023-10077-3

Pascoe, M., Parker, A., & Van Vliet, H.. (2021). Individualized Exercise in the Treatment of Depression: The IDEA Randomized Controlled Trial Protocol. *Contemporary Clinical Trials, 105*, 106389.

Paulus, W. (2011). Transcranial electrical stimulation (tES–tDCS; tRNS, tACS) methods. *Neuropsychological Rehabilitation, 21*(5), 602–617. DOI: 10.1080/09602011.2011.557292 PMID: 21819181

Pereira, C. S., Padoan, C. S., Garcia, L. F., Patusco, L., & Magalhães, P. V. S. (2019). Barriers and facilitators perceived by people with bipolar disorder for the practice of exercise: A qualitative study. *Trends in Psychiatry and Psychotherapy, 41*(1), 1–8. DOI: 10.1590/2237-6089-2017-0069 PMID: 30994778

Petersen, R. C., & Jack, C. R. (2009). Alzheimer's Disease and Dementia: The Future of Early Detection and Intervention. The Lancet Neurology, 8(7), 563-572. doi:DOI: 10.1016/S1474-4422(09)70142-7

Pinioti, E., Glarou, E., Lappas, A. S., Fober, I., Helfer, B., Siafis, S., Christodoulou, N., Nikolakopoulou, A., Leucht, S., & Samara, M. (2025). Examining the safety profile of clozapine versus other antipsychotics: Systematic review and meta-analysis. *The British Journal of Psychiatry*, •••, 1–10. DOI: 10.1192/bjp.2025.10421 PMID: 41146456

Portigliatti Pomeri, A., La Salvia, A., Carletto, S., Oliva, F., & Ostacoli, L. (2021). EMDR in cancer patients: A systematic review. *Frontiers in Psychology, 11*, 590204. DOI: 10.3389/fpsyg.2020.590204

Rattay, B., & Benndorf, R. A. (2021). Drug-Induced Idiosyncratic Agranulocytosis - Infrequent but Dangerous. *Frontiers in Pharmacology, 12*, 727717. Advance online publication. DOI: 10.3389/fphar.2021.727717 PMID: 34483939

Rechenberg, K., & Koerner, K. (2021). Cognitive behavioral therapy in adolescents with type 1 diabetes: An integrative review. *Journal of Pediatric Nursing, 60*, 190–197. DOI: 10.1016/j.pedn.2021.03.021

Richards, A., Horwood, J., Boden, J., Kennedy, M., Sellers, R., Riglin, L., Mistry, S., Jones, H., Smith, D. J., Zammit, S., Owen, M., O'Donovan, M. C., & Harold, G. T. (2019). Associations between schizophrenia genetic risk, anxiety disorders and manic/hypomanic episode in a longitudinal population cohort study. *The British Journal of Psychiatry*, *214*(2), 96–102. Advance online publication. DOI: 10.1192/bjp.2018.227 PMID: 30472973

Riehl, L., Fürst, J., Kress, M., & Rykalo, N. (2024). The importance of the gut microbiome and its signals for a healthy nervous system and the multifaceted mechanisms of neuropsychiatric disorders. *Frontiers in Neuroscience*, *17*, 1302957. DOI: 10.3389/fnins.2023.1302957 PMID: 38249593

Roldán, A., Monteagudo, P., Cordellat, A., Sanchis-Soler, G., & Blasco-Lafarga, C. (2021). Inspiratory Muscle Strength and Cardiorespiratory Fitness Association With Health-Related Quality of Life in Healthy Older Adults. *Frontiers in Sports and Active Living*, *3*, 624947. DOI: 10.3389/fspor.2021.624947 PMID: 33817635

Romer, L. M., Polkey, M. I., & Verges, S. (2022). Respiratory muscle training and cardiovascular health: Current evidence and future directions. *Journal of Applied Physiology*, *132*(4), 1191–1202.

Rosenbaum, S., Tiedemann, A., Sherrington, C., Curtis, J., & Ward, P. B. (2022). Physical activity interventions for people with mental illness: A systematic review and meta-analysis. *Journal of Psychiatric Research*, *153*, 25–35.

Rubio, J. M., Kane, J. M., Tanskanen, A., Tiihonen, J., & Taipale, H. (2024). Long-term persistence of the risk of agranulocytosis with clozapine compared with other antipsychotics: A nationwide cohort and case–control study in Finland. *The Lancet. Psychiatry*, *11*(6), 443–450. DOI: 10.1016/S2215-0366(24)00097-X PMID: 38697177

Ruiz-Rull, C., Jaén-Moreno, M. J., Del Pozo, G. I., Gómez, C., Montiel, F. J., Alcántara, M., Carrión, L., Chauca, G. M., Feu, N., Guler, I., Rico-Villademoros, F., Camacho-Rodríguez, C., Gutierrez-Rojas, L., Mannino, D., & Sarramea, F. (2024). Low lung function in Bipolar Disorder and Schizophrenia: A hidden risk. *Frontiers in Physiology*, *15*, 1335798. DOI: 10.3389/fphys.2024.1335798 PMID: 38737830

Saliba, M., Drapeau, N., Skime, M., Hu, X., Accardi, C. J., Athreya, A. P., Kolacz, J., Shekunov, J., Jones, D. P., Croarkin, P. E., & Romanowicz, M. (2023). PISTACHIo (PreemptIon of diSrupTive behAvior in CHIldren): Real-time monitoring of sleep and behavior of children 3–7 years old receiving parent–child interaction therapy augment with artificial intelligence — the study protocol, pilot study. *Pilot and Feasibility Studies*, *9*(1), 23. Advance online publication. DOI: 10.1186/s40814-023-01254-w PMID: 36759915

Sampogna, G., Di Vincenzo, M., Giuliani, L., Menculini, G., Mancuso, E., Arsenio, E., Cipolla, S., Della Rocca, B., Martiadis, V., Signorelli, M. S., & Fiorillo, A. (2023). A systematic review on the effectiveness of antipsychotic drugs on the quality of life of patients with schizophrenia. *Brain Sciences*, *13*(11), 1577. DOI: 10.3390/brainsci13111577 PMID: 38002537

Sarizadeh, M. S., Boogar, I. R., Talepasand, S., & Gharemanfard, F. (2021). Acceptance and commitment therapy for demoralization syndrome and cancer-related trauma: A randomized clinical trial. *International Journal of Cancer Management*, *14*(11), e114637. DOI: 10.5812/ijcm.114637

Schneider, A., Zeiler, M., Kopp, K., Wagner, G., & Karwautz, A. (2023). The Therapeutic Potential of Prebiotics and Probiotics in Child and Adolescent Psychiatric Disorders. In *Zeitschrift fur Kinder- und Jugendpsychiatrie und Psychotherapie* (Vol. 51, Issue 6). DOI: 10.1024/1422-4917/a000930

Schuch, F. B., Vancampfort, D., Firth, J., Rosenbaum, S., Ward, P. B., Silva, E. S., & Stubbs, B. (2020). Physical activity and sedentary behavior in people with major depressive disorder: A systematic review and meta-analysis. Jaffray E. *Physical Therapy in Mental Health*, *15*(1), 62–74.

Schulte, P. F. J., Veerman, S. R. T., Bakker, B., Bogers, J. P. A. M., Jongkind, A., & Cohen, D. (2024). Risk of clozapine-associated agranulocytosis and mandatory white blood cell monitoring: Can the regulations be relaxed? *Schizophrenia Research*, *268*, 74–81. DOI: 10.1016/j.schres.2023.09.024 PMID: 37770377

Serafim, S. D., da Ponte, F. D. R., Lima, F. M., Martins, D. S., Rosa, A. R., & Kunz, M. (2019). Effects of deep breathing in patients with bipolar disorder. *Perspectives in Psychiatric Care*, *55*(1), 119–125. DOI: 10.1111/ppc.12325 PMID: 30189115

Shad, M. U. (2023). Pharmacogenomic screening for agranulocytosis and efficacy with clozapine. *Journal of Translational Genetics and Genomics*, *7*(3), 141–165. DOI: 10.20517/jtgg.2023.11

Shafik, W. (2024c). Generative AI for Social Good and Sustainable Development. In *Generative AI: Current Trends and Applications* (pp. 185–217). Springer. DOI: 10.1007/978-981-97-8460-8_10

Shafik, W. (2024e). Towards Trustworthy and Explainable AI Educational Systems. In *Explainable AI for Education: Recent Trends and Challenges* (pp. 17–41). Springer. DOI: 10.1007/978-3-031-72410-7_2

Shafik, W. (2025). Human-Computer Interaction (HCI) Technologies in Socially-Enabled Artificial Intelligence. In *Future of Digital Technology and AI in Social Sectors* (pp. 121–150). IGI Global.

Shafik, W. (2024a). Connected healthcare—the impact of Internet of Things on medical services. In *Artificial Intelligence and Internet of Things based Augmented Trends for Data Driven Systems* (pp. 181–217). CRC Press., DOI: 10.1201/9781003497318-10

Shafik, W. (2024b). Deep Learning Impacts in the Field of Artificial Intelligence. In *Deep Learning Concepts in Operations Research* (pp. 9–26). Auerbach Publications., DOI: 10.1201/9781003433309-2

Shafik, W. (2024d). Science of Emotional Intelligence. In *Enhancing and Predicting Digital Consumer Behavior with AI* (pp. 284–310). IGI Global. DOI: 10.4018/979-8-3693-4453-8.ch015

Shafik, W., Kalinaki, K., Fahim, K. E., & Adam, M. (2024). Safeguarding Data Privacy and Security in Federated Learning Systems. In *Federated Deep Learning for Healthcare* (pp. 170–190). CRC Press., DOI: 10.1201/9781032694870-13

Shahid, S., Mubin, O., Al Mahmud, A., Iftikhar, Z., & Arshad, R. (2021). Child-Computer Interaction in the Global South: Designing for Children on the Margins. *Proceedings of Interaction Design and Children, IDC, 2021*, 655–657. Advance online publication. DOI: 10.1145/3459990.3460518

Shao, L., Li, Y., Yuan, Z., Guo, X., Zeng, G., & Liu, J. (2024). The effect of clozapine on immune-related biomarkers in schizophrenia patients. *Brain Research Bulletin, 218*, 111104. DOI: 10.1016/j.brainresbull.2024.111104 PMID: 39424000

Sharma, P., Jain, S., Gupta, S., & Chamola, V. (2021). Role of machine learning and deep learning in securing 5G-driven industrial IoT applications. *Ad Hoc Networks, 123*, 102685. Advance online publication. DOI: 10.1016/j.adhoc.2021.102685

Shei, R. J., Paris, H. L., Sogard, A. S., & Mickleborough, T. D. (2022). Time to Move Beyond a "One-Size Fits All" Approach to Inspiratory Muscle Training. *Frontiers in Physiology, 12*, 766346. DOI: 10.3389/fphys.2021.766346 PMID: 35082689

Shei, R. J., Paris, H. L., Wilhite, D. P., Chapman, R. F., & Mickleborough, T. D. (2016). The role of inspiratory muscle training in athletic performance: A systematic review. *Sports Medicine (Auckland, N.Z.)*, *46*(5), 707–717.

Sidtis, D. V. L., Rogers, T., Godier, V., Tagliati, M., & Sidtis, J. J. (2010). Voice and fluency changes as a function of speech task and deep brain stimulation. *Journal of Speech, Language, and Hearing Research: JSLHR*, *53*(5), 1167–1177. DOI: 10.1044/1092-4388(2010/09-0154) PMID: 20643796

Simon, J., Luetzow, A., & Conte, J. R. (2020). Thirty years of the convention on the rights of the child: Developments in child sexual abuse and exploitation. *Child Abuse & Neglect*, *110*, 104399. Advance online publication. DOI: 10.1016/j.chiabu.2020.104399 PMID: 32122640

Singto, T., Sergeeva, A., Filor, V., Vidak, J., Kleuser, B., Belik, V.,...Bäumer, W. (2025). Immune cells in dorsal root ganglia are associated with pruritus in a mouse model of allergic contact dermatitis and co-culture study. (1872-8421 (Electronic)).

Siqueira-Campos, V. A.-O., de Deus, M. A.-O., Poli-Neto, O. A.-O., Rosa, E. S. J. C. A.-O., de Deus, J. A.-O., & Conde, D. A.-O. X. Current Challenges in the Management of Chronic Pelvic Pain in Women: From Bench to Bedside. (1179-1411 (Print)).

Siskind, D., Sharma, M., Pawar, M., Pearson, E., Wagner, E., Warren, N., & Kisely, S. (2021). Clozapine levels as a predictor for therapeutic response: A systematic review and meta-analysis. *Acta Psychiatrica Scandinavica*, *144*(5), 422–432. DOI: 10.1111/acps.13361 PMID: 34374073

Skaper, S. D., Facci, L., Zusso, M., & Giusti, P. (2018). An inflammation-centric view of neurological disease: Beyond the neuron. *Frontiers in Cellular Neuroscience*, *12*, 72. DOI: 10.3389/fncel.2018.00072 PMID: 29618972

Stanos, S. P., Tyburski, M. D., & Harden, R. N. (2021). 37 - Chronic Pain. In Cifu, D. X. (Ed.), *Braddom's Physical Medicine and Rehabilitation* (6th ed., pp. 748–773. e745). Elsevier., https://doi.org/https://doi.org/10.1016/B978-0-323-62539-5.00037-0 DOI: 10.1016/B978-0-323-62539-5.00037-0

Stein, R. E. K. (2022). Mental health concerns and childhood chronic physical health conditions: A narrative review. *Pediatric Medicine*, *5*, 8. DOI: 10.21037/pm-20-107

Stein, R., Garay, M., & Nguyen, A. (2024). It Matters: Early Childhood Mental Health, Educator Stress, and Burnout. *Early Childhood Education Journal*, *52*(2), 333–344. Advance online publication. DOI: 10.1007/s10643-022-01438-8 PMID: 36619683

Stubbs, B., Koyanagi, A., Schuch, F. B., Firth, J., Rosenbaum, S., Veronese, N., Solmi, M., Mugisha, J., & Vancampfort, D. (2016). Physical activity and depression: A large cross-sectional, population-based study across 36 low- and middle-income countries. *Acta Psychiatrica Scandinavica*, *134*(6), 546–556. DOI: 10.1111/acps.12654 PMID: 27704532

Stubbs, B., Vancampfort, D., Firth, J., Hallgren, M., Schuch, F. B., Mugisha, J., & Rosenbaum, S. (2018). Physical activity and serious mental illness: A systematic review and meta-analysis of cardiorespiratory fitness. *Acta Psychiatrica Scandinavica*, *138*(6), 464–478.

Stubbs, B., Vancampfort, D., Hallgren, M., Firth, J., Veronese, N., Solmi, M., Brand, S., Cordes, J., Malchow, B., Gerber, M., Schmitt, A., Correll, C. U., De Hert, M., Gaughran, F., Schneider, F., Kinnafick, F., Falkai, P., Möller, H. J., & Kahl, K. G. (2018). EPA guidance on physical activity as a treatment for severe mental illness: A meta-review of the evidence and Position Statement from the European Psychiatric Association (EPA), supported by the International Organization of Physical Therapists in Mental Health (IOPTMH). *European Psychiatry : the Journal of the Association of European Psychiatrists*, *54*, 124–144. DOI: 10.1016/j.eurpsy.2018.07.004 PMID: 30257806

Sullivan, S. A., Hamilton, W., Tilling, K., Redaniel, T., Moran, P., & Lewis, G. (2018). Association of primary care consultation patterns with early signs and symptoms of psychosis. *JAMA Network Open*, *1*(7), e185174. DOI: 10.1001/jamanetworkopen.2018.5174 PMID: 30646393

Sutherland, S., Grace Kelly, A., Ryden, A., Dmochowski, R. R., Reynolds, W. S., & McKernan, L. C. (2023). Compensatory coping and depression in women with interstitial cystitis/bladder pain syndrome. *Neurourology and Urodynamics*, *42*(1), 322–329. DOI: 10.1002/nau.25089 PMID: 36378850

Svensson, M., Erhardt, S., Hållmarker, U., James, S., & Deierborg, T. (2022). A physically active lifestyle is associated with lower long-term incidence of bipolar disorder in a population-based, large-scale study. *International Journal of Bipolar Disorders*, *10*(1), 26. DOI: 10.1186/s40345-022-00272-6 PMID: 36316595

Swartz, H. A., & Swanson, J. (2014). Psychotherapy for Bipolar Disorder in Adults: A Review of the Evidence. *Focus - American Psychiatric Publishing*, *12*(3), 251–266. DOI: 10.1176/appi.focus.12.3.251 PMID: 26279641

Sylvia, L. G., Friedman, E. S., Kocsis, J. H., Bernstein, E. E., Brody, B. D., Kinrys, G., Kemp, D. E., Shelton, R. C., McElroy, S. L., Bobo, W. V., Kamali, M., McInnis, M. G., Tohen, M., Bowden, C. L., Ketter, T. A., Deckersbach, T., Calabrese, J. R., Thase, M. E., Reilly-Harrington, N. A., & Nierenberg, A. A. (2013). Association of exercise with quality of life and mood symptoms in a comparative effectiveness study of bipolar disorder. *Journal of Affective Disorders*, *151*(2), 722–727. DOI: 10.1016/j.jad.2013.07.031 PMID: 23993440

Szypłowska, M., Tarkowski, R., & Kułak, K. (2023). The impact of endometriosis on depressive and anxiety symptoms and quality of life: A systematic review. *Frontiers in Public Health*, *11*, 1230303. DOI: 10.3389/fpubh.2023.1230303 PMID: 37744486

Tabari, F., Berger, J. I., Flouty, O., Copeland, B., Greenlee, J. D., & Johari, K. (2024). Speech, voice, and language outcomes following deep brain stimulation: A systematic review. *PLoS One*, *19*(5), e0302739. DOI: 10.1371/journal.pone.0302739 PMID: 38728329

The WERCAP Screen and the WERC Stress Screen: Psychometrics of self-rated i instruments for assessing bipolar and psychotic disorder risk and perceived stress burden. *Comprehensive Psychiatry*, *55*(7), 1757–1771. https://doi.org/DOI: 10.1016/j.comppsych.2014.07.004

Thomson, D., Turner, A., Lauder, S., Gigler, M. E., Berk, L., Singh, A. B., Pasco, J. A., Berk, M., & Sylvia, L. (2015). A brief review of exercise, bipolar disorder, and mechanistic pathways. *Frontiers in Psychology*, *6*, 147. DOI: 10.3389/fpsyg.2015.00147 PMID: 25788889

Tizenberg, B. N., Brenner, L. A., Lowry, C. A., Okusaga, O. O., Benavides, D. R., Hoisington, A. J.,... Postolache, T. A.-O. (2021). Biological and Psychological Factors Determining Neuropsychiatric Outcomes in COVID-19. (1535-1645 (Electronic)).

Tralongo, F., Konecki, C., Feliu, C., Kaladjian, A., & Djerada, Z. (2023). Association between clozapine plasma concentrations and treatment response: A systematic review, meta-analysis and individual participant data meta-analysis. *Clinical Pharmacokinetics*, *62*(6), 807–818. DOI: 10.1007/s40262-023-01247-1 PMID: 37145296

Uludag, K. (2024a). Brain imaging studies on Tardive Dyskinesia in schizophrenia patients and animal models: A comprehensive review. *Future Neurology*, *19*(1), 2433936. DOI: 10.1080/14796708.2024.2433936

Uludag, K. (2024b). Predicting Gender Based on Severity of Symptoms of Schizophrenia and Cognitive Parameters. In *Applications of Parallel Data Processing for Biomedical Imaging* (pp. 276–287). IGI Global. DOI: 10.4018/979-8-3693-2426-4.ch014

Uludag, K., & Kara, F. (2024). The impact of oxidative stress biomarkers on memory in individuals with schizophrenia and antioxidant use. In *Nutrition Controversies and Advances in Autoimmune Disease* (pp. 477–500). IGI Global. DOI: 10.4018/979-8-3693-5528-2.ch018

Uludag, K., Wang, D. M., Goodman, C., Wang, L., & Zhang, X. (2021). Prevalence, clinical correlates and risk factors associated with Tardive Dyskinesia in Chinese patients with schizophrenia. *Asian Journal of Psychiatry*, *66*, 102877. DOI: 10.1016/j.ajp.2021.102877 PMID: 34638091

van Barneveld, E., Manders, J., van Osch, F. H., van Poll, M., Visser, L., van Hanegem, N., Lim, A. C., Bongers, M. Y., & Leue, C. (2022). Depression, anxiety, and correlating factors in endometriosis: A systematic review and meta-analysis. *Journal of Women's Health*, *31*(2), 219–230. DOI: 10.1089/jwh.2021.0021 PMID: 34077695

Van Dixhoorn, J. (2007). Whole-body breathing: A systems perspective on respiratory retraining. In Lehrer, P. M., Woolfolk, R. L., & Sime, W. E. (Eds.), *Principles and practice of stress management* (3rd ed., pp. 291–332). The Guilford Press.

Van Meijel, B., van der Gaag, M., Kahn, R. S., & Grypdonck, M. H. F. (2004). Recognition of early warning signs in patients with schizophrenia: A review of the literature. *International Journal of Mental Health Nursing*, *13*(2), 107–116. DOI: 10.1111/j.1440-0979.2004.00314.x PMID: 15318905

Vancampfort, D., Hagemann, N., Wyckaert, S., Rosenbaum, S., Stubbs, B., Firth, J., Schuch, F. B., Probst, M., & Sienaert, P. (2017). Higher cardio-respiratory fitness is associated with increased mental and physical quality of life in people with bi polar disorder: A controlled pilot study. *Psychiatry Research*, *256*, 219–224. DOI: 10.1016/j.psychres.2017.06.066 PMID: 28646785

Vancampfort, D., Rosenbaum, S., Schuch, F., Ward, P. B., Richards, J., Mugisha, J., Probst, M., & Stubbs, B. (2017). Cardiorespiratory Fitness in Severe Mental Illness: A Systematic Review and Meta-analysis. *Sports Medicine (Auckland, N.Z.)*, *47*(2), 343–352. DOI: 10.1007/s40279-016-0574-1 PMID: 27299747

Ventura, A. M. B., Hayes, R. D., & Fonseca de Freitas, D. (2022). Ethnic disparities in clozapine prescription for service-users with schizophrenia-spectrum disorders: A systematic review. *Psychological Medicine*, *52*(12), 2212–2223. DOI: 10.1017/S0033291722001878 PMID: 35787301

Walker, A. K., Kavelaars A Fau - Heijnen, C. J., Heijnen Cj Fau - Dantzer, R., & Dantzer, R. (2013). Neuroinflammation and comorbidity of pain and depression. (1521-0081 (Electronic)).

Wang, Y., Li, B., Zhou, Y., Wang, Y., Han, X., Zhang, S., He, Z., & Ouyang, L. (2021). Does endometriosis disturb mental health and quality of life? A systematic review and meta-analysis. *Gynecologic and Obstetric Investigation*, *86*(4), 315–335. DOI: 10.1159/000516517 PMID: 34352799

Wan, J., Shin, D. B., Syed, M. N., Abuabara, K., Lemeshow, A. R., & Gelfand, J. M. (2023). Atopic dermatitis and risk of major neuropsychiatric disorders in children: A population-based cohort study. *Journal of the European Academy of Dermatology and Venereology*, *37*(1), 114–122. Advance online publication. DOI: 10.1111/jdv.18564 PMID: 36018560

Wei, J., & Dong, T. (2025). The Effect of Clozapine on Immune-Related Biomarkers in Schizophrenia Patients. *Journal of Biochemical and Molecular Toxicology*, *39*(9), e70503. DOI: 10.1002/jbt.70503 PMID: 40965598

Weiner, M., Warren, L., & Fiedorowicz, J. G. (2011). Cardiovascular morbidity and mortality in bipolar disorder. *Annals of Clinical Psychiatry*, *23*(1), 40–47. DOI: 10.1177/104012371102300107 PMID: 21318195

Wenke, S., Jung, N., Forthmann, B., Maier, C., Hirschfeld, G., & Muehlan, H. (2022). Rare pediatric diseases and pathways to psychosocial care: A qualitative interview study with professional experts in Germany. *Orphanet Journal of Rare Diseases*, *17*(1), 361. DOI: 10.1186/s13023-021-02127-2

Wheeler, A., Humberstone, V., & Robinson, G. (2009). Outcomes for schizophrenia patients with clozapine treatment: How good does it get? *Journal of Psychopharmacology (Oxford, England)*, *23*(8), 957–965. DOI: 10.1177/0269881108093588 PMID: 18635713

Willcocks, I. R., Legge, S. E., Nalmpanti, M., Mazzeo, L., King, A., Jansen, J., & Walters, J. T. (2021). Clozapine metabolism is associated with absolute neutrophil count in individuals with treatment-resistant schizophrenia. *Frontiers in Pharmacology*, *12*, 658734. DOI: 10.3389/fphar.2021.658734 PMID: 33959025

Wilson, C. A., Newham, J., Rankin, J., Ismail, K., Simonoff, E., Reynolds, R. M., Stoll, N., & Howard, L. M. (2022). Systematic review and meta-analysis of risk of gestational diabetes in women with preconception mental disorders. In *Journal of Psychiatric Research* (Vol. 149). DOI: 10.1016/j.jpsychires.2022.03.013

World Health Organization (WHO). (2021). Dementia. [WHO Fact Sheet]. Retrieved from https://www.who.int/news-room/fact-sheets/detail/dementia

Wu, C., Wang, L., Zhou, X., Zhou, Y., Han, S., Dong, X., & Liu, H. (2025). Using structural equation modelling to explore the relationship between insomnia, anxiety and depression to the severity of BPS/IC: A cross-sectional study in Chongqing, China. *BMJ Open, 15*(12), e099604. DOI: 10.1136/bmjopen-2025-099604 PMID: 41407415

Yamamoto, M. P., Carillo, J. F., & Howard, F. M. (2014). Chronic Abdominal Pain of Gynecologic Causes: Diagnosis and Treatment. In *Chronic Abdominal Pain: An Evidence-Based, Comprehensive Guide to Clinical Management* (pp. 103-113). Springer.

Yang, F. C., Zhou, Y., Zhang, S. Y., & Ma, R. (2025). Depression and anxiety in patients with endometriosis-associated chronic pain: Neuroimmune mechanisms mediated by inflammatory factors. (2220-3206 (Print)).

Yang, M.-H., Huang, J.-Y., Chen, S.-L., & Wei, J. C.-C. (2021). Association of interstitial cystitis/bladder pain syndrome with stress-related diseases: A nationwide population-based study. *Journal of Clinical Medicine, 10*(23), 5669. DOI: 10.3390/jcm10235669 PMID: 34884371

Yang, Y., Wei, P., Shi, J., Mao, Y., Zhang, J., Lei, D., & Li, W. (2025). Early assessment of responsive neurostimulation for drug-resistant epilepsy in China: A multicenter, self-controlled study. *Chinese Medical Journal, 138*(4), 430–440. DOI: 10.1097/CM9.0000000000003292 PMID: 39593204

Young-Hyman, D., de Groot, M., Hill-Briggs, F., Gonzalez, J. S., Hood, K. K., & Peyrot, M. (2016). Psychosocial care for people with diabetes: A position statement of the American Diabetes Association. *Diabetes Care, 39*(12), 2126–2140. DOI: 10.2337/dc16-2053

Young, W. (2009). Review of Lithium Effects on Brain and Blood. *Cell Transplantation, 18*(9), 951–975. DOI: 10.3727/096368909X471251 PMID: 19523343

Yuan, X., Wang, S., Shi, Y., Yang, Y., Zhang, Y., Xia, L., Zhang, K., & Liu, H. (2022). Pro-inflammatory cytokine levels are elevated in female patients with schizophrenia treated with clozapine. *Psychopharmacology, 239*(3), 765–771. DOI: 10.1007/s00213-022-06067-y PMID: 35080634

Zhang, L., Luo, Y., Wei, T., Wang, D., He, Z. A.-O., Lan, L., & Zeng, F. A.-O. (2025). Acupuncture's Multisystem Neuroimmunomodulation: Central-Peripheral Interactions in Gastroenteric, Psychiatric, and Chronic Pain Disorders. (1755-5949 (Electronic)).

Zhang, W., & Liu, Q. (2023). Investigation and analysis of digital demand for children's books. *Nurture*, *17*(4), 653–663. Advance online publication. DOI: 10.55951/nurture.v17i4.450

Zhang, Y., Tao, S., Coid, J., Wei, W., Wang, Q., Yue, W., & Yang, G. (2024). The role of total white blood cell count in antipsychotic treatment for patients with schizophrenia. *Current Neuropharmacology*, *22*(1), 159–167. DOI: 10.2174/1570159X21666230104090046 PMID: 36600620

Zhixiang, C., Yan, L., Liu, X., Lingjie, X., Dong, H., Tao, S., & Yanqing, L. (2025). A Chinese Guideline for the Diagnosis and Treatment of Neuropathic Pain. *International Journal of Plant Research*, *1*(4), 56–86. DOI: 10.11648/j.ijpr.20250104.12

Zhou, Y., Zheng, W., Guo, F., Wu, S., & Zhong, C. (2025). The anti-inflammation pharmacodynamics of lithium: Therapy of bipolar disorder. *Journal of Psychopharmacology (Oxford, England)*, *39*(6), 533–544. DOI: 10.1177/02698811251326942 PMID: 40138498

Related References

To continue our tradition of advancing information science and technology research, we have compiled a list of recommended IGI Global readings. These references will provide additional information and guidance to further enrich your knowledge and assist you with your own research and future publications.

Abu Seman, S. A., & Ramayah, T. (2017). Are We Ready to App?: A Study on mHealth Apps, Its Future, and Trends in Malaysia Context. In Pelet, J. (Ed.), *Mobile Platforms, Design, and Apps for Social Commerce* (pp. 69–83). Hershey, PA: IGI Global. DOI: 10.4018/978-1-5225-2469-4.ch005

Adeleke, I. T., & Abdul, Q. B. (2020). Opinions on Cyber Security, Electronic Health Records, and Medical Confidentiality: Emerging Issues on Internet of Medical Things From Nigeria. In Pankajavalli, P., & Karthick, G. (Eds.), *Incorporating the Internet of Things in Healthcare Applications and Wearable Devices* (pp. 199–211). IGI Global. https://doi.org/10.4018/978-1-7998-1090-2.ch012

Aggarwal, S., & Azad, V. (2017). A Hybrid System Based on FMM and MLP to Diagnose Heart Disease. In Bhattacharyya, S., De, S., Pan, I., & Dutta, P. (Eds.), *Intelligent Multidimensional Data Clustering and Analysis* (pp. 293–325). Hershey, PA: IGI Global. DOI: 10.4018/978-1-5225-1776-4.ch011

Al-Busaidi, S. S. (2018). Interdisciplinary Relationships Between Medicine and Social Sciences. In Al-Suqri, M., Al-Kindi, A., AlKindi, S., & Saleem, N. (Eds.), *Promoting Interdisciplinarity in Knowledge Generation and Problem Solving* (pp. 124–137). Hershey, PA: IGI Global. DOI: 10.4018/978-1-5225-3878-3.ch009

Al Kareh, T., & Thoumy, M. (2018). The Impact of Health Information Digitization on the Physiotherapist-Patient Relationship: A Pilot Study of the Lebanese Community. *International Journal of Healthcare Information Systems and Informatics, 13*(2), 29–53. DOI: 10.4018/IJHISI.2018040103

Alenzuela, R. (2017). Research, Leadership, and Resource-Sharing Initiatives: The Role of Local Library Consortia in Access to Medical Information. In Ram, S. (Ed.), *Library and Information Services for Bioinformatics Education and Research* (pp. 199–211). Hershey, PA: IGI Global. DOI: 10.4018/978-1-5225-1871-6.ch012

Ali, S., Samie, A. U., Ali, A., Bhat, A. H., Mir, T., & Prasad, B. V. (2020). Mental Health: A Global Issue Affecting the Pattern of Life in Kashmir. In Taukeni, S. (Ed.), *Biopsychosocial Perspectives and Practices for Addressing Communicable and Non-Communicable Diseases* (pp. 18–29). IGI Global. https://doi.org/10.4018/978-1-7998-2139-7.ch002

Almpani, S., Stefaneas, P., Boley, H., Mitsikas, T., & Frangos, P. (2019). A Rule-Based Model for Compliance of Medical Devices Applied to the European Market. *International Journal of Extreme Automation and Connectivity in Healthcare*, *1*(2), 56–78. https://doi.org/10.4018/IJEACH.2019070104

Alnakhi, W. K. (2021). Medical Travel and Public Health: Definitions, Frameworks, and Future Research. In Singh, M., & Kumaran, S. (Eds.), *Growth of the Medical Tourism Industry and Its Impact on Society: Emerging Research and Opportunities* (pp. 74–94). IGI Global. https://doi.org/10.4018/978-1-7998-3427-4.ch004

Ameri, H., Alizadeh, S., & Noughabi, E. A. (2017). Application of Data Mining Techniques in Clinical Decision Making: A Literature Review and Classification. In Noughabi, E., Raahemi, B., Albadvi, A., & Far, B. (Eds.), *Handbook of Research on Data Science for Effective Healthcare Practice and Administration* (pp. 257–295). Hershey, PA: IGI Global. DOI: 10.4018/978-1-5225-2515-8.ch012

Anand, S. (2017). Medical Image Enhancement Using Edge Information-Based Methods. In Singh, B. (Ed.), *Computational Tools and Techniques for Biomedical Signal Processing* (pp. 123–148). Hershey, PA: IGI Global. DOI: 10.4018/978-1-5225-0660-7.ch006

Anton, J. L., Soriano, J. V., Martinez, M. I., & Garcia, F. B. (2018). Comprehensive E-Learning Appraisal System. In M. Khosrow-Pour, D.B.A. (Ed.), *Encyclopedia of Information Science and Technology, Fourth Edition* (pp. 5787-5799). Hershey, PA: IGI Global. https://doi.org/DOI: 10.4018/978-1-5225-2255-3.ch503

Aslan, F. (2021). Could There Be an Alternative Method of Media Literacy in Promoting Health in Children and Adolescents? Media Literacy and Health Promotion. In G. Sarı (Eds.), *Handbook of Research on Representing Health and Medicine in Modern Media* (pp. 191-199). IGI Global. https://doi.org/10.4018/978-1-7998-6825-5.ch013

Atzori, B., Hoffman, H. G., Vagnoli, L., Messeri, A., & Grotto, R. L. (2018). Virtual Reality as Distraction Technique for Pain Management in Children and Adolescents. In M. Khosrow-Pour, D.B.A. (Ed.), *Encyclopedia of Information Science and Technology, Fourth Edition* (pp. 5955-5965). Hershey, PA: IGI Global. DOI: 10.4018/978-1-5225-2255-3.ch518

Audibert, M., Mathonnat, J., Pélissier, A., & Huang, X. X. (2018). The Impact of the New Rural Cooperative Medical Scheme on Township Hospitals' Utilization and Income Structure in Weifang Prefecture, China. In I. Management Association (Ed.), *Health Economics and Healthcare Reform: Breakthroughs in Research and Practice* (pp. 109-121). Hershey, PA: IGI Global. https://doi.org/DOI: 10.4018/978-1-5225-3168-5.ch007

Aulia, A., & Pratiti, B. (2022). Cyberchondria and Medical Student Syndrome: An Anxious Path to Be an Anxiety Healer? In Aker, H., & Aiken, M. (Eds.), *Handbook of Research on Cyberchondria, Health Literacy, and the Role of Media in Society's Perception of Medical Information* (pp. 98–113). IGI Global. https://doi.org/10.4018/978-1-7998-8630-3.ch006

Babu, A., & Ayyappan, S. (2017). A Methodological Evaluation of Crypto-Watermarking System for Medical Images. In Bhatt, C., & Peddoju, S. (Eds.), *Cloud Computing Systems and Applications in Healthcare* (pp. 189–217). Hershey, PA: IGI Global. DOI: 10.4018/978-1-5225-1002-4.ch010

Bakke, A. (2017). Ethos in E-Health: From Informational to Interactive Websites. In Folk, M., & Apostel, S. (Eds.), *Establishing and Evaluating Digital Ethos and Online Credibility* (pp. 85–103). Hershey, PA: IGI Global. DOI: 10.4018/978-1-5225-1072-7.ch005

Bali, S. (2018). Enhancing the Reach of Health Care Through Telemedicine: Status and New Possibilities in Developing Countries. In Pandey, U., & Indrakanti, V. (Eds.), *Open and Distance Learning Initiatives for Sustainable Development* (pp. 339–354). Hershey, PA: IGI Global. DOI: 10.4018/978-1-5225-2621-6.ch019

Balls-Berry, J. E., & Albold, C. (2019). Asynchronous Education for Graduate Medical Trainees to Reduce Health Disparities and Address Social Determinants of Health: Online Education for Graduate Medical Trainees. In Demiroz, E., & Waldman, S. (Eds.), *Optimizing Medical Education With Instructional Technology* (pp. 1–20). IGI Global. https://doi.org/10.4018/978-1-5225-6289-4.ch001

Barrett, T. E. (2018). Essentials for Education and Training for Tomorrow's Physicians. In Smith, C. (Ed.), *Exploring the Pressures of Medical Education From a Mental Health and Wellness Perspective* (pp. 230–252). Hershey, PA: IGI Global. DOI: 10.4018/978-1-5225-2811-1.ch010

Bazan, V., Jax, M. D., & Zwischenberger, J. B. (2020). Alice in Simulation-Land: Surgical Simulation in Medical Education. In Gotian, R., Kang, Y., & Safdieh, J. (Eds.), *Handbook of Research on the Efficacy of Training Programs and Systems in Medical Education* (pp. 449–458). IGI Global. https://doi.org/10.4018/978-1-7998-1468-9.ch023

Beaudoin, S. (2019). The Hidden Face of Medical Intervention. In C. Albuquerque (Eds.), *Emerging Trends and Innovations in Privacy and Health Information Management* (pp. 188-211). IGI Global. https://doi.org/10.4018/978-1-5225-8470-4.ch008

Bernardes, O., Amorim, V., & Usman, B. (2021). The Good, the Bad, and the Ugly: Don't Blame COVID-19 for Health System Inefficiencies. In J. Santos, & I. Pereira (Ed.), *Management and Marketing for Improved Competitiveness and Performance in the Healthcare Sector* (pp. 115-139). IGI Global. https://doi.org/10.4018/978-1-7998-7263-4.ch006

Berrahal, S., & Boudriga, N. (2017). The Risks of Wearable Technologies to Individuals and Organizations. In Marrington, A., Kerr, D., & Gammack, J. (Eds.), *Managing Security Issues and the Hidden Dangers of Wearable Technologies* (pp. 18–46). Hershey, PA: IGI Global. DOI: 10.4018/978-1-5225-1016-1.ch002

Bhargava, P. (2018). Blended Learning: An Effective Application to Clinical Teaching. In Tang, S., & Lim, C. (Eds.), *Preparing the Next Generation of Teachers for 21st Century Education* (pp. 302–320). Hershey, PA: IGI Global. DOI: 10.4018/978-1-5225-4080-9.ch018

Bird, J. L. (2017). Writing Healing Narratives. In Bryan, V., & Bird, J. (Eds.), *Healthcare Community Synergism between Patients, Practitioners, and Researchers* (pp. 1–28). Hershey, PA: IGI Global. DOI: 10.4018/978-1-5225-0640-9.ch001

Bougoulias, K., Kouris, I., Prasinos, M., Giokas, K., & Koutsouris, D. (2017). Ob/Gyn EMR Software: A Solution for Obstetricians and Gynecologists. In Moumtzoglou, A. (Ed.), *Design, Development, and Integration of Reliable Electronic Healthcare Platforms* (pp. 101–111). Hershey, PA: IGI Global. DOI: 10.4018/978-1-5225-1724-5.ch006

Bouslimi, R., Ayadi, M. G., & Akaichi, J. (2018). Medical Image Retrieval in Healthcare Social Networks. *International Journal of Healthcare Information Systems and Informatics, 13*(2), 13–28. DOI: 10.4018/IJHISI.2018040102

Bouzaabia, O., Bouzaabia, R., & Mejri, K. (2017). Role of Internet in the Development of Medical Tourism Service in Tunisia. In Capatina, A., & Rancati, E. (Eds.), *Key Challenges and Opportunities in Web Entrepreneurship* (pp. 211–241). Hershey, PA: IGI Global. DOI: 10.4018/978-1-5225-2466-3.ch009

Brown-Jackson, K. L. (2018). Telemedicine and Telehealth: Academics Engaging the Community in a Call to Action. In Burton, S. (Ed.), *Engaged Scholarship and Civic Responsibility in Higher Education* (pp. 166–193). Hershey, PA: IGI Global. DOI: 10.4018/978-1-5225-3649-9.ch008

Bwalya, K. J. (2017). Next Wave of Tele-Medicine: Virtual Presence of Medical Personnel. In Moahi, K., Bwalya, K., & Sebina, P. (Eds.), *Health Information Systems and the Advancement of Medical Practice in Developing Countries* (pp. 168–180). Hershey, PA: IGI Global. DOI: 10.4018/978-1-5225-2262-1.ch010

Celik, G. (2018). Determining Headache Diseases With Genetic Algorithm. In Kose, U., Guraksin, G., & Deperlioglu, O. (Eds.), *Nature-Inspired Intelligent Techniques for Solving Biomedical Engineering Problems* (pp. 249–262). Hershey, PA: IGI Global. DOI: 10.4018/978-1-5225-4769-3.ch012

Chakraborty, S., Chatterjee, S., Ashour, A. S., Mali, K., & Dey, N. (2018). Intelligent Computing in Medical Imaging: A Study. In Dey, N. (Ed.), *Advancements in Applied Metaheuristic Computing* (pp. 143–163). Hershey, PA: IGI Global. DOI: 10.4018/978-1-5225-4151-6.ch006

Chandra, L., Downey, C. L., Svavarsdottir, H. S., Skinner, H., & Young, A. L. (2020). Gender Equity in Medical Leadership. In Bellini, M., & Papalois, V. (Eds.), *Gender Equity in the Medical Profession* (pp. 94–109). IGI Global. https://doi.org/10.4018/978-1-5225-9599-1.ch007

Chandran, S. (2019). Medical Data Storage and Compression. In Swarnambiga, A. (Ed.), *Medical Image Processing for Improved Clinical Diagnosis* (pp. 140–154). IGI Global. https://doi.org/10.4018/978-1-5225-5876-7.ch007

Chavez, A., & Kovarik, C. (2017). Open Source Technology for Medical Practice in Developing Countries. In Moahi, K., Bwalya, K., & Sebina, P. (Eds.), *Health Information Systems and the Advancement of Medical Practice in Developing Countries* (pp. 33–59). Hershey, PA: IGI Global. DOI: 10.4018/978-1-5225-2262-1.ch003

Chen, S., Traba, C., Lamba, S., & Soto-Greene, M. (2020). Professional and Career Development of Medical Students. In Gotian, R., Kang, Y., & Safdieh, J. (Eds.), *Handbook of Research on the Efficacy of Training Programs and Systems in Medical Education* (pp. 305–326). IGI Global. https://doi.org/10.4018/978-1-7998-1468-9.ch016

Chien, G. C., Haroutunian, A., England, B., & Candido, K. D. (2019). Optimizing Medical Education With Instructional Technology: Technology to Optimize Teaching Human Anatomy. In Demiroz, E., & Waldman, S. (Eds.), *Optimizing Medical Education With Instructional Technology* (pp. 71–78). IGI Global. https://doi.org/10.4018/978-1-5225-6289-4.ch005

Choudhari, R. H. (2021). Multidimensional Impact of Climate Change on Human Reproduction and Fertility: A Medical Perspective on Changing Dynamics. In K. Wani, & N. Naha (Eds.), *Climate Change and Its Impact on Fertility* (pp. 278-315). IGI Global. https://doi.org/10.4018/978-1-7998-4480-8.ch014

Ciufudean, C. (2018). Innovative Formalism for Biological Data Analysis. In M. Khosrow-Pour, D.B.A. (Ed.), *Encyclopedia of Information Science and Technology, Fourth Edition* (pp. 1814-1824). Hershey, PA: IGI Global. DOI: 10.4018/978-1-5225-2255-3.ch158

Colaguori, R., & Danesi, M. (2017). Medical Semiotics: A Revisitation and an Exhortation. *International Journal of Semiotics and Visual Rhetoric*, *1*(1), 11–18. DOI: 10.4018/IJSVR.2017010102

Cole, A. W., & Salek, T. A. (2017). Adopting a Parasocial Connection to Overcome Professional Kakoethos in Online Health Information. In Folk, M., & Apostel, S. (Eds.), *Establishing and Evaluating Digital Ethos and Online Credibility* (pp. 104–120). Hershey, PA: IGI Global. DOI: 10.4018/978-1-5225-1072-7.ch006

Deperlioglu, O. (2018). Intelligent Techniques Inspired by Nature and Used in Biomedical Engineering. In Kose, U., Guraksin, G., & Deperlioglu, O. (Eds.), *Nature-Inspired Intelligent Techniques for Solving Biomedical Engineering Problems* (pp. 51–77). Hershey, PA: IGI Global. DOI: 10.4018/978-1-5225-4769-3.ch003

Desai, K. P., Shah, M. A., Lapasia, M. C., Patil, S. A., & Pathak, S. P. (2022). Applied Intelligence for Mental Health Detection: ManoVaidya – A Mental Health Therapist. In Thakare, A., Wagh, S., Bhende, M., Anter, A., & Gao, X. (Eds.), *Handbook of Research on Applied Intelligence for Health and Clinical Informatics* (pp. 80–91). IGI Global. https://doi.org/10.4018/978-1-7998-7709-7.ch005

Dey, N., & Ashour, A. S. (2018). Meta-Heuristic Algorithms in Medical Image Segmentation: A Review. In Dey, N. (Ed.), *Advancements in Applied Metaheuristic Computing* (pp. 185–203). Hershey, PA: IGI Global. DOI: 10.4018/978-1-5225-4151-6.ch008

Dey, N., Ashour, A. S., & Althoupety, A. S. (2017). Thermal Imaging in Medical Science. In Santhi, V. (Ed.), *Recent Advances in Applied Thermal Imaging for Industrial Applications* (pp. 87–117). Hershey, PA: IGI Global. DOI: 10.4018/978-1-5225-2423-6.ch004

Di Virgilio, F., Camillo, A. A., & Camillo, I. C. (2017). The Impact of Social Network on Italian Users' Behavioural Intention for the Choice of a Medical Tourist Destination. *International Journal of Tourism and Hospitality Management in the Digital Age, 1*(1), 36–49. DOI: 10.4018/IJTHMDA.2017010103

Dobani, F., Pennington, M. L., Coe, E., Morrison, P., & Gulliver, S. B. (2020). Bridging the Gaps: Toward Effective Collaboration Between Peer Supporters and Behavioral Health Professionals. In Bowers, C., Beidel, D., & Marks, M. (Eds.), *Mental Health Intervention and Treatment of First Responders and Emergency Workers* (pp. 190–204). IGI Global. https://doi.org/10.4018/978-1-5225-9803-9.ch011

Dogra, A. K., & Dogra, P. (2017). The Medical Tourism Industry in the BRIC Nations: An Indian Analysis. In Dhiman, M. (Ed.), *Opportunities and Challenges for Tourism and Hospitality in the BRIC Nations* (pp. 320–336). Hershey, PA: IGI Global. DOI: 10.4018/978-1-5225-0708-6.ch020

Doublestein, B. A., Lee, W. T., & Pfohl, R. M. (2020). Overview of Professionalism Competence: Bringing Balance to the Medical Education Continuum. In Selladurai, R., Hobson, C., Selladurai, R., & Greer, A. (Eds.), *Evaluating Challenges and Opportunities for Healthcare Reform* (pp. 215–231). IGI Global. https://doi.org/10.4018/978-1-7998-2949-2.ch010

Drowos, J. L., & Wood, S. K. (2017). Preparing Future Physicians to Adapt to the Changing Health Care System: Promoting Humanism through Curricular Design. In Bryan, V., & Bird, J. (Eds.), *Healthcare Community Synergism between Patients, Practitioners, and Researchers* (pp. 106–125). Hershey, PA: IGI Global. DOI: 10.4018/978-1-5225-0640-9.ch006

Dulam, K. (2017). Medical Patents and Impact on Availability and Affordability of Essential Medicines in India. In Aggarwal, R., & Kaur, R. (Eds.), *Patent Law and Intellectual Property in the Medical Field* (pp. 41–57). Hershey, PA: IGI Global. DOI: 10.4018/978-1-5225-2414-4.ch003

Dutta, P. (2017). Decision Making in Medical Diagnosis via Distance Measures on Interval Valued Fuzzy Sets. *International Journal of System Dynamics Applications, 6*(4), 63–83. DOI: 10.4018/IJSDA.2017100104

Dutta, P. (2021). Medical Pre-Screening of Common Diseases: An Interval-Valued Fuzzy Set Approach. In Azar, A., & Kamal, N. (Eds.), *Handbook of Research on Modeling, Analysis, and Control of Complex Systems* (pp. 267–292). IGI Global. https://doi.org/10.4018/978-1-7998-5788-4.ch011

Dwivedi, M. K., Pandey, S. K., & Singh, P. K. (2021). Public Health Surveillance System: Infectious Diseases. In Yadav, D., Bansal, A., Bhatia, M., Hooda, M., & Morato, J. (Eds.), *Diagnostic Applications of Health Intelligence and Surveillance Systems* (pp. 201–220). IGI Global. https://doi.org/10.4018/978-1-7998-6527-8.ch010

El Guemhioui, K., & Demurjian, S. A. (2017). Semantic Reconciliation of Electronic Health Records Using Semantic Web Technologies. *International Journal of Information Technology and Web Engineering, 12*(2), 26–48. DOI: 10.4018/IJITWE.2017040102

Etim, A., Etim, D. N., & Scott, J. (2020). Mobile Health and Telemedicine: Awareness, Adoption and Importance of Health Study. *International Journal of Healthcare Information Systems and Informatics, 15*(1), 81–96. https://doi.org/10.4018/IJHISI.2020010105

Fino, E., & Hanna-Khalil, B. (2020). Psychometric Post-Examination Analysis in Medical Education Training Programs. In Gotian, R., Kang, Y., & Safdieh, J. (Eds.), *Handbook of Research on the Efficacy of Training Programs and Systems in Medical Education* (pp. 221–242). IGI Global. https://doi.org/10.4018/978-1-7998-1468-9.ch012

Fishback, J. L., & Klein, R. M. (2019). Collaborative Learning for Histopathology Education. In Demiroz, E., & Waldman, S. (Eds.), *Optimizing Medical Education With Instructional Technology* (pp. 177–193). IGI Global. https://doi.org/10.4018/978-1-5225-6289-4.ch010

Fisher, J. (2018). Sociological Perspectives on Improving Medical Diagnosis Emphasizing CAD. In M. Khosrow-Pour, D.B.A. (Ed.), *Encyclopedia of Information Science and Technology, Fourth Edition* (pp. 1017-1024). Hershey, PA: IGI Global. DOI: 10.4018/978-1-5225-2255-3.ch088

Franco Santos, D., Branco Silva, A. R., Novo, M. D., & Vaz de Almeida, C. (2022). Medical Burnout: Is Mindfulness an Effective Coping Strategy? In Gupta, S. (Ed.), *Handbook of Research on Clinical Applications of Meditation and Mindfulness-Based Interventions in Mental Health* (pp. 184–194). IGI Global. https://doi.org/10.4018/978-1-7998-8682-2.ch012

Frank, E. M. (2018). Healthcare Education: Integrating Simulation Technologies. In Bryan, V., Musgrove, A., & Powers, J. (Eds.), *Handbook of Research on Human Development in the Digital Age* (pp. 163–182). Hershey, PA: IGI Global. DOI: 10.4018/978-1-5225-2838-8.ch008

Gambhir, P. (2021). Enhancing Mental Health: A Role for Technology. In Hooke, A. (Ed.), *Technological Breakthroughs and Future Business Opportunities in Education, Health, and Outer Space* (pp. 264–269). IGI Global. https://doi.org/10.4018/978-1-7998-6772-2.ch017

Garcia-Santa, N., San Miguel, B., & Ugai, T. (2019). Converging Semantic Knowledge and Deep Learning for Medical Coding. *International Journal of Privacy and Health Information Management*, *7*(2), 33–52. https://doi.org/10.4018/IJPHIM.2019070103

Garner, G. (2018). Foundations for Yoga Practice in Rehabilitation. In Telles, S., & Singh, N. (Eds.), *Research-Based Perspectives on the Psychophysiology of Yoga* (pp. 263–307). Hershey, PA: IGI Global. DOI: 10.4018/978-1-5225-2788-6.ch015

Garrote Andújar, S. A., Araújo Vila, N., Brea, J. A., & de Araújo, A. F. (2021). Medical Tourism: Analysis and Expectations Worldwide. In Borges, A., & Rodrigues, P. (Eds.), *New Techniques for Brand Management in the Healthcare Sector* (pp. 84–102). IGI Global. https://doi.org/10.4018/978-1-7998-3034-4.ch006

Gavurová, B., Kováč, V., & Šoltés, M. (2018). Medical Equipment and Economic Determinants of Its Structure and Regulation in the Slovak Republic. In M. Khosrow-Pour, D.B.A. (Ed.), *Encyclopedia of Information Science and Technology, Fourth Edition* (pp. 5841-5852). Hershey, PA: IGI Global. DOI: 10.4018/978-1-5225-2255-3.ch508

Ge, X., Wang, Q., Huang, K., Law, V., & Thomas, D. C. (2017). Designing Simulated Learning Environments and Facilitating Authentic Learning Experiences in Medical Education. In Stefaniak, J. (Ed.), *Advancing Medical Education Through Strategic Instructional Design* (pp. 77–100). Hershey, PA: IGI Global. DOI: 10.4018/978-1-5225-2098-6.ch004

Gewald, H., & Gewald, C. (2018). Inhibitors of Physicians' Use of Mandatory Hospital Information Systems (HIS). *International Journal of Healthcare Information Systems and Informatics*, *13*(1), 29–44. DOI: 10.4018/IJHISI.2018010103

Ghosh, D., & Dinda, S. (2017). Health Infrastructure and Economic Development in India. In Das, R. (Ed.), *Social, Health, and Environmental Infrastructures for Economic Growth* (pp. 99–119). Hershey, PA: IGI Global. DOI: 10.4018/978-1-5225-2364-2.ch006

Ghosh, K., & Sen, K. C. (2017). The Potential of Crowdsourcing in the Health Care Industry. In Wickramasinghe, N. (Ed.), *Handbook of Research on Healthcare Administration and Management* (pp. 418–427). Hershey, PA: IGI Global. DOI: 10.4018/978-1-5225-0920-2.ch024

Gonzalez-Urquijo, M., Macias-Rodriguez, Y., & Davila-Rivas, J. A. (2022). The Role of Telemedicine and Globalization in Medical Education. In Lopez, M. (Ed.), *Advancing Health Education With Telemedicine* (pp. 288–295). IGI Global. https://doi.org/10.4018/978-1-7998-8783-6.ch015

Gopalan, V., Chan, E., & Ho, D. T. (2018). Deliberate Self-Harm and Suicide Ideology in Medical Students. In Smith, C. (Ed.), *Exploring the Pressures of Medical Education From a Mental Health and Wellness Perspective* (pp. 122–143). Hershey, PA: IGI Global. DOI: 10.4018/978-1-5225-2811-1.ch005

Goswami, N. (2021). Effects of Spaceflight, Aging, and Bedrest on Falls: Aging Meets Spaceflight! In Eklund, P. (Ed.), *Integrated Care and Fall Prevention in Active and Healthy Aging* (pp. 91–106). IGI Global. https://doi.org/10.4018/978-1-7998-4411-2.ch005

Goswami, S., Dey, U., Roy, P., Ashour, A., & Dey, N. (2017). Medical Video Processing: Concept and Applications. In Dey, N., Ashour, A., & Patra, P. (Eds.), *Feature Detectors and Motion Detection in Video Processing* (pp. 1–17). Hershey, PA: IGI Global. DOI: 10.4018/978-1-5225-1025-3.ch001

Goswami, S., Mahanta, K., Goswami, S., Jigdung, T., & Devi, T. P. (2018). Ageing and Cancer: The Epigenetic Basis, Alternative Treatment, and Care. In Prasad, B., & Akbar, S. (Eds.), *Handbook of Research on Geriatric Health, Treatment, and Care* (pp. 206–235). Hershey, PA: IGI Global. DOI: 10.4018/978-1-5225-3480-8.ch012

Gouva, M. I. (2017). The Psychological Impact of Medical Error on Patients, Family Members, and Health Professionals. In Riga, M. (Ed.), *Impact of Medical Errors and Malpractice on Health Economics, Quality, and Patient Safety* (pp. 171–196). Hershey, PA: IGI Global. DOI: 10.4018/978-1-5225-2337-6.ch007

Gündüz, U., & Pembecioğlu, N. (2021). Case Study of Gender and Career Choices: Being and Becoming Medical People. In G. Sarı (Ed.), *Handbook of Research on Representing Health and Medicine in Modern Media* (pp. 269-307). IGI Global. https://doi.org/10.4018/978-1-7998-6825-5.ch018

Gupta, A. (2021). Artificial Intelligence Approaches to Detect Neurodegenerative Disease From Medical Records: A Perspective. In Rani, G., & Tiwari, P. (Eds.), *Handbook of Research on Disease Prediction Through Data Analytics and Machine Learning* (pp. 254–267). IGI Global. https://doi.org/10.4018/978-1-7998-2742-9.ch013

Gürcü, M., & Tengilimoğlu, D. (2017). Health Tourism-Based Destination Marketing. In Bayraktar, A., & Uslay, C. (Eds.), *Strategic Place Branding Methodologies and Theory for Tourist Attraction* (pp. 308–331). Hershey, PA: IGI Global. DOI: 10.4018/978-1-5225-0579-2.ch015

Gürsel, G. (2017). For Better Healthcare Mining Health Data. In Bhattacharyya, S., De, S., Pan, I., & Dutta, P. (Eds.), *Intelligent Multidimensional Data Clustering and Analysis* (pp. 135–158). Hershey, PA: IGI Global. DOI: 10.4018/978-1-5225-1776-4.ch006

Gyaase, P. O., Darko-Lartey, R., William, H., & Borkloe, F. (2017). Towards an Integrated Electronic Medical Records System for Quality Healthcare in Ghana: An Exploratory Factor Analysis. *International Journal of Computers in Clinical Practice*, *2*(2), 38–55. DOI: 10.4018/IJCCP.2017070103

Hagle, H. N., Liu, Y., Murphy, D. M., & Krom, L. (2022). Innovative Adaptation of Training and Technical Assistance: Education for the Behavioral Health Workforce. In Ford, C., & Garza, K. (Eds.), *Handbook of Research on Updating and Innovating Health Professions Education: Post-Pandemic Perspectives* (pp. 239–264). IGI Global. https://doi.org/10.4018/978-1-7998-7623-6.ch011

Halis, M., & Halis, M. (2021). The Relationship Between Organizational Culture and Organizational Commitment: A Research in Private Health Institutions. In G. Sarı (Ed.), *Handbook of Research on Representing Health and Medicine in Modern Media* (pp. 308-329). IGI Global. https://doi.org/10.4018/978-1-7998-6825-5.ch019

Halis, M., Tepret, S., Çamlibel, Z., & Halis, M. (2021). Competitiveness in Medical Tourism: An Evaluation on Kocaeli Medical Tourism Market. In G. Sarı (Ed.), *Handbook of Research on Representing Health and Medicine in Modern Media* (pp. 239-268). IGI Global. https://doi.org/10.4018/978-1-7998-6825-5.ch017

Hanel, P. (2017). Is China Catching Up?: Health-Related Applications of Biotechnology. In Bas, T., & Zhao, J. (Eds.), *Comparative Approaches to Biotechnology Development and Use in Developed and Emerging Nations* (pp. 465–520). Hershey, PA: IGI Global. DOI: 10.4018/978-1-5225-1040-6.ch016

Hartman, A., & Brown, S. (2017). Synergism through Therapeutic Visual Arts. In Bryan, V., & Bird, J. (Eds.), *Healthcare Community Synergism between Patients, Practitioners, and Researchers* (pp. 29–48). Hershey, PA: IGI Global. DOI: 10.4018/978-1-5225-0640-9.ch002

Heck, A. J., Cross, C. E., & Tatum, V. Y. (2020). Early Medical Education Readiness Interventions: Enhancing Undergraduate Preparedness. In Gotian, R., Kang, Y., & Safdieh, J. (Eds.), *Handbook of Research on the Efficacy of Training Programs and Systems in Medical Education* (pp. 283–304). IGI Global. https://doi.org/10.4018/978-1-7998-1468-9.ch015

Hemant, B., Arasappa, R. G. I., Udupa, K., & Varambally, S. (2021). Yoga for Mental Health Disorders: Research and Practice. In Telles, S., & Gupta, R. (Eds.), *Handbook of Research on Evidence-Based Perspectives on the Psychophysiology of Yoga and Its Applications* (pp. 179–198). IGI Global. https://doi.org/10.4018/978-1-7998-3254-6.ch011

Herdeiro, M. T., Gouveia, N., & Roque, F. (2021). Clinical Research and Regulatory Affairs: Skills and Tools in Pharmacy Education. In Figueiredo, I., & Cavaco, A. (Eds.), *Pedagogies for Pharmacy Curricula* (pp. 160–184). IGI Global. https://doi.org/10.4018/978-1-7998-4486-0.ch008

Hosoda, M., & Hosoda, M. (2019). Supporting Patient-led Initiatives to Improve Healthcare: An Investigation of Cancer and ME/CFS Support Groups and Prefectural Medical Councils in Japan. *International Journal of Patient-Centered Healthcare*, *9*(2), 44–56. https://doi.org/10.4018/IJPCH.20190701.oa2

Iqbal, S., Ahmad, S., & Willis, I. (2017). Influencing Factors for Adopting Technology Enhanced Learning in the Medical Schools of Punjab, Pakistan. *International Journal of Information and Communication Technology Education*, *13*(3), 27–39. DOI: 10.4018/IJICTE.2017070103

Jagiello, K., Sosnowska, A., Mikolajczyk, A., & Puzyn, T. (2017). Nanomaterials in Medical Devices: Regulations' Review and Future Perspectives. *Journal of Nanotoxicology and Nanomedicine*, *2*(2), 1–11. DOI: 10.4018/JNN.2017070101

Jagtap, R., Phulare, K., Kurhade, M., & Gawande, K. S. (2021). Healthcare Conversational Chatbot for Medical Diagnosis. In Patil, B., & Vohra, M. (Eds.), *Handbook of Research on Engineering, Business, and Healthcare Applications of Data Science and Analytics* (pp. 401–415). IGI Global. https://doi.org/10.4018/978-1-7998-3053-5.ch020

Janosek, D. M. (2022). What Is the "Public Good" in a Pandemic? Who Decides?: Policy Makers and the Need for Leadership in Society's Perception of Medical Information. In Aker, H., & Aiken, M. (Eds.), *Handbook of Research on Cyberchondria, Health Literacy, and the Role of Media in Society's Perception of Medical Information* (pp. 1–15). IGI Global. https://doi.org/10.4018/978-1-7998-8630-3.ch001

Jena, T. K. (2018). Skill Training Process in Medicine Through Distance Mode. In Pandey, U., & Indrakanti, V. (Eds.), *Optimizing Open and Distance Learning in Higher Education Institutions* (pp. 228–243). Hershey, PA: IGI Global. DOI: 10.4018/978-1-5225-2624-7.ch010

Joseph, V., & Miller, J. M. (2018). Medical Students' Perceived Stigma in Seeking Care: A Cultural Perspective. In Smith, C. (Ed.), *Exploring the Pressures of Medical Education From a Mental Health and Wellness Perspective* (pp. 44–67). Hershey, PA: IGI Global. DOI: 10.4018/978-1-5225-2811-1.ch002

Joyce, B. L., & Swanberg, S. M. (2017). Using Backward Design for Competency-Based Undergraduate Medical Education. In Stefaniak, J. (Ed.), *Advancing Medical Education Through Strategic Instructional Design* (pp. 53–76). Hershey, PA: IGI Global. DOI: 10.4018/978-1-5225-2098-6.ch003

Kalder, M., & Kostev, K. (2021). Epidemiology of Gynaecological and Breast Cancers: Incidence, Survival, and Mental Health. In Dinas, K., Petousis, S., Kalder, M., & Mavromatidis, G. (Eds.), *Handbook of Research on Oncological and Endoscopical Dilemmas in Modern Gynecological Clinical Practice* (pp. 1–21). IGI Global. https://doi.org/10.4018/978-1-7998-4213-2.ch001

Kaljo, K., & Jacques, L. (2018). Flipping the Medical School Classroom. In M. Khosrow-Pour, D.B.A. (Ed.), *Encyclopedia of Information Science and Technology, Fourth Edition* (pp. 5800-5809). Hershey, PA: IGI Global. DOI: 10.4018/978-1-5225-2255-3.ch504

Karanfiloglu, M. (2021). The Role of Social Media Use in Health Communication: Digitized Health Communication During COVID-19 Pandemic. In G. Sarı (Eds.), *Handbook of Research on Representing Health and Medicine in Modern Media* (pp. 84-104). IGI Global. https://doi.org/10.4018/978-1-7998-6825-5.ch006

Karthikeyan, P., Vasuki, S., & Karthik, K. (2019). Non-Subsampled Contourlet Transform-Based Effective Denoising of Medical Images: Denoising of Medical Images Using Contourlet. In Swarnambiga, A. (Ed.), *Medical Image Processing for Improved Clinical Diagnosis* (pp. 155–183). IGI Global. https://doi.org/10.4018/978-1-5225-5876-7.ch008

Kashyap, R., & Rahamatkar, S. (2019). Medical Image Segmentation: An Advanced Approach. In Paul, S., Bhattacharya, P., & Bit, A. (Eds.), *Early Detection of Neurological Disorders Using Machine Learning Systems* (pp. 292–321). IGI Global. https://doi.org/10.4018/978-1-5225-8567-1.ch015

Kasina, H., Bahubalendruni, M. V., & Botcha, R. (2017). Robots in Medicine: Past, Present and Future. *International Journal of Manufacturing, Materials, and Mechanical Engineering*, 7(4), 44–64. DOI: 10.4018/IJMMME.2017100104

Katehakis, D. G. (2018). Electronic Medical Record Implementation Challenges for the National Health System in Greece. *International Journal of Reliable and Quality E-Healthcare*, 7(1), 16–30. DOI: 10.4018/IJRQEH.2018010102

Katehakis, D. G., & Kouroubali, A. (2022). Digital Transformation Challenges for the Development of Quality Electronic Medical Records in Greece. In Moumtzoglou, A. (Ed.), *Quality of Healthcare in the Aftermath of the COVID-19 Pandemic* (pp. 112–134). IGI Global. https://doi.org/10.4018/978-1-7998-9198-7.ch007

Kaur, P. D., & Sharma, P. (2017). Success Dimensions of ICTs in Healthcare. In Singh, B. (Ed.), *Computational Tools and Techniques for Biomedical Signal Processing* (pp. 149–173). Hershey, PA: IGI Global. DOI: 10.4018/978-1-5225-0660-7.ch007

Kaushik, P. (2018). Comorbidity of Medical and Psychiatric Disorders in Geriatric Population: Treatment and Care. In Prasad, B., & Akbar, S. (Eds.), *Handbook of Research on Geriatric Health, Treatment, and Care* (pp. 448–474). Hershey, PA: IGI Global. DOI: 10.4018/978-1-5225-3480-8.ch025

Khachane, M. Y. (2017). Organ-Based Medical Image Classification Using Support Vector Machine. *International Journal of Synthetic Emotions*, 8(1), 18–30. DOI: 10.4018/IJSE.2017010102

Kharbanda, V., Madaan, R., & Bhatia, K. K. (2021). Incautious Usage of Social Media: Impact on Emotional Intelligence and Health Concerns. In Yadav, D., Bansal, A., Bhatia, M., Hooda, M., & Morato, J. (Eds.), *Diagnostic Applications of Health Intelligence and Surveillance Systems* (pp. 172–186). IGI Global. https://doi.org/10.4018/978-1-7998-6527-8.ch008

Kirci, P. (2018). Intelligent Techniques for Analysis of Big Data About Healthcare and Medical Records. In Shah, N., & Mittal, M. (Eds.), *Handbook of Research on Promoting Business Process Improvement Through Inventory Control Techniques* (pp. 559–582). Hershey, PA: IGI Global. DOI: 10.4018/978-1-5225-3232-3.ch029

Kldiashvili, E. (2018). Cloud Approach for the Medical Information System: MIS on Cloud. In Khosrow-Pour, M. (Ed.), *Incorporating Nature-Inspired Paradigms in Computational Applications* (pp. 238–261). Hershey, PA: IGI Global. DOI: 10.4018/978-1-5225-5020-4.ch008

Ko, H., Mesicek, L., Choi, J., Choi, J., & Hwang, S. (2018). A Study on Secure Contents Strategies for Applications With DRM on Cloud Computing. *International Journal of Cloud Applications and Computing*, *8*(1), 143–153. DOI: 10.4018/IJCAC.2018010107

Komendziński, T., Mikołajewska, E., & Mikołajewski, D. (2018). Cross-Cultural Decision-Making in Healthcare: Theory and Practical Application in Real Clinical Conditions. In Rosiek-Kryszewska, A., & Leksowski, K. (Eds.), *Healthcare Administration for Patient Safety and Engagement* (pp. 276–298). Hershey, PA: IGI Global. DOI: 10.4018/978-1-5225-3946-9.ch015

Konecny, L. T. (2018). Medical School Wellness Initiatives. In Smith, C. (Ed.), *Exploring the Pressures of Medical Education From a Mental Health and Wellness Perspective* (pp. 209–228). Hershey, PA: IGI Global. DOI: 10.4018/978-1-5225-2811-1.ch009

Kromrei, H., Solomonson, W. L., & Juzych, M. S. (2017). Teaching Residents How to Teach. In Stefaniak, J. (Ed.), *Advancing Medical Education Through Strategic Instructional Design* (pp. 164–185). Hershey, PA: IGI Global. DOI: 10.4018/978-1-5225-2098-6.ch008

Kulkarni, S., Savyanavar, A., Kulkarni, P., Stranicri, A., & Ghorpade, V. (2018). Framework for Integration of Medical Image and Text-Based Report Retrieval to Support Radiological Diagnosis. In Kolekar, M., & Kumar, V. (Eds.), *Biomedical Signal and Image Processing in Patient Care* (pp. 86–122). Hershey, PA: IGI Global. DOI: 10.4018/978-1-5225-2829-6.ch006

Kumar, A., & Sarkar, B. K. (2018). Performance Analysis of Nature-Inspired Algorithms-Based Bayesian Prediction Models for Medical Data Sets. In Singh, U., Tiwari, A., & Singh, R. (Eds.), *Soft-Computing-Based Nonlinear Control Systems Design* (pp. 134–155). Hershey, PA: IGI Global. DOI: 10.4018/978-1-5225-3531-7.ch007

Labbadi, W., & Akaichi, J. (2017). Efficient Algorithm for Answering Fuzzy Medical Requests in Pervasive Healthcare Information Systems. *International Journal of Healthcare Information Systems and Informatics*, *12*(2), 46–64. DOI: 10.4018/IJHISI.2017040103

Lagumdzija, A., & Swing, V. K. (2017). Health, Digitalization, and Individual Empowerment. In Topor, F. (Ed.), *Handbook of Research on Individualism and Identity in the Globalized Digital Age* (pp. 380–402). Hershey, PA: IGI Global. DOI: 10.4018/978-1-5225-0522-8.ch017

Lamey, T. W., & Davidson-Shivers, G. V. (2017). Instructional Strategies and Sequencing. In Stefaniak, J. (Ed.), *Advancing Medical Education Through Strategic Instructional Design* (pp. 30–52). Hershey, PA: IGI Global. DOI: 10.4018/978-1-5225-2098-6.ch002

Lee, D. C., & Gefen, D. (2020). Promises and Challenges of Medical Patient Healthcare Portals in Underserved Communities: The Case of Einstein Medical Center Philadelphia (EMCP). In McHaney, R., Reychev, I., Azuri, J., McHaney, M., & Moshonov, R. (Eds.), *Impacts of Information Technology on Patient Care and Empowerment* (pp. 219–251). IGI Global. https://doi.org/10.4018/978-1-7998-0047-7.ch012

Leon, G. (2017). The Role of Forensic Medicine in Medical Errors. In Riga, M. (Ed.), *Impact of Medical Errors and Malpractice on Health Economics, Quality, and Patient Safety* (pp. 144–170). Hershey, PA: IGI Global. DOI: 10.4018/978-1-5225-2337-6.ch006

Leung, L. Y. (2020). Representation of Gender Equality From the Perspective of the Medical Trainee and its Ripple Effect: Highlighting Gender Inequality in Medical Student Experiences. In Bellini, M., & Papalois, V. (Eds.), *Gender Equity in the Medical Profession* (pp. 29–50). IGI Global. https://doi.org/10.4018/978-1-5225-9599-1.ch003

Lopes, M. J., Fonseca, C., & Barbosa, P. (2020). The Individual Care Plan as Electronic Health Record: A Tool for Management, Integration of Care, and Better Health Results. In Mendes, D., Fonseca, C., Lopes, M., García-Alonso, J., & Murillo, J. (Eds.), *Exploring the Role of ICTs in Healthy Aging* (pp. 1–12). IGI Global. https://doi.org/10.4018/978-1-7998-1937-0.ch001

Love, L., & McDowelle, D. (2018). Developing a Comprehensive Wellness Program for Medical Students. In Smith, C. (Ed.), *Exploring the Pressures of Medical Education From a Mental Health and Wellness Perspective* (pp. 190–208). Hershey, PA: IGI Global. DOI: 10.4018/978-1-5225-2811-1.ch008

Lovell, K. L. (2017). Development and Evaluation of Neuroscience Computer-Based Modules for Medical Students: Instructional Design Principles and Effectiveness. In Stefaniak, J. (Ed.), *Advancing Medical Education Through Strategic Instructional Design* (pp. 262–276). Hershey, PA: IGI Global. DOI: 10.4018/978-1-5225-2098-6.ch013

Lubin, R., & Hamlin, M. D. (2018). Medical Student Burnout: A Social Cognitive Learning Perspective on Medical Student Mental Health and Wellness. In Smith, C. (Ed.), *Exploring the Pressures of Medical Education From a Mental Health and Wellness Perspective* (pp. 92–121). Hershey, PA: IGI Global. DOI: 10.4018/978-1-5225-2811-1.ch004

Luk, C. Y. (2018). Moving Towards Universal Health Coverage: Challenges for the Present and Future in China. In Fong, B., Ng, A., & Yuen, P. (Eds.), *Sustainable Health and Long-Term Care Solutions for an Aging Population* (pp. 19–45). Hershey, PA: IGI Global. DOI: 10.4018/978-1-5225-2633-9.ch002

Mackintosh, S. E., & Katsaros, E. (2020). Building Interprofessional Competencies Into Medical Education and Assessment. In Waldman, S., & Bowlin, S. (Eds.), *Building a Patient-Centered Interprofessional Education Program* (pp. 84–112). IGI Global. https://doi.org/10.4018/978-1-7998-3066-5.ch005

Magalhães, J. L., Quoniam, L., Hartz, Z., Silveira, H., & Rito, P. D. (2022). Knowledge Management in Big Data Times for Global Health: Challenges for Quality in One Health. In Lima de Magalhães, J., Hartz, Z., Jamil, G., Silveira, H., & Jamil, L. (Eds.), *Handbook of Research on Essential Information Approaches to Aiding Global Health in the One Health Context* (pp. 149–163). IGI Global. https://doi.org/10.4018/978-1-7998-8011-0.ch008

Mahat, M., & Pettigrew, A. (2017). The Regulatory Environment of Non-Profit Higher Education and Research Institutions and Its Implications for Managerial Strategy: The Case of Medical Education and Research. In West, L., & Worthington, A. (Eds.), *Handbook of Research on Emerging Business Models and Managerial Strategies in the Nonprofit Sector* (pp. 336–351). Hershey, PA: IGI Global. DOI: 10.4018/978-1-5225-2537-0.ch017

Maitra, I. K., & Bandhyopadhyaay, S. K. (2017). Adaptive Edge Detection Method towards Features Extraction from Diverse Medical Imaging Technologies. In Bhattacharyya, S., De, S., Pan, I., & Dutta, P. (Eds.), *Intelligent Multidimensional Data Clustering and Analysis* (pp. 159–192). Hershey, PA: IGI Global. DOI: 10.4018/978-1-5225-1776-4.ch007

Mane, V. M., Patki, S., Dhumma, A. V., & Apte, K. J. (2022). Telehealth System for Effective Treatment in COVID-19 Pandemics. In Thakare, A., Wagh, S., Bhende, M., Anter, A., & Gao, X. (Eds.), *Handbook of Research on Applied Intelligence for Health and Clinical Informatics* (pp. 328–339). IGI Global. https://doi.org/10.4018/978-1-7998-7709-7.ch019

Mangu, V. P. (2017). Mobile Health Care: A Technology View. In Bhatt, C., & Peddoju, S. (Eds.), *Cloud Computing Systems and Applications in Healthcare* (pp. 1–18). Hershey, PA: IGI Global. DOI: 10.4018/978-1-5225-1002-4.ch001

Manirabona, A., Fourati, L. C., & Boudjit, S. (2017). Investigation on Healthcare Monitoring Systems: Innovative Services and Applications. *International Journal of E-Health and Medical Communications*, *8*(1), 1–18. DOI: 10.4018/IJEHMC.2017010101

Martins, C. L., Martinho, D., Marreiros, G., Conceição, L., Faria, L., & Simões de Almeida, R. (2022). Artificial Intelligence in Digital Mental Health. In Marques, A., & Queirós, R. (Eds.), *Digital Therapies in Psychosocial Rehabilitation and Mental Health* (pp. 201–225). IGI Global. https://doi.org/10.4018/978-1-7998-8634-1.ch010

Marwan, M., Kartit, A., & Ouahmane, H. (2018). A Framework to Secure Medical Image Storage in Cloud Computing Environment. *Journal of Electronic Commerce in Organizations*, *16*(1), 1–16. DOI: 10.4018/JECO.2018010101

Mason, A., Bhati, S., Jiang, R., & Spencer, E. A. (2020). Medical Tourism Patient Mortality: Considerations From a 10-Year Review of Global News Media Representations. In Merviö, M. (Ed.), *Global Issues and Innovative Solutions in Healthcare, Culture, and the Environment* (pp. 206–225). IGI Global. https://doi.org/10.4018/978-1-7998-3576-9.ch011

Masoud, M. P., Nejad, M. K., Darebaghi, H., Chavoshi, M., & Farahani, M. (2018). The Decision Support System and Conventional Method of Telephone Triage by Nurses in Emergency Medical Services: A Comparative Investigation. *International Journal of E-Business Research*, *14*(1), 77–88. DOI: 10.4018/IJEBR.2018010105

Mathew, N. E., Walter, A., & Eapen, V. (2020). Mental Health Challenges in Children With Intellectual Disabilities. In Gopalan, R. (Ed.), *Developmental Challenges and Societal Issues for Individuals With Intellectual Disabilities* (pp. 13–39). IGI Global. https://doi.org/10.4018/978-1-7998-1223-4.ch002

Mazzola, A. (2020). The Social Mandate to Deal With Mental Health: A Comparison Between Interventions in a Mental Health Center, a School, and a Psychoanalytic Office. In Padmanaban, S., & Subudhi, C. (Eds.), *Psycho-Social Perspectives on Mental Health and Well-Being* (pp. 234–254). IGI Global. https://doi.org/10.4018/978-1-7998-1185-5.ch012

McDonald, W. G., Martin, M., & Salzberg, L. D. (2018). From Medical Student to Medical Resident: Graduate Medical Education and Mental Health in the United States. In Smith, C. (Ed.), *Exploring the Pressures of Medical Education From a Mental Health and Wellness Perspective* (pp. 145–169). Hershey, PA: IGI Global. DOI: 10.4018/978-1-5225-2811-1.ch006

McGrowder, D. A., Miller, F. G., Nwokocha, C., Wilson-Clarke, C. F., Anderson, M., Anderson-Jackson, L., Williams, L., & Alexander-Lindo, R. (2021). Medical Herbs and the Treatment of Diabetes Mellitus: Mechanisms of Action. In Hussain, A., & Behl, S. (Eds.), *Treating Endocrine and Metabolic Disorders With Herbal Medicines* (pp. 48–73). IGI Global. https://doi.org/10.4018/978-1-7998-4808-0.ch003

Medhekar, A. (2017). The Role of Social Media for Knowledge Dissemination in Medical Tourism: A Case of India. In Chugh, R. (Ed.), *Harnessing Social Media as a Knowledge Management Tool* (pp. 25–54). Hershey, PA: IGI Global. DOI: 10.4018/978-1-5225-0495-5.ch002

Medhekar, A. (2020). Digital Health Innovation Enhancing Patient Experience in Medical Travel. In Sandhu, K. (Ed.), *Opportunities and Challenges in Digital Healthcare Innovation* (pp. 13–35). IGI Global. https://doi.org/10.4018/978-1-7998-3274-4.ch002

Medhekar, A., & Haq, F. (2018). Urbanization and New Jobs Creation in Healthcare Services in India: Challenges and Opportunities. In Benna, U., & Benna, I. (Eds.), *Urbanization and Its Impact on Socio-Economic Growth in Developing Regions* (pp. 198–218). Hershey, PA: IGI Global. DOI: 10.4018/978-1-5225-2659-9.ch010

Mehta, P. (2017). Framework of Indian Healthcare System and its Challenges: An Insight. In Bryan, V., & Bird, J. (Eds.), *Healthcare Community Synergism between Patients, Practitioners, and Researchers* (pp. 247–271). Hershey, PA: IGI Global. DOI: 10.4018/978-1-5225-0640-9.ch011

Mendes, E., Sousa, B. B., & Gonçalves, M. (2021). The Role of Technologies in Relationship Management and Internal Marketing: An Approach in the Health Sector. In J. Santos, & I. Pereira (Ed.), *Management and Marketing for Improved Competitiveness and Performance in the Healthcare Sector* (pp. 213-237). IGI Global. https://doi.org/10.4018/978-1-7998-7263-4.ch010

Meyer, T. M., & Simen, J. H. (2020). Geriatric Interprofessional Education: A Practical Guide for Health Professions Educators. In Waldman, S., & Bowlin, S. (Eds.), *Building a Patient-Centered Interprofessional Education Program* (pp. 120–136). IGI Global. https://doi.org/10.4018/978-1-7998-3066-5.ch007

Mi, M. (2017). Informal Learning in Medical Education. In Stefaniak, J. (Ed.), *Advancing Medical Education Through Strategic Instructional Design* (pp. 225–244). Hershey, PA: IGI Global. DOI: 10.4018/978-1-5225-2098-6.ch011

Mishra, K., & Thomas, R. (2022). Low Cost, User-Controlled Peroneal Stimulator for Foot Drop in Patients With Stroke: An Experiment in Indian Rehabilitation Set-Up. In Stasolla, F. (Ed.), *Assistive Technologies for Assessment and Recovery of Neurological Impairments* (pp. 279–303). IGI Global. https://doi.org/10.4018/978-1-7998-7430-0.ch014

Mishra, S., & Panda, M. (2019). Artificial Intelligence in Medical Science. In Bouchemal, N. (Ed.), *Intelligent Systems for Healthcare Management and Delivery* (pp. 306–330). IGI Global. https://doi.org/10.4018/978-1-5225-7071-4.ch014

Mosadeghrad, A. M., & Woldemichael, A. (2017). Application of Quality Management in Promoting Patient Safety and Preventing Medical Errors. In Riga, M. (Ed.), *Impact of Medical Errors and Malpractice on Health Economics, Quality, and Patient Safety* (pp. 91–112). Hershey, PA: IGI Global. DOI: 10.4018/978-1-5225-2337-6.ch004

Moumtzoglou, A. (2017). Digital Medicine: The Quality Standpoint. In Moumtzoglou, A. (Ed.), *Design, Development, and Integration of Reliable Electronic Healthcare Platforms* (pp. 179–195). Hershey, PA: IGI Global. DOI: 10.4018/978-1-5225-1724-5.ch011

Moumtzoglou, A., & Pouliakis, A. (2018). Population Health Management and the Science of Individuality. *International Journal of Reliable and Quality E-Healthcare*, 7(2), 1–26. DOI: 10.4018/IJRQEH.2018040101

Mukhtar, W. F., & Abuelyaman, E. S. (2017). Opportunities and Challenges of Big Data in Healthcare. In Wickramasinghe, N. (Ed.), *Handbook of Research on Healthcare Administration and Management* (pp. 47–58). Hershey, PA: IGI Global. DOI: 10.4018/978-1-5225-0920-2.ch004

Munugala, S., Brar, G. K., Syed, A., Mohammad, A., & Halgamuge, M. N. (2018). The Much Needed Security and Data Reforms of Cloud Computing in Medical Data Storage. In Lytras, M., & Papadopoulou, P. (Eds.), *Applying Big Data Analytics in Bioinformatics and Medicine* (pp. 99–113). Hershey, PA: IGI Global. DOI: 10.4018/978-1-5225-2607-0.ch005

Naha, N., & Manickavachagam, G. (2021). Textile Industry and Health Hazards: Impact of Climate Change Issues and Fertility Potential. In K. Wani, & N. Naha (Ed.), *Climate Change and Its Impact on Fertility* (pp. 42-69). IGI Global. https://doi.org/10.4018/978-1-7998-4480-8.ch003

Nair, L. D. (2019). Childhood Neurodegenerative Disorders. In Uddin, M., & Amran, M. (Eds.), *Handbook of Research on Critical Examinations of Neurodegenerative Disorders* (pp. 385–412). IGI Global. https://doi.org/10.4018/978-1-5225-5282-6.ch018

Nayak, S. R., & Mishra, J. (2019). Analysis of Medical Images Using Fractal Geometry. In Dey, N., Ashour, A., Kalia, H., Goswami, R., & Das, H. (Eds.), *Histopathological Image Analysis in Medical Decision Making* (pp. 181–201). IGI Global. https://doi.org/10.4018/978-1-5225-6316-7.ch008

Netto, J. T., Hartz, Z., & de Magalhães, J. L. (2022). One Health and Information Management Using Big Data in Health: A Brazilian Case Study for COVID-19. In Lima de Magalhães, J., Hartz, Z., Jamil, G., Silveira, H., & Jamil, L. (Eds.), *Handbook of Research on Essential Information Approaches to Aiding Global Health in the One Health Context* (pp. 36–51). IGI Global. https://doi.org/10.4018/978-1-7998-8011-0.ch003

Ngara, R. (2017). Multiple Voices, Multiple Paths: Towards Dialogue between Western and Indigenous Medical Knowledge Systems. In Ngulube, P. (Ed.), *Handbook of Research on Theoretical Perspectives on Indigenous Knowledge Systems in Developing Countries* (pp. 332–358). Hershey, PA: IGI Global. DOI: 10.4018/978-1-5225-0833-5.ch015

Nikumbh, D. D., Sayyad, S., Joshi, R. R., Dubey, K. S., Mehta, D. V., & Matta, D. K. (2022). Applied Intelligence for Medical Diagnosing. In Thakare, A., Wagh, S., Bhende, M., Anter, A., & Gao, X. (Eds.), *Handbook of Research on Applied Intelligence for Health and Clinical Informatics* (pp. 44–79). IGI Global. https://doi.org/10.4018/978-1-7998-7709-7.ch004

O'Connor, Y., & Heavin, C. (2018). Defining and Characterising the Landscape of eHealth. In M. Khosrow-Pour, D.B.A. (Ed.), *Encyclopedia of Information Science and Technology, Fourth Edition* (pp. 5864-5875). Hershey, PA: IGI Global. DOI: 10.4018/978-1-5225-2255-3.ch510

Ochonogor, W. C., & Okite-Amughoro, F. A. (2018). Building an Effective Digital Library in a University Teaching Hospital (UTH) in Nigeria. In Tella, A., & Kwanya, T. (Eds.), *Handbook of Research on Managing Intellectual Property in Digital Libraries* (pp. 184–204). Hershey, PA: IGI Global. DOI: 10.4018/978-1-5225-3093-0.ch010

Olivares, S. L., Cruz, A. G., Cabrera, M. V., Regalado, A. I., & García, J. E. (2017). An Assessment Study of Quality Model for Medical Schools in Mexico. In Mukerji, S., & Tripathi, P. (Eds.), *Handbook of Research on Administration, Policy, and Leadership in Higher Education* (pp. 404–439). Hershey, PA: IGI Global. DOI: 10.4018/978-1-5225-0672-0.ch016

Omoruyi, E. A., & Omidele, F. (2018). Resident Physician and Medical Academic Faculty Burnout: A Review of Current Literature. In Smith, C. (Ed.), *Exploring the Pressures of Medical Education From a Mental Health and Wellness Perspective* (pp. 171–189). Hershey, PA: IGI Global. DOI: 10.4018/978-1-5225-2811-1.ch007

Pandey, A., Singh, B., Saini, B. S., & Sood, N. (2019). Medical Data Security Tools and Techniques in E-Health Applications. In Singh, B., Saini, B., Singh, D., & Pandey, A. (Eds.), *Medical Data Security for Bioengineers* (pp. 124–131). IGI Global. https://doi.org/10.4018/978-1-5225-7952-6.ch006

Papadopoulou, P., Lytras, M., & Marouli, C. (2018). Bioinformatics as Applied to Medicine: Challenges Faced Moving from Big Data to Smart Data to Wise Data. In Lytras, M., & Papadopoulou, P. (Eds.), *Applying Big Data Analytics in Bioinformatics and Medicine* (pp. 1–25). Hershey, PA: IGI Global. DOI: 10.4018/978-1-5225-2607-0.ch001

Paraskou, A., & George, B. P. (2018). An Overview of Reproductive Tourism. In *Legal and Economic Considerations Surrounding Reproductive Tourism: Emerging Research and Opportunities* (pp. 1–17). Hershey, PA: IGI Global. DOI: 10.4018/978-1-5225-2694-0.ch001

Pereira, S., Silva, L., Machado, J., & Cabral, A. (2020). The Clinical Informatization in Portugal: An Approach to the National Health Service Certification. *International Journal of Reliable and Quality E-Healthcare*, *9*(2), 34–47. https://doi.org/10.4018/IJRQEH.2020040103

Phuritsabam, B., & Devi, A. B. (2017). Information Seeking Behavior of Medical Scientists at Jawaharlal Nehru Institute of Medical Science: A Study. In Ram, S. (Ed.), *Library and Information Services for Bioinformatics Education and Research* (pp. 177–187). Hershey, PA: IGI Global. DOI: 10.4018/978-1-5225-1871-6.ch010

Pieczka, B. (2018). Management of Risk and Adverse Events in Medical Entities. In Rosiek-Kryszewska, A., & Leksowski, K. (Eds.), *Healthcare Administration for Patient Safety and Engagement* (pp. 31–46). Hershey, PA: IGI Global. DOI: 10.4018/978-1-5225-3946-9.ch003

Poduval, J. (2017). Medical Errors: Impact on Health Care Quality. In Riga, M. (Ed.), *Impact of Medical Errors and Malpractice on Health Economics, Quality, and Patient Safety* (pp. 33–60). Hershey, PA: IGI Global. DOI: 10.4018/978-1-5225-2337-6.ch002

Politis, D., Stagiopoulos, P., Aidona, S., Kyriafinis, G., & Constantinidis, I. (2018). Autonomous Learning and Skill Accreditation: A Paradigm for Medical Studies. In Kumar, A. (Ed.), *Optimizing Student Engagement in Online Learning Environments* (pp. 266–296). Hershey, PA: IGI Global. DOI: 10.4018/978-1-5225-3634-5.ch012

Pomares-Quimbaya, A., González, R. A., Sierra, A., Daza, J. C., Muñoz, O., García, A., & Bohórquez, W. R. (2017). ICT for Enabling the Quality Evaluation of Health Care Services: A Case Study in a General Hospital. In Moumtzoglou, A. (Ed.), *Design, Development, and Integration of Reliable Electronic Healthcare Platforms* (pp. 196–210). Hershey, PA: IGI Global. DOI: 10.4018/978-1-5225-1724-5.ch012

Ponnuswamy, P., Paul, A. S., & Jose, A. B. (2021). Pre-, Peri-, and Post-Natal Risk Factors in ADHD. In Gopalan, R. (Ed.), *New Developments in Diagnosing, Assessing, and Treating ADHD* (pp. 43–54). IGI Global. https://doi.org/10.4018/978-1-7998-5495-1.ch003

Pouliakis, A., Margari, N., Karakitsou, E., Archondakis, S., & Karakitsos, P. (2018). Emerging Technologies Serving Cytopathology: Big Data, the Cloud, and Mobile Computing. In El Naqa, I. (Ed.), *Emerging Developments and Practices in Oncology* (pp. 114–152). Hershey, PA: IGI Global. DOI: 10.4018/978-1-5225-3085-5.ch005

Praveenkumar, P., Santhiyadevi, R., & Amirtharajan, R. (2019). Medical Data Are Safe: An Encrypted Quantum Approach. In Singh, B., Saini, B., Singh, D., & Pandey, A. (Eds.), *Medical Data Security for Bioengineers* (pp. 142–165). IGI Global. https://doi.org/10.4018/978-1-5225-7952-6.ch008

Punhani, R., Saini, S., Varun, N., & Rustagi, R. (2021). mHealth: A Resolution in Improving Global Health. In D. Yadav, A. Bansal, M. Bhatia, M. Hooda, & J. Morato (Ed.), *Diagnostic Applications of Health Intelligence and Surveillance Systems* (pp. 86-105). IGI Global. https://doi.org/10.4018/978-1-7998-6527-8.ch004

Quintela, A., & Veiga, A. (2022). An Integrated Approach (Social and Health) in the Elderly With Diabetes: An Increase in Health Literacy. In Vaz de Almeida, C., & Ramos, S. (Eds.), *Handbook of Research on Assertiveness, Clarity, and Positivity in Health Literacy* (pp. 134–142). IGI Global. https://doi.org/10.4018/978-1-7998-8824-6.ch008

Rai, A., Kothari, R., & Singh, D. P. (2017). Assessment of Available Technologies for Hospital Waste Management: A Need for Society. In Singh, R., Singh, A., & Srivastava, V. (Eds.), *Environmental Issues Surrounding Human Overpopulation* (pp. 172–188). Hershey, PA: IGI Global. DOI: 10.4018/978-1-5225-1683-5.ch010

Rajagopalan, S., Janakiraman, S., & Rengarajan, A. (2019). Medical Image Encryption: Microcontroller and FPGA Perspective. In Singh, B., Saini, B., Singh, D., & Pandey, A. (Eds.), *Medical Data Security for Bioengineers* (pp. 278–304). IGI Global. https://doi.org/10.4018/978-1-5225-7952-6.ch014

Ramamoorthy, S., & Sivasubramaniam, R. (2018). Image Processing Including Medical Liver Imaging: Medical Image Processing from Big Data Perspective, Ultrasound Liver Images, Challenges. In Lytras, M., & Papadopoulou, P. (Eds.), *Applying Big Data Analytics in Bioinformatics and Medicine* (pp. 380–392). Hershey, PA: IGI Global. DOI: 10.4018/978-1-5225-2607-0.ch016

Rathor, G. P., & Gupta, S. K. (2017). Improving Multimodality Image Fusion through Integrate AFL and Wavelet Transform. In Tiwari, V., Tiwari, B., Thakur, R., & Gupta, S. (Eds.), *Pattern and Data Analysis in Healthcare Settings* (pp. 143–157). Hershey, PA: IGI Global. DOI: 10.4018/978-1-5225-0536-5.ch008

Rexhepi, H., & Persson, A. (2017). Challenges to Implementing IT Support for Evidence Based Practice Among Nurses and Assistant Nurses: A Qualitative Study. *Journal of Electronic Commerce in Organizations*, *15*(2), 61–76. DOI: 10.4018/JECO.2017040105

Ribeiro, A. D., Ribeiro, L. P., Silva, C. A., & Magalhães-Ribeiro, L. P. (2021). Patient Safety: The Patient's Perspective From Public Sector Health Institutions in the Algarve Region, Portugal. In Eklund, P. (Ed.), *Integrated Care and Fall Prevention in Active and Healthy Aging* (pp. 200–222). IGI Global. https://doi.org/10.4018/978-1-7998-4411-2.ch011

Rodrigues, H., & Brochado, A. (2021). Going for Silver-Senior Consumers' Reviews of Medical Tourism. In Borges, A., & Rodrigues, P. (Eds.), *New Techniques for Brand Management in the Healthcare Sector* (pp. 64–83). IGI Global. https://doi.org/10.4018/978-1-7998-3034-4.ch005

Rodrigues, J. M., Oliveira, F., Ribeiro, C. P., & Santos, R. C. (2022). Mobile Mental Health for Depression Assistance: Research Directions, Obstacles, Advantages, and Disadvantages of Implementing mHealth. In Marques, A., & Queirós, R. (Eds.), *Digital Therapies in Psychosocial Rehabilitation and Mental Health* (pp. 21–40). IGI Global. https://doi.org/10.4018/978-1-7998-8634-1.ch002

Ros, M., Weaver, L., & Neuwirth, L. S. (2020). Virtual Reality Stereoscopic 180-Degree Video-Based Immersive Environments: Applications for Training Surgeons and Other Medical Professionals. In Stefaniak, J. (Ed.), *Cases on Instructional Design and Performance Outcomes in Medical Education* (pp. 92–119). IGI Global. https://doi.org/10.4018/978-1-7998-5092-2.ch005

Rosiek, A. (2018). The Assessment of Actions of the Environment and the Impact of Preventive Medicine for Public Health in Poland. In Rosiek-Kryszewska, A., & Leksowski, K. (Eds.), *Healthcare Administration for Patient Safety and Engagement* (pp. 106–119). Hershey, PA: IGI Global. DOI: 10.4018/978-1-5225-3946-9.ch006

Rosiek, A., & Rosiek-Kryszewska, A. (2018). Managed Healthcare: Doctor Life Satisfaction and Its Impact on the Process of Communicating With the Patient. In Rosiek-Kryszewska, A., & Leksowski, K. (Eds.), *Healthcare Administration for Patient Safety and Engagement* (pp. 244–261). Hershey, PA: IGI Global. DOI: 10.4018/978-1-5225-3946-9.ch013

Rosiek-Kryszewska, A., & Rosiek, A. (2018). The Involvement of the Patient and his Perspective Evaluation of the Quality of Healthcare. In Rosiek-Kryszewska, A., & Leksowski, K. (Eds.), *Healthcare Administration for Patient Safety and Engagement* (pp. 121–144). Hershey, PA: IGI Global. DOI: 10.4018/978-1-5225-3946-9.ch007

Rosiek-Kryszewska, A., & Rosiek, A. (2018). The Impact of Management and Leadership Roles in Building Competitive Healthcare Units. In Rosiek-Kryszewska, A., & Leksowski, K. (Eds.), *Healthcare Administration for Patient Safety and Engagement* (pp. 13–30). Hershey, PA: IGI Global. DOI: 10.4018/978-1-5225-3946-9.ch002

Rouzbehani, K. (2017). Health Policy Implementation: Moving Beyond Its Barriers in United States. In Wickramasinghe, N. (Ed.), *Handbook of Research on Healthcare Administration and Management* (pp. 541–552). Hershey, PA: IGI Global. DOI: 10.4018/978-1-5225-0920-2.ch032

Sajjad, N., Hassan, S., Qadir, J., Ali, R., & Shah, D. (2020). Analyses of the Recycling Potential of Medical Plastic Wastes. In Wani, K., Ariana, L., & Zuber, S. (Eds.), *Handbook of Research on Environmental and Human Health Impacts of Plastic Pollution* (pp. 178–199). IGI Global. https://doi.org/10.4018/978-1-5225-9452-9.ch010

Sam, S. (2017). Mobile Phones and Expanding Human Capabilities in Plural Health Systems. In Moahi, K., Bwalya, K., & Sebina, P. (Eds.), *Health Information Systems and the Advancement of Medical Practice in Developing Countries* (pp. 93–114). Hershey, PA: IGI Global. DOI: 10.4018/978-1-5225-2262-1.ch006

Santos-Trigo, M., Suaste, E., & Figuerola, P. (2018). Technology Design and Routes for Tool Appropriation in Medical Practices. In M. Khosrow-Pour, D.B.A. (Ed.), *Encyclopedia of Information Science and Technology, Fourth Edition* (pp. 3794-3804). Hershey, PA: IGI Global. DOI: 10.4018/978-1-5225-2255-3.ch329

Sarivougioukas, J., Vagelatos, A., Parsopoulos, K. E., & Lagaris, I. E. (2018). Home UbiHealth. In M. Khosrow-Pour, D.B.A. (Ed.), *Encyclopedia of Information Science and Technology, Fourth Edition* (pp. 7765-7774). Hershey, PA: IGI Global. DOI: 10.4018/978-1-5225-2255-3.ch675

Sarkar, B. K. (2017). Big Data and Healthcare Data: A Survey. *International Journal of Knowledge-Based Organizations, 7*(4), 50–77. DOI: 10.4018/IJKBO.2017100104

Sarkar, K., & Li, B. (2021). Deep Learning for Medical Image Segmentation. In Saxena, S., & Paul, S. (Eds.), *Deep Learning Applications in Medical Imaging* (pp. 40–77). IGI Global. https://doi.org/10.4018/978-1-7998-5071-7.ch002

Savani, M. M. (2021). Commitment Devices for Health: Theory and Evidence on Weight Loss. In Mihaila, V. (Ed.), *Behavioral-Based Interventions for Improving Public Policies* (pp. 35–54). IGI Global. https://doi.org/10.4018/978-1-7998-2731-3.ch003

Saxena, K., & Banodha, U. (2017). An Essence of the SOA on Healthcare. In Bhadoria, R., Chaudhari, N., Tomar, G., & Singh, S. (Eds.), *Exploring Enterprise Service Bus in the Service-Oriented Architecture Paradigm* (pp. 283–304). Hershey, PA: IGI Global. DOI: 10.4018/978-1-5225-2157-0.ch018

Saxena, N. (2020). Considerations for Stakeholders of Medical Tourism: A Comprehensive Examination. In Paul, S., & Kulshreshtha, S. (Eds.), *Global Developments in Healthcare and Medical Tourism* (pp. 23–37). IGI Global. https://doi.org/10.4018/978-1-5225-9787-2.ch002

Segura-Azuara, N. D., Guzman-Segura, J. G., Guzmán-Segura, N. M., & Guzmán-Segura, J. P. (2022). Disease Awareness Campaigns: Education for Citizenship in Medical Schools. In Lopez, M. (Ed.), *Advancing Health Education With Telemedicine* (pp. 113–122). IGI Global. https://doi.org/10.4018/978-1-7998-8783-6.ch006

Sekaran, P. A. (2022). Smart Medical Kit in Chronic Kidney Disease Management. In Jeya Mala, D. (Ed.), *Integrating AI in IoT Analytics on the Cloud for Healthcare Applications* (pp. 24–40). IGI Global. https://doi.org/10.4018/978-1-7998-9132-1.ch002

Sen, K., & Ghosh, K. (2018). Incorporating Global Medical Knowledge to Solve Healthcare Problems: A Framework for a Crowdsourcing System. *International Journal of Healthcare Information Systems and Informatics*, *13*(1), 1–14. DOI: 10.4018/IJHISI.2018010101

Senanayake, B., Tyagi, N., Zhou, X., & Edirippulige, S. (2020). Workforce Readiness and Digital Health Integration. In Sandhu, K. (Ed.), *Opportunities and Challenges in Digital Healthcare Innovation* (pp. 170–185). IGI Global. https://doi.org/10.4018/978-1-7998-3274-4.ch010

Shakdher, A., & Pandey, K. (2017). REDAlert+: Medical/Fire Emergency and Warning System using Android Devices. *International Journal of E-Health and Medical Communications*, *8*(1), 37–51. DOI: 10.4018/IJEHMC.2017010103

Shekarian, E., Abdul-Rashid, S. H., & Olugu, E. U. (2017). An Integrated Fuzzy VIKOR Method for Performance Management in Healthcare. In Tavana, M., Szabat, K., & Puranam, K. (Eds.), *Organizational Productivity and Performance Measurements Using Predictive Modeling and Analytics* (pp. 40–61). Hershey, PA: IGI Global. DOI: 10.4018/978-1-5225-0654-6.ch003

Shijina, V., & John, S. J. (2017). Multiple Relations and its Application in Medical Diagnosis. *International Journal of Fuzzy System Applications*, *6*(4), 47–62. DOI: 10.4018/IJFSA.2017100104

Shipley, N., & Chakraborty, J. (2018). Big Data and mHealth: Increasing the Usability of Healthcare Through the Customization of Pinterest – Literary Perspective. In Machado, J., Abelha, A., Santos, M., & Portela, F. (Eds.), *Next-Generation Mobile and Pervasive Healthcare Solutions* (pp. 46–66). Hershey, PA: IGI Global. DOI: 10.4018/978-1-5225-2851-7.ch004

Shridevi, S., & Saleena, B. (2019). Semantic Technologies for Medical Knowledge Representation. In Puratchikody, A., Prabu, S., & Umamaheswari, A. (Eds.), *Computer Applications in Drug Discovery and Development* (Vol. 5, pp. 260–275). IGI Global. https://doi.org/10.4018/978-1-5225-7326-5.ch012

Simões de Almeida, R. (2022). Mobile Mental Health: Opportunities and Challenges. In Marques, A., & Queirós, R. (Eds.), *Digital Therapies in Psychosocial Rehabilitation and Mental Health* (pp. 1–20). IGI Global. https://doi.org/10.4018/978-1-7998-8634-1.ch001

Simões de Almeida, R., & da Silva, T. P. (2022). AI Chatbots in Mental Health: Are We There Yet? In Marques, A., & Queirós, R. (Eds.), *Digital Therapies in Psychosocial Rehabilitation and Mental Health* (pp. 226–243). IGI Global. https://doi.org/10.4018/978-1-7998-8634-1.ch011

Singh, A., & Dutta, M. K. (2017). A Reversible Data Hiding Scheme for Efficient Management of Tele-Ophthalmological Data. *International Journal of E-Health and Medical Communications, 8*(3), 38–54. DOI: 10.4018/IJEHMC.2017070103

Skourti, P. K., & Pavlakis, A. (2017). The Second Victim Phenomenon: The Way Out. In Riga, M. (Ed.), *Impact of Medical Errors and Malpractice on Health Economics, Quality, and Patient Safety* (pp. 197–222). Hershey, PA: IGI Global. DOI: 10.4018/978-1-5225-2337-6.ch008

Smith, C. R. (2018). Medical Students' Quest Towards the Long White Coat: Impact on Mental Health and Well-Being. In Smith, C. (Ed.), *Exploring the Pressures of Medical Education From a Mental Health and Wellness Perspective* (pp. 1–42). Hershey, PA: IGI Global. DOI: 10.4018/978-1-5225-2811-1.ch001

Smith, S. I., & Dandignac, M. (2018). Perfectionism: Addressing Lofty Expectations in Medical School. In Smith, C. (Ed.), *Exploring the Pressures of Medical Education From a Mental Health and Wellness Perspective* (pp. 68–91). Hershey, PA: IGI Global. DOI: 10.4018/978-1-5225-2811-1.ch003

Soczywko, J., & Rutkowska, D. (2018). The Patient/Provider Relationship in Emergency Medicine: Organization, Communication, and Understanding. In Rosiek-Kryszewska, A., & Leksowski, K. (Eds.), *Healthcare Administration for Patient Safety and Engagement* (pp. 74–105). Hershey, PA: IGI Global. DOI: 10.4018/978-1-5225-3946-9.ch005

Soni, P. (2018). Implications of HIPAA and Subsequent Regulations on Information Technology. In Gupta, M., Sharman, R., Walp, J., & Mulgund, P. (Eds.), *Information Technology Risk Management and Compliance in Modern Organizations* (pp. 71–98). Hershey, PA: IGI Global. DOI: 10.4018/978-1-5225-2604-9.ch004

Souza, T. de V. I. E. (2020). Certifications for Medical Interpreters: A Comparative Analysis. In I. Souza, & E. Fragkou (Eds.), *Handbook of Research on Medical Interpreting* (pp. 26-53). IGI Global. https://doi.org/10.4018/978-1-5225-9308-9.ch002

Srivastava, A., & Aggarwal, A. K. (2018). Medical Image Fusion in Spatial and Transform Domain: A Comparative Analysis. In Anwar, M., Khosla, A., & Kapoor, R. (Eds.), *Handbook of Research on Advanced Concepts in Real-Time Image and Video Processing* (pp. 281–300). Hershey, PA: IGI Global. DOI: 10.4018/978-1-5225-2848-7.ch011

Srivastava, S. K., & Roy, S. N. (2018). Recommendation System: A Potential Tool for Achieving Pervasive Health Care. In Machado, J., Abelha, A., Santos, M., & Portela, F. (Eds.), *Next-Generation Mobile and Pervasive Healthcare Solutions* (pp. 111–127). Hershey, PA: IGI Global. DOI: 10.4018/978-1-5225-2851-7.ch008

Stanimirovic, D. (2017). Digitalization of Death Certification Model: Transformation Issues and Implementation Concerns. In Saeed, S., Bamarouf, Y., Ramayah, T., & Iqbal, S. (Eds.), *Design Solutions for User-Centric Information Systems* (pp. 22–43). Hershey, PA: IGI Global. DOI: 10.4018/978-1-5225-1944-7.ch002

Subbaraman, K., Singh, M., & Johar, I. P. (2021). Medical Tourism: History, Global Scenario, and Indian Perspectives. In Singh, M., & Kumaran, S. (Eds.), *Growth of the Medical Tourism Industry and Its Impact on Society: Emerging Research and Opportunities* (pp. 1–18). IGI Global. https://doi.org/10.4018/978-1-7998-3427-4.ch001

Sukkird, V., & Shirahada, K. (2018). E-Health Service Model for Asian Developing Countries: A Case of Emergency Medical Service for Elderly People in Thailand. In Khosrow-Pour, M. (Ed.), *Optimizing Current Practices in E-Services and Mobile Applications* (pp. 214–232). Hershey, PA: IGI Global. DOI: 10.4018/978-1-5225-5026-6.ch011

Talbot, T. B. (2017). Making Lifelike Medical Games in the Age of Virtual Reality: An Update on "Playing Games with Biology" from 2013. In Dubbels, B. (Ed.), *Transforming Gaming and Computer Simulation Technologies across Industries* (pp. 103–119). Hershey, PA: IGI Global. DOI: 10.4018/978-1-5225-1817-4.ch006

Tarver, E. (2022). Virtual Simulation: A Flipped Classroom Teaching Tool for Healthcare Education. In Coelho, L., Queirós, R., & Reis, S. (Eds.), *Emerging Advancements for Virtual and Augmented Reality in Healthcare* (pp. 65–81). IGI Global. https://doi.org/10.4018/978-1-7998-8371-5.ch005

Tripathi, S., & Musiolik, T. H. (2022). Fairness and Ethics in Artificial Intelligence-Based Medical Imaging. In Musiolik, T., & Dingli, A. (Eds.), *Ethical Implications of Reshaping Healthcare With Emerging Technologies* (pp. 71–85). IGI Global. https://doi.org/10.4018/978-1-7998-7888-9.ch004

Turcu, C. E., & Turcu, C. O. (2017). Social Internet of Things in Healthcare: From Things to Social Things in Internet of Things. In Reis, C., & Maximiano, M. (Eds.), *Internet of Things and Advanced Application in Healthcare* (pp. 266–295). Hershey, PA: IGI Global. DOI: 10.4018/978-1-5225-1820-4.ch010

Tutgun Ünal, A., Ekinci, Y., & Tarhan, N. (2022). Health Literacy and Cyberchondria. In Aker, H., & Aiken, M. (Eds.), *Handbook of Research on Cyberchondria, Health Literacy, and the Role of Media in Society's Perception of Medical Information* (pp. 276–297). IGI Global. https://doi.org/10.4018/978-1-7998-8630-3.ch015

Unwin, D. W., Sanzogni, L., & Sandhu, K. (2017). Developing and Measuring the Business Case for Health Information Technology. In Moahi, K., Bwalya, K., & Sebina, P. (Eds.), *Health Information Systems and the Advancement of Medical Practice in Developing Countries* (pp. 262–290). Hershey, PA: IGI Global. DOI: 10.4018/978-1-5225-2262-1.ch015

Ustun, A. B., Yilmaz, R., & Yilmaz, F. G. (2020). Virtual Reality in Medical Education. In Umair, S. (Ed.), *Mobile Devices and Smart Gadgets in Medical Sciences* (pp. 56–73). IGI Global. https://doi.org/10.4018/978-1-7998-2521-0.ch004

Vamsi, D., & Reddy, P. (2020). Electronic Health Record Security in Cloud: Medical Data Protection Using Homomorphic Encryption Schemes. In Chakraborty, C. (Ed.), *Smart Medical Data Sensing and IoT Systems Design in Healthcare* (pp. 22–47). IGI Global. https://doi.org/10.4018/978-1-7998-0261-7.ch002

Vartholomaios, P., Ramdani, N., Christophorou, C., Georgiadis, D., Guilcher, T., Blouin, M., Rebiai, M., Panayides, A. S., Pattichis, C. S., Sarafidis, M., Costarides, V., Vellidou, E., & Koutsouris, D. (2019). ENDORSE Concept: An Integrated Indoor Mobile Robotic System for Medical Diagnostic Support. *International Journal of Reliable and Quality E-Healthcare*, *8*(3), 47–59. https://doi.org/10.4018/IJRQEH.2019070104

Vasant, P. (2018). A General Medical Diagnosis System Formed by Artificial Neural Networks and Swarm Intelligence Techniques. In Kose, U., Guraksin, G., & Deperlioglu, O. (Eds.), *Nature-Inspired Intelligent Techniques for Solving Biomedical Engineering Problems* (pp. 130–145). Hershey, PA: IGI Global. DOI: 10.4018/978-1-5225-4769-3.ch006

Vaz de Almeida, C. (2022). ACP Model-Assertiveness, Clarity, and Positivity: A Communication and Health Literacy Model for Health Professionals. In Vaz de Almeida, C., & Ramos, S. (Eds.), *Handbook of Research on Assertiveness, Clarity, and Positivity in Health Literacy* (pp. 1–22). IGI Global. https://doi.org/10.4018/978-1-7998-8824-6.ch001

Verma, K. (2022). Modeling Digital Healthcare Services Using NLP and IoT in Smart Cities. In Thomas, J., Geropanta, V., Karagianni, A., Panchenko, V., & Vasant, P. (Eds.), *Smart Cities and Machine Learning in Urban Health* (pp. 138–155). IGI Global. https://doi.org/10.4018/978-1-7998-7176-7.ch007

Viswanathan, J., Saranya, N., & Inbamani, A. (2021). Deep Learning Applications in Medical Imaging: Introduction to Deep Learning-Based Intelligent Systems for Medical Applications. In Saxena, S., & Paul, S. (Eds.), *Deep Learning Applications in Medical Imaging* (pp. 156–177). IGI Global. https://doi.org/10.4018/978-1-7998-5071-7.ch007

Wang, X., Su, K., & Su, L. (2019). Research on Improved Apriori Algorithm Based on Data Mining in Electronic Cases. *International Journal of Healthcare Information Systems and Informatics, 14*(3), 16–28. https://doi.org/10.4018/IJHISI.2019070102

Wickramasinghe, N. (2020). Minority Health and Wellness: A Digital Health Opportunity. In Wickramasinghe, N. (Ed.), *Handbook of Research on Optimizing Healthcare Management Techniques* (pp. 116–126). IGI Global. https://doi.org/10.4018/978-1-7998-1371-2.ch008

Wickramasinghe, N., Geholt, V., Sloane, E., Smart, P. J., & Schaffer, J. L. (2021). Using Health 4.0 to Enable Post-Operative Wellness Monitoring: The Case of Colorectal Surgery. In Wickramasinghe, N. (Ed.), *Optimizing Health Monitoring Systems With Wireless Technology* (pp. 233–247). IGI Global. https://doi.org/10.4018/978-1-5225-6067-8.ch016

Wilcox, S., Huzo, O., Minhas, A., Walters, N., Adada, J. E., Pennington, M., Roseme, L., Mohammed, D., Dusic, A., & Zeine, R. (2022). The Impact of Medical or Health-Related Internet Searches on Patient Compliance: The Dr. Net Study. In Aker, H., & Aiken, M. (Eds.), *Handbook of Research on Cyberchondria, Health Literacy, and the Role of Media in Society's Perception of Medical Information* (pp. 72–97). IGI Global. https://doi.org/10.4018/978-1-7998-8630-3.ch005

Witzke, K., & Specht, O. (2017). M Health Telemedicine and Telepresence in Oral and Maxillofacial Surgery: An Innovative Prehospital Healthcare Concept in Structurally Weak Areas. *International Journal of Reliable and Quality E-Healthcare, 6*(4), 37–48. DOI: 10.4018/IJRQEH.2017100105

Wong, A. K., & Lo, M. F. (2018). Using Pervasive Computing for Sustainable Healthcare in an Aging Population. In Fong, B., Ng, A., & Yuen, P. (Eds.), *Sustainable Health and Long-Term Care Solutions for an Aging Population* (pp. 187–202). Hershey, PA: IGI Global. DOI: 10.4018/978-1-5225-2633-9.ch010

Wu, W., Martin, B. C., & Ni, C. (2017). A Systematic Review of Competency-Based Education Effort in the Health Professions: Seeking Order Out of Chaos. In Rasmussen, K., Northrup, P., & Colson, R. (Eds.), *Handbook of Research on Competency-Based Education in University Settings* (pp. 352–378). Hershey, PA: IGI Global. DOI: 10.4018/978-1-5225-0932-5.ch018

Yadav, S., Ekbal, A., Saha, S., Pathak, P. S., & Bhattacharyya, P. (2017). Patient Data De-Identification: A Conditional Random-Field-Based Supervised Approach. In S. Saha, A. Mandal, A. Narasimhamurthy, S. V, & S. Sangam (Eds.), *Handbook of Research on Applied Cybernetics and Systems Science* (pp. 234-253). Hershey, PA: IGI Global. DOI: 10.4018/978-1-5225-2498-4.ch011

Yu, B., Wijesekera, D., & Costa, P. C. (2017). Informed Consent in Healthcare: A Study Case of Genetic Services. In Moumtzoglou, A. (Ed.), *Design, Development, and Integration of Reliable Electronic Healthcare Platforms* (pp. 211–242). Hershey, PA: IGI Global. DOI: 10.4018/978-1-5225-1724-5.ch013

Yu, B., Wijesekera, D., & Costa, P. C. (2017). Informed Consent in Electronic Medical Record Systems. In I. Management Association (Ed.), *Healthcare Ethics and Training: Concepts, Methodologies, Tools, and Applications* (pp. 1029-1049). Hershey, PA: IGI Global. DOI: 10.4018/978-1-5225-2237-9.ch049

Yu, M., Li, J., & Wang, W. (2017). Creative Life Experience among Students in Medical Education. In Zhou, C. (Ed.), *Handbook of Research on Creative Problem-Solving Skill Development in Higher Education* (pp. 158–184). Hershey, PA: IGI Global. DOI: 10.4018/978-1-5225-0643-0.ch008

Zanetti, C. A., George, A., Stiegmann, R. A., & Phelan, D. (2020). Digital Health. In Gotian, R., Kang, Y., & Safdieh, J. (Eds.), *Handbook of Research on the Efficacy of Training Programs and Systems in Medical Education* (pp. 404–426). IGI Global. https://doi.org/10.4018/978-1-7998-1468-9.ch021

Zangão, M. O. (2020). Self-Perceived Health Status. In Fonseca, C., Lopes, M., Mendes, D., Mendes, F., & García-Alonso, J. (Eds.), *Handbook of Research on Health Systems and Organizations for an Aging Society* (pp. 1–11). IGI Global. DOI: 10.4018/978-1-5225-9818-3.ch001

Zarour, K. (2017). Towards a Telehomecare in Algeria: Case of Diabetes Measurement and Remote Monitoring. *International Journal of E-Health and Medical Communications*, *8*(4), 61–80. DOI: 10.4018/IJEHMC.2017100104

Zavyalova, Y. V., Korzun, D. G., Meigal, A. Y., & Borodin, A. V. (2017). Towards the Development of Smart Spaces-Based Socio-Cyber-Medicine Systems. *International Journal of Embedded and Real-Time Communication Systems*, *8*(1), 45–63. DOI: 10.4018/IJERTCS.2017010104

Zeinali, A. A. (2018). Word Formation Study in Developing Naming Guidelines in the Translation of English Medical Terms Into Persian. In M. Khosrow-Pour, D.B.A. (Ed.), *Encyclopedia of Information Science and Technology, Fourth Edition* (pp. 5136-5147). Hershey, PA: IGI Global. DOI: 10.4018/978-1-5225-2255-3.ch446

Zineldin, M., & Vasicheva, V. (2018). Reducing Medical Errors and Increasing Patient Safety: TRM and 5 Q's Approaches for Better Quality of Life. In *Technological Tools for Value-Based Sustainable Relationships in Health: Emerging Research and Opportunities* (pp. 87–115). Hershey, PA: IGI Global. DOI: 10.4018/978-1-5225-4091-5.ch005

About the Contributors

Samet Uludag is an expert in family medicine. He graduated from well-known Istanbul University's Faculty of Medicine and possesses over 5 years of experience as a physician.

Kadir Uludag holds Ph.D. in Applied psychology (Chinese Academy of Sciences). He is currently doing postdoc in Shanghai Jiaotong University Mental Health Center. His research interest includes schizophrenia research, drug addiction and educational psychology. In addition, he runs a website to share and comment on peer-reviewed articles (ifx0.com).

***

Jennifer Schulz is a professor in the Psychology, Social Work, Criminal Justice, and Sociology Department at Ashland University in North Central Ohio. She teaches courses on human rights, social welfare, human behavior, abnormal psychology, research methods, and social policy. She maintains an active clinical license and performs contract work as a crisis therapist, in addition to providing writing and consultation services related to evidence-based practices in social work and psychology. Her research interests focus on eating disorders and other mental health topics. Dr. Schulz taught for five years at Mount Vernon Nazarene University before accepting her current position at Ashland University. She holds a Doctor of Philosophy in Psychology from National University and a Master of Social with with an emphasis on mental health and substance abuse counseling from The Ohio State University.

Wasswa Shafik (Member, IEEE) received a Bachelor of Science degree in information technology from Ndejje University, Uganda, a Master of Engineering degree in Information Technology (Computer and Communication Networks) from Yazd University, Iran, and a PhD in Computer Science with the School of Digital

Science, Universiti Brunei Darussalam, Brunei Darussalam. He is also the Founder and Research Director of the Dig Connectivity Research Laboratory (DCRLab) after serving as a Research Associate at the Network Interconnectivity Research Laboratory at Yazd University. Prior to this, he worked as a Community Data Analyst at Population Services International (PSI-Uganda), a Community Data Officer at the Programme for Accessible Health Communication (PACE-Uganda), a Research Assistant at the Socio-Economic Data Centre (SEDC-Uganda), Uganda, an Assistant Data Officer at TechnoServe, Kampala, Uganda, and Asmaah Charity Organization as Cheif Executive Officer. He has hundreds of publications with renowned publishers. His research interests include Artificial Intelligence, Neural Networks, Computer Vision, Smart Agriculture, Digital Health, and Green Computing.

Index

T

V

www.ingramcontent.com/pod-product-compliance
Lightning Source LLC
LaVergne TN
LVHW081521300926
849161LV00006B/1258